BSAVA Manual of Small Animal Anaesthesia and Analgesia

formerly
Manual of Anaesthesia for Small Animal Practice

Editors:

Chris Seymour
MA VetMB DVA MRCVS
Forty Hill, Enfield, Middx EN1 4DF

and

Robin Gleed
BVSc DVA DipACVA DipECVA MRCVS
Department of Clinical Sciences,
ollege of Veterinary Medicine, Cornell University,
Ithaca, NY 14853, USA

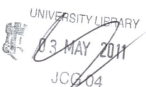

A catalogue record for this book is available from the British Library

ISBN 0 905214 48 X

The publishers and contributors cannot take responsibility for information
provided on dosages and methods of application of drugs mentioned in this
publication. Details of this kind must be verified by individual users from the
appropriate literature.

Typeset by: Fusion Design, Fordingbridge, Hampshire, UK

Printed by: Stephens & George, Merthyr Tydfil, Mid Glamorgan, UK

Andrea M. Nolan MVB PhD DVA
Department of Veterinary Clinical Studies, University of Glasgow Veterinary School, Bearsden Road, Bearsden, Glasgow, G61 1QH

Peter Pascoe BVSc PhD DVA DipACVA MRCVS
Department of Veterinary Medicine, University of California – Davis, Davis, CA 95616, USA

Jacky Reid BVMS PhD DVA
Department of Veterinary Clinical Studies, University of Glasgow Veterinary School, Bearsden Road, Bearsden, Glasgow, G61 1QH

Hamish D. Rodger BVMS MSc PhD MRCVS
Department of Clinical Studies, School of Veterinary Medicine, University of Pennsylvania, New Bolton Center, 382 West Street Road, Kennett Square, PA 19348-1692, USA

Chris Seymour MA VetMB DVA MRCVS
23 Mahon Close, Forty Hill, Enfield, Middx, EN1 4DF

Karen Walsh BVetMed CertVA MRCVS
Animal Health Trust, Lanwades Park, Kentford, Newmarket, Suffolk CB8 7UU

Avril E. Waterman-Pearson PhD BVSc DVA DipECVA MRCA FRCVS
University of Bristol, Department of Clinical Veterinary Science, Langford House, Langford, Bristol, BS40 5DT

Foreword

Because of my specialist interest in anaesthesia it gives me particular pleasure to write the Foreword for the new *Manual of Anaesthesia and Analgesia*. This new edition of one of our most popular manuals has been completely rewritten to encompass a practice-orientated clinical approach. The joint Editors have assembled a formidable group of experts to write individual chapters, with several international contributors. The subject of analgesia is covered in depth, and in response to changing trends in pet ownership there is a much expanded section on anaesthesia of exotic species. Recent innovations in both the pharmacology of new drugs and the introduction of new equipment are fully discussed.

I am sure that practitioners will give a big welcome to the section on anaesthesia in the clinical setting, in which the regimens appropriate for different types of surgery are discussed. In addition, the chapter dealing with the hazards of caesarean section will provide both reassurance and the answers to the most commonly asked anaesthetic questions.

As with the previous editions I am confident that this Manual will be a bestseller and become part of every practice library. It will undoubtedly prove of immense value to both veterinary surgeons and nurses alike.

John F.R. Hird
BSAVA President 1998-99

Preface

A sound understanding of general anaesthesia is vital for all practitioners, whatever their primary area of expertise. In addition, adequate pain control after injury, either traumatic or surgical, is one of the most important responsibilities of all veterinary surgeons.

This manual, with contributions from a distinguished panel of international experts, offers the clinician a practical and easily accessible guide to anaesthesia and analgesia in small animals. Basic principles and pharmacology are clearly explained, followed by anaesthetic management in the clinical setting. With increasing specialization in practice and increased client expectations, the complexity of surgical techniques and the types of patient they are performed upon have grown apace. One aim of this manual, therefore, has been to describe the perioperative management of patients with pre-existing pathology and its influence on the course of anaesthesia. An understanding of these special requirements is essential for a successful outcome.

Uniquely, the manual includes information on differences between UK and North American practice. Although the text retains British Pharmacopoeia names for drugs, where these are different from their North American counterparts the US Pharmacopoeia name is given at first use in each chapter.

In a multi-author book such as this, there is necessarily material that is covered more than once. The Editors have decided not to eliminate this overlap on the grounds that there is value in seeing how different authorities view similar clinical problems. This approach has also reduced the need for extensive cross-referencing between chapters.

The many significant developments in the fields of anaesthesia and patient monitoring that have occurred since the first edition in 1989 are described, and there is a substantially expanded section on exotic species.

This manual is primarily aimed at veterinary practitioners and students. However, the close involvement of veterinary nurses in the care of anaesthetized patients means that they will also find much of relevance in this book, particularly those studying for the RCVS Diploma in Advanced Veterinary Nursing.

Chris Seymour, Enfield, Middlesex, UK
Robin Gleed, Ithaca, New York, USA

March 1999

Basic Principles

CHAPTER ONE

The Practice of Veterinary Anaesthesia and Analgesia

Ronald S. Jones

INTRODUCTION

The origins of veterinary anaesthesia are unclear. It is recorded, however, that Paracelsus administered ether to chickens in 1540. Henry Hill Hickman administered carbon dioxide to experimental animals and showed that it alleviated the pain of surgery. It was not until Morton's demonstration of the effects of ether in Boston, in 1846, that its use as an anaesthetic came to the public's attention. In the United Kingdom, ether was first given to human patients in Dumfries and London. Within a year it was being used in cats and dogs. Chloroform was discovered a year later and became more popular than ether in medical and veterinary anaesthesia. Cocaine was used as a local anaesthetic, and its use in animals was highlighted by Hobday, who published the first book on veterinary anaesthesia in 1915. This was followed by legislation – the Animals Anaesthetics Act, 1919. In the 1930s there was considerable development in barbiturate anaesthesia, with the use of intravenous pentobarbitone and thiopentone. This was mainly popularized by Professor J. G. Wright. At that time, work was also being carried out on extradural (epidural) anaesthesia by Dr G. B. Brook.

In the past 50 years there have been considerable advances in veterinary anaesthesia, mainly linked to developments in human medical anaesthesia. These include endotracheal intubation, closed circuit anaesthesia, the introduction of fluorinated inhalational agents e.g. halothane and isoflurane, and new injectable agents, e.g. ketamine and propofol for the induction of anaesthesia. One development that has been specific to veterinary anaesthesia is the use of α_2-adrenoceptor agonist drugs.

DEFINITIONS

Anaesthesia

Anaesthesia was proposed by Oliver Wendell Holmes to describe the reversible process of depression of the central nervous system (CNS) with drugs that produce unconsciousness and a reduced or absent response to noxious stimuli, which the patient does not recall.

Hypnosis

Hypnosis is a condition of artificially induced sleep which, in animals, is usually produced by drugs. Some authorities consider hypnosis to be synonymous with anaesthesia. Confusion also surrounds hypnosis, as it was originally considered, along with muscle relaxation and analgesia, to be a component of anaesthesia.

Analgesia

Analgesia implies a diminished or abolished perception of pain, or the relief of pain. If some analgesic drugs are given in sufficient doses they can produce anaesthesia.

TYPES OF ANAESTHESIA

There are two types of anaesthesia: general anaesthesia and local, or regional, anaesthesia.

General anaesthesia

General anaesthetic agents normally produce a controlled and reversible intoxication of the CNS of the animal. All methods of preventing awareness of pain, which involve loss of consciousness and the inability to recall traumatic events from diagnostic or surgical procedures, are referred to as general anaesthesia. General anaesthetic agents are given either by inhalation or by injection.

Inhalational anaesthetics

This type of general anaesthesia involves the addition of an anaesthetic gas or vapour to the gases inspired by the animal. The majority of these agents undergo a minimal amount of metabolism within the animal's body. Hence the greater part of the inhaled agent is excreted via the lungs in an unchanged state. This contributes to the relatively high degree of safety when using this type of anaesthesia. If an overdose does occur, the animal can be ventilated with oxygen, and the expired gases can be vented, which means that resuscitation is usually rapid and effective. The term minimum alveolar concentration (MAC) is used to describe the end-tidal concentration of any inhalational agent that needs to be given to a population of animals to prevent a response to a painful stimulus in 50% of that population. It has been determined for all of the commonly used agents, and the value varies from species to species. Familiarity with this concept and the values enables inhalational agents to be given with considerable safety, particularly when non-rebreathing circuits and accurately calibrated and temperature-compensated (Tec) vaporizers are used.

Injectable anaesthetics

A number of anaesthetic agents such as ketamine can be administered by the subcutaneous, intramuscular or intravenous routes. In contrast, some agents e.g. thiopentone, are extremely irritant when injected by routes other than intravenous. Compared with anaesthetic agents given by the inhalational route, those given by injection cannot be removed from the body, and elimination of these drugs and the cessation of their action depends on detoxification and/or excretion, which is usually via the bile and/or the urine. With some drugs, e.g. thiopentone, there is a major redistribution of the drug throughout the body, and metabolism is relatively slow. The safety of injectable agents depends on strict control of the dose and the accurate estimation of the weight of the animal. Considerable care and skill are always required when using injectable anaesthetic agents in animals to assess the dose. Although there are guidelines for the doses of all commonly used agents, those that are safe and effective in a young healthy animal may constitute an overdose in an elderly and/or sick animal. It is relatively easy to overdose an elderly or sick animal. Overdose with injectable agents can be fatal in the absence of simple equipment for resuscitation and the administration of oxygen. Recovery from injectable anaesthesia depends on the kinetic profile of the drug and the manner in which the drug is dealt with by the body. If the drug is rapidly cleared, recovery can sometimes be as fast as that with an inhalational agent. One of the advantages of injectable anaesthetic techniques is that the amount of anaesthetic agent given to the patient is accurately known at any particular time. With experience of patients' reactions to an agent in particular situations, it is possible to obtain a fairly accurate forecast of the effects of that agent in other patients.

The use of injectable anaesthetics for maintenance of anaesthesia is increasing in popularity. The technique usually involves giving an agent by intravenous infusion, together with supplementary analgesic agents. This route has the distinct advantage that no potentially hazardous substances are exhaled into the environment.

Local anaesthesia

This results from temporary blockade of sensory nerves and is often accompanied by a concurrent block of motor nerves. All of the commonly available local anaesthetic drugs have the potential to produce toxic effects on the CNS or cardiorespiratory system. Toxic effects occur when large doses of the drug are absorbed into the circulation from the site of injection.

Local anaesthesia can take a variety of different forms:

Topical application

This has limited use and is usually confined to the eye and mucous membranes of the nasopharynx, larynx, penis, vagina, rectum and urethra. Topical anaesthetics are applied as a gel or solution, or by aerosol, depending on the area.

Infiltration

This involves the injection of the agent at the site of operation. Unless the procedure is minor and the volume of solution small, local toxicity of the agent may impair healing.

Regional anaesthesia

This involves the injection of local anaesthetic solutions around a nerve, to produce a temporary sensory and motor blockade.

Extradural (epidural) analgesia

This involves the injection of drugs into the spinal canal at the lumbosacral space. It is normally used in dogs but can be used in cats. The technique has undergone a resurgence in popularity in recent years, with the use of several agents, such as opioid analgesics, for the production of longer term analgesia.

Intravenous regional anaesthesia

This involves the injection of a local anaesthetic solution distal to the site of a tourniquet on a limb. Analgesia occurs in a few minutes and lasts while the tourniquet occludes the arterial blood supply to the limb.

LEGAL ASPECTS (UNITED KINGDOM)

In several countries, including the United Kingdom, there is legislation governing the administration of anaesthetic agents to animals. This is the Protection of Animals (Anaesthetics) Act, 1964, which has a number of minor amendments. The act specifies that very few procedures can be carried out on certain species without anaesthesia. Procedures include castration under a certain age in some species, docking of tails, removal of dewclaws and disbudding of calves under 1 week of age.

Several agents that are used for anaesthesia and analgesia in the dog and cat are governed by the Misuse of Drugs Act, 1971, and its associated regulations. Over 100 substances are listed in the Act, and they are placed in four schedules that relate mainly to their potential for misuse by humans. The regulations impose a legal obligation on all practitioners prescribing and giving controlled drugs. Separate registers must be kept for all controlled drugs that are used and supplied. Veterinary surgeons are required to keep these drugs in a locked receptacle that can be opened only by an authorized person or someone with the authorized person's consent. A locked car is not classed as a locked receptacle.

Duty of care

The veterinary surgeon has a duty of care (taken from Halsbury's Laws of England) towards the client: in deciding whether the animal can be safely anaesthetized; in deciding on the appropriate type of anaesthesia; in the administration of the anaesthetic; and in consultation with other veterinary surgeons to ensure that the client is properly advised about the recommended course and any special considerations. The veterinary surgeon must also bring to the task a reasonable degree of skill and knowledge and must exercise a reasonable degree of care. Failure to do so, which results in the death or injury of an animal, gives the owner the right to bring a legal action against the veterinary surgeon for recovery of damages. In recent years there have been two high profile court cases involving anaesthetized animals being returned to the owners before they were fully recovered. Both animals subsequently died. The Courts found the veterinary surgeons negligent.

Negligence

An error of judgement does not necessarily amount to negligence. Whether or not the degree of competence, skill and knowledge has been exercised in any particular case is normally tested against what is seen to be normal accepted practice. In such a situation, the veterinary surgeon in general practice will be judged against the standard of the good, careful and competent practising veterinary surgeon. However, veterinary surgeons of specialist or consultant status in anaesthesia will be judged against the standards set by their peers.

There is often confusion between negligence and disgraceful professional conduct that could lead to disciplinary action by the Royal College of Veterinary Surgeons (RCVS). Negligence *per se* does not amount to disgraceful professional conduct, unless it is so gross and excessive that it is liable to bring the veterinary profession into disrepute. It is only then that a disciplinary action may ensue.

Consent

In every case involving anaesthesia, it is essential to ensure that the owners or, in their absence, adult agents, sign a consent form for the anaesthesia. It is not sufficient for them to just sign a blank piece of paper – it is essential that the surgical, or diagnostic, procedure and the anaesthetic technique and their associated risks are explained to the owners. They are not only indicating that they are giving their consent but also that they have understood what has been explained to them.

AIMS OF ANAESTHESIA

Generally, the aims of anaesthesia are to:

- Prevent awareness of, and response to, pain
- Provide restraint and immobility of the animal and relaxation of muscles, when this is required for a particular procedure
- Achieve both of the above without jeopardizing the life and safety of the animal before, during and after anaesthesia.

It was considered that a single anaesthetic agent could achieve these aims and, occasionally, this is true today. However, as new agents become available and new techniques are developed, a combination of agents with specific actions is more likely to be used to produce safe and relatively trouble-free anaesthesia.

ANAESTHETIC RISK

While the mortality in fit healthy cats and dogs is around 1 in 679, it decreases to around 1 in 31 in animals that have disease (Clarke and Hall, 1990). Anaesthesia is an unnatural state, and the induction of anaesthesia always carries a risk. The degree of risk can vary widely and, as indicated above, this should always be explained to owners. Even experienced anaesthetists sometimes have difficulty in assessing the risk of a specific procedure in a particular animal. However, there are a number of important factors which need to be considered before informing an owner. These are that:

- The skill and competence of the anaesthetist have a pronounced effect on the degree of risk to which a patient is exposed. Good and comprehensive training is essential, but the art of anaesthesia can only be developed with experience
- When presented for anaesthesia, the animals' state of health has a significant effect on outcome. Animals may be young and healthy or old and moribund, or their condition may be between the two. In addition, animals may be presented as emergencies from trauma of varying severity. In an attempt to quantify risks, the American Society of Anaesthesiologists has produced five categories:
  1. Normal healthy patient with no disease
  2. Slight or moderate systemic disease causing no obvious incapacity

3. Slight to moderate systemic disease causing mild symptoms, e.g. moderate pyrexia, hypovolaemia or anaemia
4. Extreme systemic disease constituting a threat to life, e.g. toxaemia, uraemia, severe hypovolaemia, cardiac failure
5. Moribund or dying patients.

While it is accepted that this classification is a useful aid, it should be appreciated that it applies only to the physical state of the patient, and a number of other factors must be considered in order to categorize the risk fully.

The skill and competence of the surgeon has an obvious influence on the anaesthetic risk. Inexperienced surgeons are likely to take longer to carry out a procedure, and to produce greater trauma than more experienced surgeons.

The influence of facilities is also important. A well equipped and staffed unit is likely to produce better results than a less organized unit.

CHOICE OF ANAESTHETIC TECHNIQUE

A variety of factors influence the choice of a particular technique. These include:

- Facilities: If facilities are poor and likely to prejudice the outcome of the anaesthetic procedure, they should not be used. For example, a well administered intravenous technique may be much safer than an inhalational agent given with inferior equipment
- Skill and experience of the anaesthetist and surgeon: These are extremely important in choosing a technique (particularly noticeable if they are used to working as a team)
- Facilities for postoperative recovery and care: These will be influenced by whether the animal is to be hospitalized or returned to the owner (see legal aspects above). It is important to ensure that adequate postoperative analgesia is provided
- Temperament of patient: This can have an important influence on the choice of technique. In animals of good temperament, a minimum amount of sedative premedication may be required before the intravenous induction of anaesthesia. Competent assistance in restraint can be of extreme value. Some cats may be so unruly that crush cages or inhalational anaesthetic induction chambers are needed. Vicious dogs may require a heavy sedative premedication before anaesthesia, which can influence the subsequent doses of anaesthetic agents

- Species and breed of animal: These can influence the choice of technique. Some breeds respond adversely to some intravenous agents. Some Boxers are sensitive to acepromazine
- Age and general health: These are important influences on the choice of agents and the doses used. Doses of anaesthetic agents need to be reduced in both young and elderly animals. In puppies and kittens of a very young age, inhalational agents are the drugs of choice. Such patients are also very susceptible to hypothermia. Most animals can be anaesthetized relatively safely, provided adequate preparation is practised. Problems with fluid balance should be corrected, and diabetic patients should be stabilized before anaesthesia. Even if anaesthesia is deferred for some days, it is essential to ensure that patients are healthy before anaesthesia
- Site and nature of the surgery: These influence the choice of technique. Operations on the head and neck require endotracheal intubation. Special care must be taken during oral, dental and pharyngeal surgery to prevent the accumulation of any material that could be inhaled after removal of the endotracheal tube. The use of an endoscope within the respiratory tract presents problems because of competition for the airway, and anaesthetic techniques need to be adapted to deal with this problem
- Use of muscle relaxant drugs. Intermittent positive-pressure ventilation is required when such drugs are used to provide profound muscle relaxation during anaesthetic techniques for surgery of the thorax and abdomen or for some orthopaedic procedures
- Anaesthesia for Caesarian section: This requires special techniques because multiple lives are involved
- Examination under anaesthesia: Although this normally requires only short periods of anaesthesia, considerable care is still required. The old adage that 'there may be minor procedures but never minor anaesthetics' certainly applies
- Proposed duration of surgery: This must always be considered when selecting an anaesthetic technique. Short procedures can be carried out with a single dose of thiopentone, and slightly longer ones with multiple doses of propofol. Even under these circumstances, equipment must be readily available to carry out endotracheal intubation and intermittent positive-pressure ventilation. In situations where procedures are likely to be prolonged, it is important to ensure that proper inhalational anaesthetic techniques are used.

PERSONNEL

The role of veterinary nurses and technicians in anaesthesia is currently the subject of debate within the veterinary profession in the United Kingdom and elsewhere. It is well accepted that both the maintenance of anaesthetic equipment and preparation for anaesthesia can be delegated to veterinary nurses. They also play a major role in the restraint and management of animals during induction. However, current legal advice to the RCVS indicates that the induction and maintenance of anaesthesia is an act of veterinary surgery, as defined under the Veterinary Surgeons Act, 1966.

The current role of the veterinary nurse in veterinary anaesthesia in the United Kingdom is such that: 'Provided the veterinary surgeon is physically present during anaesthesia and immediately available for consultation, it would be in order for a veterinary nurse, whose name is on the list held by the RCVS, to provide assistance by:

- Administering the selected pre- and postoperative sedative, analgesic or other agents
- Administering prescribed non-incremental anaesthetic agents on the instruction of the directing veterinary surgeon
- Monitoring clinical signs and maintaining an anaesthetic record
- Maintaining anaesthesia by administering supplementary incremental doses of intravenous anaesthetic agents or adjusting the delivered concentration of anaesthetic agents, under the direct instruction of the supervising veterinary surgeon'.

REFERENCE AND FURTHER READING

Clarke KW and Hall LW (1990) A survey of anaesthesia in small animal practice: AVA/BSAVA report. *Journal of the Association for Veterinary Anaesthesia* **17**, 4–10

Hall LW and Clarke KW (1991) *Veterinary Anaesthesia, 9th edn.* Baillière Tindall, London

CHAPTER TWO

Preoperative Assessment

Robin Gleed

INTRODUCTION

All patients should be evaluated before undergoing anaesthesia. This evaluation should be directed towards the detection and investigation of conditions that may interfere with anaesthesia. It should not be restricted to an investigation of the reason for anaesthetizing the animal. Necessarily, it will focus on the nervous, cardiovascular, pulmonary, hepatic and renal systems. An accurate preanaesthetic evaluation helps in appropriate choice of anaesthetic protocol, forewarns of possible complications and permits an assessment of risk.

Ideally, preanaesthetic assessment should occur in two stages: first, a thorough evaluation 1–7 days before anaesthesia, giving time for further diagnostic procedures that may be needed and for treatment of any significant abnormalities that are found; and second, an abbreviated evaluation on admission of the patient. For practical reasons, assessment is often carried out in one stage at the time of admission of the patient and may, of necessity, be shortened for patients presented for emergency procedures.

The fundamental components of this preanaesthetic evaluation are the history and physical examination. Extensive assessment of blood samples and other diagnostic procedures should be carried out only when indicated by the findings of the history and physical examination.

A trained veterinary nurse or animal health technician can obtain a satisfactory history and physical examination. Nevertheless, many veterinarians who delegate these responsibilities to a nurse/technician also feel an obligation to talk in person with the owners of patients that they are going to anaesthetize. In any case, if the history and physical examination reveal something that may interfere with anaesthesia, veterinarians should communicate directly with their clients. Anaesthetic mishaps are a common cause of litigation in both the UK and the USA. Experience suggests that most law suits and much ill feeling can be forestalled by good communication with clients before the event.

All of the results of the preoperative assessment should be recorded and stored in the patient's record, either in a computer database or on paper. A prepared form for this record expedites the process and helps ensure that all of the necessary information is collected and the appropriate procedures are carried out. The headings given below may be used as the basis for a comprehensive record of the preanaesthetic evaluation.

HISTORY

The following components of the history are usually gathered by interviewing the owner and are based on those identified by Poffenbarger (1991).

Signalment

The basic details should include species, breed, sex and age of the patient. Verification of the client's address and availability by telephone should also happen at this time. The latter is useful because it is not unusual to need to communicate with a client while a procedure is underway (e.g. to obtain permission for euthanasia of an animal with an inoperable tumour) and delay at such times is frustrating at best. The patient's unique identifier, for example, clinic number, should also be recorded.

Main complaint

Although the major goal of the history is to detect any conditions that may interfere with a normal anaesthetic, experience suggests that most clients prefer to discuss first the reason for which the anaesthesia is being performed, for example, ovariohysterectomy or repair of a fractured femur.

History of the present illness

The severity, onset and duration of relevant clinical signs should be determined. This may be important for animals that have recently been traumatized or are vomiting.

Medical history

This should include details of puppy or kitten diseases, adult illnesses, traumatic injuries and previous surgeries. Any adverse responses to previous anaesthetic episodes, including delayed recovery, should be well documented and their causes identified if possible.

Current health status

Apart from the main complaint (discussed above), the animal's vaccination status should be defined and a record made of all drugs presently being given.

Systems review

This is usually best attempted as a series of neutral questions worded, if possible, so that they do not encourage a specific response.

General

- Has there been any change in *name's* weight?
- Has there been any change in *name's* behaviour?
- Does *name* show any signs of pain? If so, where?

Nervous system

- Has *name* ever had seizures? If so, when and how frequently?

Cardiopulmonary system

- Does *name* cough or sneeze? If so, when?
- Does *name* exercise as usual?

Gastrointestinal system

- How is *name's* appetite?
- Has *name's* drinking changed?
- Has there been any diarrhoea or vomiting?

Genitourinary system

- Has *name* been spayed/castrated? If so, when?
- Have *name's* urinary habits changed?
- Has there been any vaginal/preputial discharge or excessive licking of those areas?

Musculoskeletal system

- Does *name* seem weak?
- Does *name* favour any leg when walking or running?

Integument

- Has *name* been chewing or scratching him/ herself a lot? If so, where?

To reduce the risk of regurgitation and aspiration, it is usual to fast adult dogs and cats for at least 6 hours before anaesthesia for elective surgery. Young animals and very small patients (e.g. many bird species, guinea pigs) may be fasted for a shorter period or not at all. Admission to the hospital is an appropriate time to ask when the animal last ate and to confirm that instructions for fasting have been followed.

PHYSICAL EXAMINATION

The physical examination, comprising observation, palpation, auscultation and percussion, enables the veterinary surgeon to gather information (Poffenbarger, 1991). Most practitioners further develop their own routine for physical examination that encompasses all important organ systems and can be applied to all patients. Often this routine starts with a general observation of the patient without disturbing it, followed by measurement of breathing rate, heart rate and rectal temperature. Patients should then be weighed for accurate dosing of drugs. An accurate bodyweight is crucial for small patients (<5 kg) where the error in estimated bodyweight is relatively greater than it is in larger animals. Thereafter, it is usual to examine the patient in orderly fashion, from front to back: mouth, head, neck, thorax, abdomen and limbs. The preanaesthetic physical examination rarely requires equipment more sophisticated than a set of scales, a thermometer, a stethoscope and a penlight. However, a reflex hammer and a haemostat may help in examination of reflex and sensory function.

Ordinarily the results of the physical examination are recorded by organ system on a form (e.g. general appearance, mucous membranes, the nervous, cardiovascular, pulmonary, gastrointestinal, genitourinary and musculoskeletal systems and the integument and lymph nodes). Each system should be marked as normal, abnormal or not examined. All abnormal findings should be described to the extent possible.

To minimize the chances of procedures being carried out on wrong patients, many large hospitals use the physical examination at admission as an opportunity to apply a numbered and named collar or some other individual identification system. In such hospitals it is the routine for all interventions (e.g. administration of drugs) to be preceded by a check of the patient's identity. At admission, it is also a convention in many hospitals to put a red collar on aggressive animals. This forewarns anyone who may handle the animal after admission to take special care.

The side of all lateralized signs or lesions should be clearly recorded during the physical examination. This minimizes the possibility of subsequent procedures, for example, stifle arthrotomy, being carried out on the wrong limb.

It is usual in many practices to perform basic blood tests on patients about to be anaesthetized. These quick assessment tests usually include packed cell volume (PCV) and total protein (often determined by refractometer), blood glucose and blood urea nitrogen concentrations (the last two values often determined by dipstick test). These tests provide useful baseline data and are not expensive or time consuming. Extensive blood profiles, consisting of batches of measurements, have been advocated for screening patients before anaesthesia. In practice, such profiles are expensive for the client and rarely detect disease processes that have not previously been detected in the history or physical examination. On the rare occasions when such a disease process is detected *de novo*, it is even more unlikely to require modification of the anaesthetic technique. Preanaesthetic blood profiles may even do harm because they tend to create 'red herrings.' This is because the results of most laboratory blood tests are given with a normal range for that test. This normal range is usually within ± 2 SD of the mean from a population of normal animals. This suggests that 1 in 20 normal animals have a measurement for that variable that is outside the normal range. Hence, if 10 different variables are measured on a blood sample from a normal animal, it is quite possible that at least one variable will be marked as abnormal. Time and clients' money may be wasted in investigating this spurious finding, if it is not recognized as a mistake in interpretation. As a general rule, expensive blood tests should only be undertaken when specifically indicated by findings in the history or physical examination, i.e. to confirm a finding, to measure the seriousness of a disease process or to assess the progress of treatment.

PREANAESTHETIC FINDINGS THAT MAY REQUIRE PARTICULAR ATTENTION

Breed-related factors

- Miniature Schnauzers often have sick sinus syndrome. This breed should be evaluated by electrocardiograph before and during anaesthesia
- Dobermann Pinschers often have the coagulation defect, von Willebrand's disease. Ideally, all of these dogs should have von Willebrand's factor activity measured before any surgical intervention. Buccal mucosal bleeding time should be measured before surgery; the author prefers to measure this after the patient has been premedicated, but it may be measured after induction of anaesthesia. If the buccal mucosal bleeding time is >3 minutes and bleeding is anticipated during surgery, then the patient may be treated with desmopressin acetate. Cryoprecipitate, fresh frozen plasma or whole blood may also be prepared for administration (see Chapter 11)
- Greyhounds and other sight hounds have greatly increased susceptibility to thiobarbiturates. This effect makes inadvisable the use of thiopentone in such dogs
- Boxers (at least in the UK) and large breed dogs are very susceptible to small doses of phenothiazine tranquillizers, e.g. acepromazine
- Brachycephalic breeds (e.g. Bull Dog or Pekingese) are susceptible to airway obstruction after induction of anaesthesia and are difficult to intubate. Preparation for maintaining an airway by visual placement of an endotracheal tube or tracheostomy should precede administration of any anaesthesia-related drugs. These patients require extra vigilance after extubation in case airway obstruction occurs.

Concurrent drugs

Typically, drugs that are regularly given should not be discontinued in anticipation of anaesthesia. Oral drugs should not be given in the period between anaesthetic premedication and induction of anaesthesia, because pills may be retained in the pharynx and oesophagus after premedicants have been given. Specific drug-related considerations are that:

- Aminoglycoside antibiotics (e.g. gentamicin, neomycin) may cause neuromuscular transmission block. In conjunction with inhaled anaesthetics, this may lead to significantly impaired ventilation. Gentamicin in high doses causes renal disease; hence renal function should be assessed in patients that have received this drug for more than 4 or 5 days
- Barbiturates that are being given to treat epilepsy should continue to be given on schedule. Theoretically, these barbiturates could have an additive effect with general anaesthetics. However, they rarely produce a clinically detectable decrease in anaesthetic requirement and may be responsible for hepatic enzyme induction
- Corticosteroids given for more than 2 days suppress release of adrenocorticotrophic hormone and, hence, may reduce the normal stress response to surgery and anaesthesia. Hydrocortisone or dexamethasone should be given intravenously to any animal that has had glucocorticoid therapy recently (see Chapter 19)
- Digitalis treatment or treatment with other cardiac glycosides is usually best continued through anaesthesia in patients that have stable cardiovascular status
- Non-steroidal anti-inflammatory drugs (NSAIDs) are legitimate adjuncts to anaesthesia and pain management. In high doses they may displace drugs such as diazepam from protein-binding sites and potentiate their activity by increasing the concentration of active drug that is available. This effect is probably of little relevance clinically. Further details of the use of NSAIDs in the perioperative period may be found in Chapter 6.

General body condition

Obesity compromises the cardiovascular system and may cause restriction of ventilatory movement; these effects are exacerbated by anaesthesia and recumbency. Both obesity and extreme thinness may interfere with normal drug disposition in the body.

History of recent trauma

Animals that have been extensively traumatized (e.g. gunshot, road traffic accident) within the preceding 4 days should be investigated for traumatic myocarditis. This may warrant electrocardiography. Ventricular premature contractions in such patients may necessitate delay of anaesthesia until they resolve (this usually occurs within 4 days of the trauma that initiated them) or specific treatment (see Chapters 14 and 21). It should be noted that chest trauma is not a prerequisite of traumatic myocarditis and that it can occur when the trauma is apparently restricted to the rear limb.

Physical examination of patients after trauma should be directed specifically towards detecting common sequelae such as ruptured diaphragm, ruptured urinary bladder and blood loss.

Respiratory disease

Evidence of respiratory disease in the history and physical examination usually requires further investigation with radiography and, if feasible, arterial blood gas analysis. Pleural effusion should be drained before induction of anaesthesia (see Chapter 14).

Cardiovascular disease

Cardiac disease is usually of most importance when it is severe enough to restrict exercise tolerance and/or produce severe cardiac dysrhythmias. Pericardial effusion should be drained before anaesthesia.

Hypertrophic cardiomyopathy is quite common in cats that are 3 to 5 years of age and should be suspected in cats with signs of hyperthyroidism. It is undoubtedly an important cause of adverse responses to anaesthesia in cats but it is notoriously difficult to detect in its early stages. The electrocardiogram of cats with cardiomyopathy is often inconclusive, as are chest radiographs; diagnosis and accurate assessment usually requires echocardiography. Cats with cardiac gallop rhythms or murmurs may be poor anaesthetic candidates because of this disease (see Chapter 14).

Hypovolaemia, dehydration and anaemia

Fluid and electrolyte deficiencies should be corrected before anaesthesia. A decrease in red cell mass is tolerated better than a decrease in blood volume, hence, a PCV of around 20% may be tolerated as long as blood volume and cardiac function are maintained.

Polydipsia and polyuria

These signs should be investigated before anaesthesia because they are commonly associated with conditions that may interfere with anaesthesia such as renal failure, diabetes and pyometra. Examination of the vulva in bitches, urine analysis, blood glucose measurement and abdominal radiography may be indicated depending on the physical examination.

Renal disease

Uraemia increases the sensitivity to anaesthetic drugs and should be corrected before anaesthesia whenever possible. Hypoperfusion of the kidney during anaesthesia may cause ischaemic damage that is sufficient to induce renal failure in patients with pre-existing subclinical disease. For this reason, elderly animals in particular should be given fluids during anaesthesia and their cardiovascular function monitored carefully (e.g. with indirect blood pressure) to avoid renal hypoperfusion (see Chapter 17).

Liver disease

Liver disease may prolong the action of anaesthetic drugs that undergo hepatic metabolism. It may also be associated with secondary conditions, for example, coagulation deficits, hypoproteinaemia and hypoglycaemia (see Chapter 16).

Diabetes

Elective surgery on diabetic patients with severe ketoacidosis should be delayed to permit regulation of the diabetic state. Even in regulated diabetic patients, blood glucose concentration should be measured immediately before anaesthesia (see Chapter 19).

Skin disease

Because of the increased risk of introducing infection into the meninges, segmental anaesthesia/analgesia by extradural (epidural) or spinal injection is contraindicated if there is pruritus at the site of injection. This is a common problem that precludes lumbosacral injection in dogs with flea-induced dermatitis.

ANAESTHETIC RISK

The findings of the history, physical examination and other investigations should be used to assess the well-being of the patient, taking into account all of the patient's medical problems and including disturbances produced by the primary presenting complaint. The American Society of Anesthesiologists (ASA) has a useful scale for formalizing this process (Figure 2.1). The advantage of this scale is that the patient assessment is summarized by a numerical value, which helps identify those patients that may warrant special attention in choice of anaesthetic protocol and in monitoring. It should be noted that the ASA scale summarizes only the patient-related factors that contribute to the risk of anaesthesia. Other factors that contribute to anaesthetic risk include the type of surgical intervention, the experience of the anaesthetist and surgeon and the anaesthetic techniques used (Guarnieri and Prevoznik, 1992). Emergency anaesthesia usually carries increased risk both because of the presumed severity of the presenting condition and also because there is less time for patient evaluation and preparation.

Category	Description	Examples
I	Healthy patient	Healthy patient for ovariohysterectomy
II	Mild systemic disease with no functional limitations	Local infection, compensated cardiac disease
III	Severe systemic disease with functional limitations	Pyrexia, moderate dehydration or anaemia
IV	Severe systemic disease that is a constant threat to life	Uncompensated heart disease
V	Moribund patient that is not expected to survive 24 hours with or without operation	Shock, severe trauma, multiple organ failure

Figure 2.1: American Society of Anesthesiologists physical status scale. The systemic disease may or may not be the condition for which the patient is undergoing anaesthesia. Emergency cases are classified as category IV and V and are marked by the addition of an 'E' to the number.

Modified from Ross and Tinker (1990) with the permission of Churchill Livingstone.

The anaesthetic assessment process is also an opportunity for communicating with the owner both to reassure them about anaesthesia and to give them a realistic appraisal of the risks associated with anaesthesia. In a university teaching hospital, <15% of dogs and cats experienced perianaesthetic complications, whereas <0.5% died in the perianaesthetic period (Gaynor *et al.*, 1999). In private practice, mortality associated with anaesthesia was 0.1–0.3% (Clarke and Hall, 1990; Dodman, 1992). Of course, these average figures are biased by many things, including the general health of the population undergoing anaesthesia. The group of patients presented to the university hospital may have included a greater proportion of sick patients than were presented in private practice. Nevertheless, these data give a baseline from which to extrapolate the particular risk for each patient.

PERMISSION FOR ANAESTHESIA AND SURGERY

It is wise to obtain permission for anaesthesia and surgery on a form, which is signed by the client at the time of admission. This should specify the individual who will be responsible for the patient while it is in the hospital. It should be noted that such forms do not provide legal protection for the veterinarian in the event that they do not fulfil their professional obligations to their patient and client.

REFERENCES

Clarke KW and Hall LW (1990) A survey of anaesthesia in small animal practice: AVA/BSAVA report. *Journal of the Association of Veterinary Anaesthesia* **17**, 4–10

Dodman NH (1992) Survey of small animal anesthetic practice in Vermont. *Journal of the Amercian Animal Hospital Association* **28**, 439–445

Gaynor JS, Dunlop CI, Wagner AE, Wertz EM, Golden AE and Demme WC (1999) Complications and mortality associated with anesthesia in dogs and cats. *Journal of the American Animal Hospital Association* **35**, 13–17

Guarnieri DM and Prevoznik SJ (1992) Preoperative evaluation. In: *Introduction to Anesthesia*, ed. DE Longnecker and FL Murphy, pp. 19–30. WB Saunders, Philadelphia

Poffenbarger EM (1991) The health history. In: *Small Animal Physical Diagnosis and Clinical Procedures*, ed. DM McCurnin and EM Poffenbarger, pp. 6–15. WB Saunders, Philadelphia

Ross AF and Tinker JH (1990) Anesthesia risk. In: *Anesthesia, 3rd edn*, ed. RD Miller, pp. 715–742. Churchill Livingstone, New York

CHAPTER THREE

Postoperative Care

Daniel Holden

INTRODUCTION

The primary goal of postoperative care is to ensure a smooth, painless and safe recovery from anaesthesia. Monitoring of the patient does not cease when the final suture is placed; this is merely the point where the recovery begins and postoperative care is provided. The patient should be monitored until a full level of consciousness is present and physiological variables have normalized. The level of sophistication of monitoring depends not only on the severity of the patient's disease, but also the surgical procedure performed. A more detailed description of monitoring equipment may be found in Chapter 5.

The area where recovery takes place should be continuously staffed by personnel who are trained and experienced in patient monitoring and are not distracted by other tasks. Rapid access to a source of oxygen, emergency equipment and drugs should be possible. The room should be well ventilated to prevent accumulation of expired volatile agents but kept at a reasonably high ambient temperature to avoid radiant heat loss from recovering patients; individually heated cages and heated water blankets should be available.

AIRWAY

Problems associated with the airway are among the most frequently encountered difficulties in the recovery period. Animals should never be left unobserved while intubated. In the vast majority of cases, the endotracheal tube (ETT) may be left in place until there is evidence of return of the cough reflex. Tube removal should be timed to occur at the end of inspiration so that removal is immediately followed by expiration, thereby assisting in the removal of debris and secretions from the trachea and larynx. Some anaesthetists prefer to extubate cats early in the recovery period to avoid the likelihood of laryngeal spasm and oedema in response to the presence of the tube. Once the ETT has been removed, the patient's neck should be gently extended and the tongue drawn forward if possible in order to maintain patency of the airway.

Common reasons for total or subtotal airway obstruction include:

- Extubation before protective laryngeal reflexes have returned
- Laryngeal paralysis/oedema/spasm
- Foreign material (blood, saliva, vomitus, teeth or swabs) obstructing the airway – especially common after nose, throat or dental procedures
- Acute palatine, parapharyngeal or retropharyngeal swellings (air, haematomas, extravasated fluid or over-tight dressings) occluding the airway
- Unobserved inhalation of all or part of the ETT
- Brachycephalic airway obstruction syndrome.

In extreme cases, inspiratory efforts against an obstructed airway may lead to pulmonary oedema. Patients with airway obstruction usually display vigorous attempts to breathe, with exaggerated thoracic and abdominal excursions that are often, but not invariably, accompanied by loud stertorous snoring respirations. Cyanosis or pallor may be evident, together with tachycardia or, in some cases, severe bradycardia. These patients are sometimes mistaken as suffering from emergence delirium (recovery-associated excitement and distress) and are given sedatives, usually with disastrous results. In many cases the patient requires oxygen therapy and may need re-anaesthetizing and intubating to resolve the obstruction (an appropriate ETT and laryngoscope should be left by the cage of any patient that might experience obstruction in the postoperative phase). The pharyngeal area should be rapidly examined and swabbed clear of debris. Some form of suction apparatus (e.g. 50 ml syringe, three-way tap, urinary catheter) or postural drainage may be required to remove more tenacious material from the upper airway.

BREATHING

Maintenance of adequate ventilation in the postoperative period is essential, not only to maintain the elimination of volatile anaesthetic agents, but also to ensure adequate oxygenation and elimination of carbon dioxide. Devices designed to measure tidal and minute volumes, such as the Wright's respirometer, may be useful to determine whether these variables are adequate after anaesthesia (especially if neuromuscular blocking techniques have been employed). In dogs and cats, minute ventilation should exceed 150 ml/kg; a value of <100 ml/kg requires ventilatory support. Measurement of end-expiratory carbon dioxide concentration is also an effective way of assessing the adequacy of ventilation; normal values should not exceed 40 mmHg (5.3 kPa).

Signs of respiratory inadequacy may vary. Respiratory rate and apparent tidal volume are usually decreased, although a high rate does not imply that ventilation is adequate. Hypoxia and hypercapnia may result in tachycardia, although this may be blunted by the bradycardic effects of opioids and α_2- agonists or by hypothermia. Central cyanosis (defined as the presence of >5 g/dl of circulating reduced haemoglobin) is a late and unreliable sign of hypoxia and a notoriously subjective phenomenon. Severe hypoxia can and does occur in the absence of cyanosis. Pulse oximetry may be useful in postoperative monitoring, but the probes are often difficult to maintain in position in recovering patients, and reduced peripheral perfusion due to hypothermia- or hypovolaemia-induced vasoconstriction may create problems in obtaining meaningful readings.

Postoperative respiratory inadequacy may be due to a number of factors. If the patient has received neuromuscular blocking drugs (e.g. pancuronium, atracurium), any residual respiratory muscle paralysis will result in ineffectual and incoordinated attempts at inspiration and potentially severe hypoventilation.

Residual effects of analgesic and anaesthetic drugs can also produce postoperative hypoventilation. Virtually all of the intravenous and volatile anaesthetic agents will obtund respiration to a greater or lesser extent. Alpha-2 agonist drugs such as xylazine and medetomidine have profound respiratory depressant effects and are commonly used in conjunction with opioid drugs that also cause depression of the respiratory system. Such depression may last well into the postoperative period if these agents are being used for postsurgical analgesia. Although both of these classes of drug have specific reversal agents, it should be remembered that drug reversal may also result in loss of analgesia. Potent µ-agonist opioids such as fentanyl may be reversed, at least in part, using partial agonist drugs such as buprenorphine to reduce respiratory depression while retaining some analgesia. This practice is known as sequential analgesia and has gained substantial popularity in rabbit and rodent anaesthesia where fentanyl is used extensively in combination with fluanisone (see Chapter 28).

Doxapram hydrochloride is used extensively as a respiratory stimulant in neonatal apnoea and in the management of ventilatory failure or inadequacy associated with anaesthesia. The drug acts on the peripheral carotid and aortic chemoreceptors as well as the respiratory centres in the medulla, and essentially increases the sensitivity to carbon dioxide, although some non-specific central nervous system stimulant properties are also recognized. This results in an increase in both tidal volume and respiratory rate. While these effects may be useful in some situations, it should be borne in mind that doxapram is not a substitute for a patent airway and positive-pressure ventilation with 100% oxygen in an unconscious apnoeic patient. The period of stimulation of respiration is usually short, and overdosage can produce side effects such as hypertension, tachycardia and seizures, all of which may be potentially dangerous in an already hypoxic animal.

Postoperative ventilatory inadequacy may also result from airway-associated complications, as previously described. In these instances signs of airway obstruction usually predominate, but in more deeply unconscious patients, apnoea may be the only presenting sign; adequate monitoring is therefore essential.

All patients undergoing surgical procedures of the thoracic cavity should have an indwelling chest drain for postoperative management. This will allow gradual restoration of intrathoracic pressure and removal of fluid and air. The chest should be drained every 15–30 minutes in the immediate postoperative phase and the volume of air and fluid removed and recorded. Alternatively, bottle drains may be used, permitting continuous drainage. Failure of the drain may result in pneumothorax, leading to profound hypoventilation. Further details may be found in Chapter 15.

Postoperative pain of the thoracic or cranial abdominal cavities may be sufficient to prevent adequate inflation of the lungs, leading to hypoventilation, hypoxia and hypercapnia. A 'multimodal' approach to analgesia should be adopted using opioid, non-opioid and local anaesthetics to reduce pain to a minimum. Despite their respiratory depressant properties, the use of opioids to relieve pain associated with the thoracic wall may in fact improve ventilation, the analgesia simply allowing greater thoracic excursion. In addition, the use of local anaesthetics such as lignocaine (lidocaine) or bupivicaine to block intercostal nerves in post-thoracotomy patients, or patients with rib fractures, is to be strongly recommended. Local anaesthetics may also be administered directly into the pleural space, providing analgesia in not only the thorax but also the cranial abdomen.

All of the above factors may occur separately or in combination; these problems may also be further compounded by the presence of postoperative hypothermia, which also acts to depress respiration, thereby delaying the elimination of volatile anaesthetic agents and significantly prolonging recovery. In a debilitated postsurgical patient, this may be sufficient to cause life-threatening respiratory insufficiency. Postoperative management of hypothermia will be discussed later in this chapter.

CIRCULATION

Management and monitoring of the circulation during the postoperative period is important to ensure a rapid smooth restoration of physiologically normal cardiovascular variables. Heart rate and rhythm, pulse rate and quality, mucous membrane colour and capillary refill time should all be regularly and frequently assessed to identify promptly any adverse trends in the patient's condition. Monitoring of central venous pressure and mean arterial pressure can be expensive but provides accurate and often invaluable information.

The most common postoperative circulatory problem is hypotension (mean arterial pressure <60 mmHg). This may be due to hypothermia, a pre-existing disease, surgical or ongoing blood loss, effects of drugs used during, or as part of, the anaesthetic, postoperative dysrhythmias, inadequate fluid administration or a combination of these factors. Signs of postoperative hypotension may include delayed recovery, pale mucous membranes, prolonged capillary refill time, poor pulse quality, tachycardia, reduced urine output, cold extremities and reduced central venous pressure. Treatment is directed at symptomatic therapy while attempting to establish and remove the underlying cause. Aggressive intravenous fluid support should be employed using balanced electrolyte solutions and/or colloids to restore pressure and perfusion. The use of hypertonic saline solutions (4 ml/kg slow bolus of 7% saline) to manage haemorrhage should be considered (for further details see Chapter 11). After the initiation of fluid therapy, the patient should be monitored closely and frequently for signs of improvement or deterioration. Any obvious sites of bleeding should have pressure dressings applied to them. Continued postsurgical haemorrhage into the abdominal cavity or retroperitoneal space may be managed successfully with abdominal and hindlimb counterpressure bandages to centralize the circulation (Figure 3.1); these bandages should be left on for up to 6 hours and then removed slowly in a caudal to cranial direction. Continued blood loss from surgical drains (e.g. chest drains) or into body cavities, should be quantified and the fluid analysed for haematocrit and total solids. Losses of fluid with a packed cell volume approaching that of the patient in excess of 10% of the patients' blood volume should be investigated surgically. Although many hypotensive patients may also be hypothermic, care should be taken with rewarming as the resultant peripheral vasodilation may precipitate a hypovolaemic crisis.

BODY TEMPERATURE

Some degree of heat loss should be anticipated in all anaesthetized patients, but profound hypothermia remains a common postoperative problem in small animals. The causes are numerous and include:

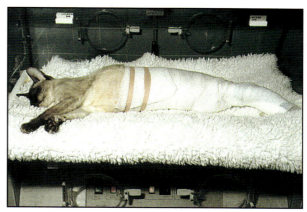

Figure 3.1: *Use of counterpressure bandaging to control intra-abdominal haemorrhage.*

- Lack of endogenous heat production due to disease, starvation, trauma or age
- Impairment of thermoregulation by drugs, disease and trauma
- Exposure to cold surfaces or environment during surgery and anaesthesia
- Radiant and evaporative heat losses due to surgical preparation and tissue exposure
- Direct delivery of cold dry gases to the lungs (bypassing normal warming and humidification mechanisms)
- Further radiant heat losses during recovery.

The pathophysiological effects of hypothermia are numerous and complex and may result in hypoventilation, arrhythmogenesis, alterations in substrate metabolism and central nervous system impairment. Shivering in the postoperative period substantially increases oxygen demand at a time when oxygen delivery to the tissues may still be impaired by the cardiopulmonary depressant effects of anaesthesia and other perioperative events. Supplying an oxygen-enriched gas mixture to high-risk patients during recovery from anaesthesia can be justified on these grounds alone. Therapy for hypothermia should be aggressive, and various rewarming techniques may be employed. As well as providing insulation, the ambient temperature should be raised (neonatal incubators are ideal for this purpose, and ex-hospital models are often available). Warming devices such as waterbeds, heat pads and 'hot hands' (surgical gloves filled with water and heated in a microwave) should not be applied directly to the patient, as burns will result. Catheterization and lavage of the urinary bladder and colon with warm 0.9% saline can be extremely effective in small patients. Progress of the patient's temperature should be carefully monitored to avoid over-heating. The best way to deal with hypothermia is to take sensible measures to minimize heat loss during anaesthesia rather than trying to rewarm patients during recovery.

EVIDENCE OF PAIN

The inability to detect postoperative pain in an animal on the part of the observer does not negate its existence. The ready availability of numerous opioid, non-opioid and local anaesthetic drugs means that the clinician has no excuse to allow postsurgical pain to go untreated. Behaviour indicating pain in animals is diverse and may vary between species, breeds or even individuals, so assessment of postoperative pain levels should be performed by careful observation, noting responses to stimuli such as stroking and gentle pressure applied onto or near the wound. Cats are far less likely to vocalize than dogs in response to a noxious stimulus and so pain may sometimes be more difficult to detect in this species.

Willingness to move, eat, drink and interact with the observer are all reasonably reliable signs of adequate analgesia. In the event of uncertainty, pain should be assumed to be present and an analgesic administered. Prolongation of recovery from anaesthesia due to postoperative opioid administration is not usually significant and is not a contraindication for use of these drugs. The perioperative use of non-steroidal analgesics (either at the time of premedication or immediately after induction) is now commonplace in veterinary analgesia, and the pre-emptive use of opioid analgesics undoubtedly improves the efficacy in the postoperative period. Assessment and management of pain is described in greater detail in Chapter 6.

CHAPTER FOUR

Anaesthetic Equipment

R. Eddie Clutton

INTRODUCTION

The popularity of injectable techniques in veterinary anaesthesia owes much to the fact that they require little equipment. However, the depression of upper airway reflexes and the hypoventilation that characterize many injectable techniques justify endotracheal intubation, oxygen (O_2) enrichment of inspired gas and intermittent lung inflation. Therefore, practitioners committed to injectable anaesthetics need to understand how some equipment operates. The advantages of inhalation techniques secure their place in companion animal anaesthesia despite reliance upon complicated equipment.

INTRAVENOUS CATHETERS

The use of intravenous catheters is warranted whether inhalation or injectable techniques are used. Properly placed, they allow the rapid administration of top-up anaesthetic doses and emergency drugs. They also lower the risk of extravascular injection (which is important when irritant drugs are used, when fluids are infused or when drugs have to be given over several minutes). A range of presterilized polythene, nylon or teflon intravenous catheters are available in various gauges and lengths. These are supplied with an inner stylet or trochar that is necessary for introduction. Several sizes should be available to cater for the range of animals encountered in clinical practice. Commercially available catheters designed for humans meet all necessary standards and safety requirements and are satisfactory in most companion animals. Consequently, problems do not result from catheters *per se*, but from inappropriate catheterization technique, e.g. venous trauma, inadvertent arterial catheterization, sepsis. However, in some subjects with abnormally resilient skin, e.g. entire male cats and dehydrated animals, the catheter fails to penetrate the dermis and 'concertinas' back upon the stylet, thus failing to enter the vein. In such cases, catheters should be passed through a small transcutaneous incision made over the vein with the tip of a number 11 scalpel blade.

INFUSION CONTROLLERS AND SYRINGE DRIVERS

Total intravenous anaesthesia maintained by incremental injections given 'to effect' is undesirable as it is characterized by fluctuations in the level of anaesthesia. In contrast, drug infusion produces more stable conditions. Water-soluble drugs, which do not react with the plastic material from which 'drip' and administration sets are made, can be mixed and infused with crystalloid solutions, e.g. alfentanil, vecuronium. However, changes in venous pressure will affect flow and necessitate constant attention to the drip rate. Infusion controllers and syringe drivers deliver fluids at a pre-set rate irrespective of changes in venous pressure.

Infusion controllers

These regulate the volume of fluid passing through a conventional fluid administration set, and are of two types: drip meters and volumetric pumps. In drip meters, a light sensor surrounds the drip chamber and counts the drips passing through. The fluid line is compressed whenever the drip rate exceeds the pre-set level. These devices are sensitive, but do not recognize that the volume of fluid per drip depends on the diameter of the drip chamber pipe, and on the hydraulic properties of the fluid itself, i.e. the drip rate, not volume delivered, is controlled. In volumetric pumps a peristaltic roller compresses the fluid line at a rate calibrated in ml/min, which is preset by the operator. Such devices deliver precise volumes and can be programmed to change the infusion rate after certain time periods have elapsed (in recognition of the different pharmacokinetic properties of different drugs). Furthermore, many automatically cease infusion when a predetermined volume has been given, when the administration set becomes occluded or when air bubbles are detected in the line. However, these devices are better suited to intensive care situations.

Syringe drivers

These consist of a chassis in which a drug-filled syringe is placed. A mains- or battery-driven electric motor turns a leadscrew which in turn depresses the syringe plunger at a constant rate. Drug delivery rate is altered by varying the motor's rate of revolution. The volume delivered depends on the cross-sectional area of the syringe. Many syringe drivers can only be used with specific makes and sizes of syringe while more sophisticated drivers automatically recognize syringe size and manufacturer. These devices are robust, simple, compact and easy to use, and are ideal when small volumes of drug or fluid need to be given, e.g. to cats.

Ideal properties of both infusion controllers and syringe drivers include: reliability, electrical safety, ease of use, accuracy, robustness, ability to use various types of administration set and syringes, respectively, clear displays and instructions and comprehensive alarm settings and controls.

ANAESTHETIC MACHINES

The essential functions of an anaesthetic machine (in combination with anaesthetic breathing systems) are to:

- Deliver safe effective concentrations of anaesthetic vapour
- Deliver O_2
- Provide a means of intermittent positive-pressure ventilation (IPPV) during apnoea or cardiopulmonary arrest
- Eliminate expired carbon dioxide (CO_2).

Anaesthetic machines also act as platforms for ancillary equipment like monitors and mechanical ventilators and scavenging and suction devices. Understanding the construction and performance of anaesthetic machines is an important prerequisite for the safe administration of anaesthetics and O_2. An improperly used anaesthetic machine can jeopardize both patients and operating room personnel.

Anaesthetic machines possess a basic pattern (Figure 4.1). The gas flow begins at a carrier gas source (A) passes through a pressure gauge (B), a pressure regulator (C) and a flowmeter assembly (D) and ends at the common gas outlet (F) where the anaesthetic breathing system (ABS) attaches. Vaporizers (E) may be incorporated within the breathing system (VIC) or, more usually, downstream from the flowmeter assembly (VOC), as in Figure 4.1. Check valves (a), emergency O_2 valves (b), low O_2 alarms (c), nitrous oxide (N_2O) cut-out devices (d), overpressure valves (e) and emergency air-intake valves (f) are useful options.

These basic components are assembled on a wheeled chassis, which may carry varying amounts of accessories.

Components

Gas supply
Gases used in anaesthesia may be stored as liquids or as compressed gases, either in banks of large cylinders or in small volume cylinders attached to the anaesthetic machine. The choice depends on gas consumption rate, which in turn depends on the practice caseload. Greater storage capacities cost more to install, but with time, costs are lower because delivery charges are reduced and larger cylinders cost proportionately less to hire and to fill.

Liquid O_2: The capacity of refrigerated liquid O_2 flasks probably exceeds the requirements of even the busiest veterinary facility and they are only practical for large teaching hospitals.

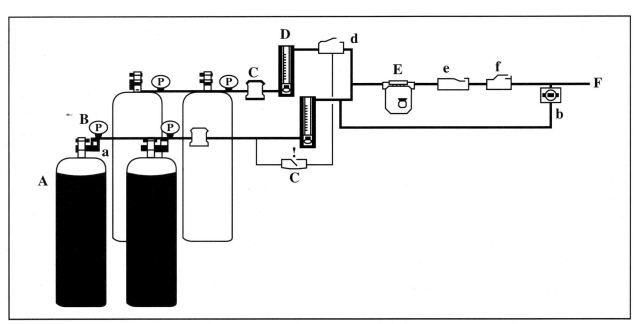

Figure 4.1: *Anaesthetic machine.*

	UK				USA		
	E	**F**	**G**	**J**	**E**	**F**	**G**
Dimensions	34 x 4	36 x 35$^1/_2$	54 x 7	56$^1/_2$ x 9	26 x 4$^1/_2$	51 x 5$^1/_2$	51 x 8$^1/_2$
Oxygen	680	1360	3400	6800	650	2062	5300
Nitrous oxide	1820	3640	9100	18200	1590	5260	13800

Figure 4.2: *Dimensions (height* x *outer diameter in inches) and approximate capacity (in litres measured at room temperature and pressure) for various commonly used gas cylinders (adapted from Ward, CS,* Anaesthetic equipment; physical principles and maintenance, *Baillière Tindall, London, 1975 and Dorsch, J.A. & Dorsch, S.E.,* Understanding anesthetic equipment; construction, care and complications, *Williams and Wilkins, Baltimore, 1984).*

Cylinder banks: Vertically standing banks of 3–5 'J'- or 'G'-sized cylinders are a convenient way to store gases in busy small animal practices. Figure 4.2 gives the capacity of commonly used cylinders. Two banks for each gas (O$_2$ and N$_2$O) are desirable; one being in use, the other in reserve. Switching between banks is performed manually or automatically. Gas flows through a manifold and series of non-return valves to the hospital through pipes inset within the walls. These end in wall-mounted gas-specific female sockets that accept gas-specific male connectors (probes) on flexible pipes that, in turn, lead to the anaesthetic machine. Cylinders are painted so that the contents are known, e.g. in the UK: O$_2$, black body and white shoulders; N$_2$O, blue; and CO$_2$, grey (in the USA, oxygen cylinders are green). Pipelines are similarly colour coded, and the connectors are size- and shape-coded so that lines cannot be accidentally crossed. In the USA, threaded medical gas pipe connections should comply with the Diameter Index Safety System (DISS).

Low-volume cylinders: Cylinder storage requires space. For most small animal practices low-volume 'E' cylinders attached to hanger yokes on the anaesthetic machine are suitable. However, when gas consumption is high, constant pressure checks and cylinder changing become tedious. Machines should hold two cylinders of O$_2$ and (optionally) N$_2$O. The cylinder valve bears holes that correspond with pins sited within the hanger yoke. The pin and hole pattern is gas specific, constitutes the pin-indexing system and aims to prevent connection of the wrong gas cylinder to the wrong yoke. The system may fail if pins are broken off by mishandling. For cost-effectiveness and convenience, anaesthetic machines should operate principally from piped gases from external stores, and machine-mounted cylinders should be used as a reserve supply.

Cylinder safety: Cylinders are filled to high pressures (at 20°C: O$_2$ 13,300 kPa (1935 p.s.i.); N$_2$O 5471 kPa (794 p.s.i.)) and so explosions are possible if they are mistreated, e.g. dropped, exposed to heat. Cylinders are submitted to tensile, impact and pressure testing at regular intervals by the manufacturer to ensure their

strength and safety. They must be stored under specific conditions (Figure 4.3). Cylinders storing liquefied gases, e.g. CO$_2$ and N$_2$O, should always be used vertically with the valve uppermost, otherwise liquid will be discharged when the valve is opened.

Before O$_2$ cylinders are connected to the hanger yoke, the cylinder valve should be opened briefly ('cracked') to flush any dust from the outlet port, which may support combustion should transfilling occur (see below).

Only sufficient force should be used to close a cylinder valve. Excessive force will damage both valve seats and spindles. Cylinder valves and associated equipment must not be lubricated and must be kept

- Cylinders should be stored:
  Under cover
  Preferably inside
  Not subjected to extremes of heat or cold
  In dry clean well ventilated storage areas
  Separately from industrial and non-medical gases

- Cylinders should not be stored:
  Near stocks of combustible material
  Near sources of heat

- Full and empty cylinders should be stored separately

- Full cylinders should be used in strict rotation (the earliest date cylinder should be used first)

- 'F'-sized and larger cylinders should be stored vertically in concrete-floored pens

- 'E'-sized and smaller cylinders should be stored horizontally

- Emergency services should be advised of the cylinder store location and the nature of gases kept there

- Warning notices prohibiting smoking and naked lights should be posted clearly on the storage compound

Figure 4.3: *Storage of medical gas cylinders.*

entirely free from carbon-based oils and greases; the combination of these with high-pressure O_2 may result in explosion. Similarly, smoking and naked lights must not be allowed within the vicinity of a cylinder or pipeline outlet, or in confined spaces where cylinders are stored or used.

Check valves

Check valves should be present on machines carrying two or more cylinders of each gas because they:

- Prevent retrograde gas flow through the inlet nipple of vacant hanger yokes when alternative gas sources (cylinder or piped supply) are in use
- Prevent gas transfer between cylinders at high and low pressures
- Allow changing of empty cylinders while gas flows from another source.

The check valves are sited within each hanger yoke assembly immediately downstream from the gas inlet nipple, and so are difficult to locate. Confirming their presence and function involves removing the cylinder from the yoke under test and opening an alternative source of the same gas. A hissing sound at the yoke indicates that the check valve is leaking or absent. When check valves are defective or missing, opening a full new cylinder before closing the old empty one will result in transfilling, where gas flows from a high pressure cylinder to a low pressure cylinder. The heat generated by this may cause the old cylinder to explode and so if the check valve function is unknown, it is safer to close the cylinder that is nearly empty before opening the full one.

Pressure/contents gauge

The pressure gauge for O_2 is indispensable as it indicates the gas volume in the cylinder. This is calculated with Boyle's law (PV = k). An 'E'-sized cylinder contains 680 litres of gas when filled to 13,300 kPa (1935 p.s.i.) at 20°C. At the same temperature, a pressure gauge registering 4500 kPa (655 p.s.i.) indicates that only 230 litres remain. The N_2O pressure gauge does not act as a contents gauge; it measures the saturated vapour pressure of gaseous N_2O in equilibrium with liquid. This remains constant until all liquid evaporates, after which pressure falls rapidly. Gas volume in N_2O cylinders is determined by weighing the cylinder and applying the formula:

Gas present (litres) = (net − tare) weight (in grams) x 22.4/44

The tare weight of an N_2O 'E' cylinder is about 5.8-6.4 kg

Pressure-reducing valves or regulators

Pressure-reducing valves (regulators) produce constant downstream pressures of 400–800 kPa (60–120 p.s.i.) and therefore constant gas flow, despite a cylinder pressure that falls with use. Without them, the cylinder valve would need to be opened incrementally to maintain constant flows. Regulators also permit safe working pressures and prevent equipment damage. Located downstream from the hanger yoke, regulators may be incorporated in the yoke itself and be impossible to identify. Machines holding two cylinders of each gas normally have one regulator per cylinder. Gases piped to the machine are regulated at source. Devices incorporating pressure gauges, regulators, flowmeters and a 'bull-nose' connector are available for the attachment of pipelines to larger cylinders (from size 'F' upwards).

Flowmeters

Flowmeters control, measure and indicate the gas flowing around them. On most anaesthetic machines, an ascending flow of gas supports a freely moving 'float' – either a ball or bobbin – in a transparent, tapered glass or plastic tube. The flow rate (in litres per minute), etched on the tube, is read from the top of bobbins and from the equator of spheres. Flowmeter accuracy is only guaranteed between the minimum and maximum calibration range. Flowmeters yield false-low readings if dirt, humidity, static electricity or non-vertical positioning makes the float rub against the tube (slots in the rim of bobbins encourage rotation and limit these problems). Flowmeters are calibrated for single gases, and so O_2 flowmeters do not accurately indicate the flow rate of N_2O. Consequently, the needle valve control knobs are colour and touch coded and bear the name of the gas.

Inappropriate settings of the O_2 and N_2O flowmeters relative to one another can cause hypoxic gas mixtures to be delivered. Old anaesthetic machines with functionally independent flow control knobs are potentially capable of delivering pure (100%) N_2O, although this risk is reduced by having colour-coded, size-coded and touch-coded flowmeter control knobs; on modern units in the UK, the O_2 control is white and is larger and has coarser convolutions than other flowmeters. Modern flowmeter assemblies catering for up to three gases (O_2, N_2O and CO_2) are available in which N_2O (and CO_2) flow is only permitted if the O_2 supply pressure exceeds 140 kPa. However, this does not preclude the delivery of hypoxic gas mixtures, which is possible when the O_2 flow control is set too low in relation to N_2O. Therefore, modern anaesthetic machines may incorporate proportioning devices, which ensure that the lowest $O_2:N_2O$ flow ratio is 1:2. The simplest device involves a chain linkage that activates the O_2 flowmeter whenever the N_2O flow control knob is switched on. A more complex (and costly) device has two controls: one sets the desired O_2 percentage (minimum value 33%); the other controls total gas flow rate from 1-20 l/min. A N_2O cut out intervenes when O_2 supply fails.

Oxygen and N_2O mix freely downstream from the flowmeter assembly to constitute the carrier gas mixture, which then enters the vaporizer.

Vaporizers

Breathing the undiluted vapour of most anaesthetics would be fatal, because their saturated vapour pressures (SVP) at room temperature produce concentrations far in excess of that required for anaesthesia. For example, the SVP for halothane at 20°C is 243 mmHg and yields a concentration given by:

$$SVP/barometric\ pressure^* \times 100 = 32\ \%$$

* Normally about 760 mmHg

This is about 40 times greater than its minimal alveolar concentration (MAC) of 0.8% (which would produce unresponsiveness in 50% of animals undergoing noxious stimulation). Vaporizers dilute the saturated vapour of volatile anaesthetics to yield a range of useful (safe) concentrations. Within the vaporizer, carrier gases flow either through a bypass channel or are diverted into a vaporization chamber, which contains anaesthetic vapour at its SVP. Here, carrier gases and anaesthetic vapour mix before rejoining gases flowing through the bypass channel. The delivered concentration (%) of anaesthetic is altered by turning the control spindle. This action changes the ratio of gas entering the vaporization chamber compared with that flowing down the bypass channel.

Vaporizers are classified according to the mechanism causing gas to flow through them. Gases flow through plenum devices because the anaesthetic machine generates a positive pressure upstream from the vaporizer. In draw-over vaporizers, gases flow because a downstream negative pressure is generated by the subject's inspiratory effort. In order that this does not restrict spontaneous ventilation, these devices must offer minimal resistance to gas flow. Consequently these devices are also known as low-resistance vaporizers.

Uncalibrated vaporizers: The Boyle bottle is a simple, inexpensive and easily maintained plenum vaporizer. However, output concentrations are not defined, drift despite constant control settings and fall as liquid anaesthetic cools or as flow rates increase over 12–25 l/min. Output increases if flow rates are reduced, but increases with increasing flow, up to a point. High concentrations are also delivered when the vaporizer is agitated, temperatures rise or back pressure, caused by IPPV, is unchecked and forces downstream gas to re-enter the vaporizer. This effect is greatest at low flow rates.

Calibrated vaporizers: Anaesthetic concentration from 'tec' (temperature compensated) and other calibrated vaporizers is similar to that selected on the dial of the spindle, provided that gas flow through the vaporizer and the temperature of liquid anaesthetic are within ranges specific for the model. In Mark III tecs, e.g. Fluotec (halothane; Ohmeda) and Fortec (isoflurane;

Ohmeda), output is constant with time and unaffected by back pressure, although the dialled concentration is only produced when the liquid anaesthetic is between 18°C and 35°C. As the temperature of liquid anaesthetic falls, a bimetallic strip opens and increases the flow rate of gas entering the vaporization chamber. Cold ambient temperatures and high gas flow rates may lower the vaporizer's temperature below 18°C and curtail output, causing difficulty in maintaining anaesthesia. Under these conditions the vaporizer requires warming. Dialled and delivered concentrations are similar at flow rates between 0.2 and 15 l/min.

Considerable attention must be paid to the selection of a vaporizer when low flow or closed system anaesthesia (see below) is used. Low-resistance vaporizers may be used either in the circuit (VIC) or out of circuit (VOC). Plenum vaporizers can only be positioned VOC. In low flow or closed systems Mark II, or preferably Mark III, Fluotecs calibrated to 8% (rather than 5%) are useful. However, discrepancies between dialled and output concentrations are high at low flow rates in some vaporizers, so a performance graph must be consulted. The Mark II Fluotec produces very high concentrations at flow rates below 4 l/min and must be used with caution.

Vaporizers are agent specific. Filling a vaporizer with the wrong anaesthetic can be prevented by keyed filling ports – the key-index vaporizer filling system. The keyed filling ports accept a key-ended tube that attaches only to the corresponding anaesthetic bottle. Used properly, the system also assists in controlling pollution because the vaporizer can be filled without spillage.

Vaporizers must always be kept in an upright position. If they are tilted, liquid anaesthetic may flow into the bypass chamber and expose the next patient to very high levels of anaesthetic vapour.

Draw-over or low-resistance vaporizers: Low-resistance vaporizers are located within the circuit either to facilitate low flow techniques or to confer portability to units designed for emergency field use in humans. They are found in the Komesaroff and Stephens' anaesthetic machines described below. They are simply constructed, inexpensive and offer little resistance to breathing, but are relatively inaccurate.

Checking plenum vaporizers before use

Before turning on the flowmeter control knobs the vaporizers should be checked to ensure they contain enough liquid anaesthetic, that the control spindle turns smoothly and that the filling port is tightly closed. If the anaesthetic machine incorporates a pressure-relief valve (see below), the vaporizer can be tested for leaks: the control spindle should be set at 0%, the O_2 flowmeter control knob set at, e.g. 8 l/min, and the common gas outlet occluded. There should be no leak from any vaporizer fittings, and the flowmeter bobbin should drop.

Back bar

The series of semi-permanent fixtures that results when flowmeters and (out of circuit) vaporizers are joined by tapered cagemount connectors and attached to a back bar, makes servicing individual components difficult. Systems such as the 'Selectatec SM' (Ohmeda) manifold are more useful as they allow rapid attachment or removal of vaporizers for refilling out of the operating room, servicing and rewarming. By accommodating up to three vaporizers, a range of volatile agents may be available. Most modern anaesthetic machines are equipped with a system that prevents more than one vaporizer at a time from being turned on (a double exclusion system).

Common gas outlet

This connects the anaesthetic machine to breathing system connectors, ventilators or O_2 supply devices. To meet these roles the outlet must be dual tapered, with a 22 mm outer male connector (to British Standard) and 15 mm inner female connector. A swivel common gas outlet (e.g. Cardiff swivel) is useful because it reduces the need to move machines, facilitates circuit positioning and reduces the risk of hoses kinking.

Oxygen flush, bypass or purge valve

The O_2 flush, bypass or purge valve receives O_2 from the pipeline inlet or cylinder regulator but bypasses the vaporizer. It is used to provide O_2 in emergency situations and may have a lock-on facility. When activated, high non-metered flow rates of pure O_2 are directed to the common gas outlet at rates of 35–60 l/min. The device is also used to flush anaesthetic from breathing systems before the patient is disconnected from the machine, thus lowering pollution. The O_2 flush valve can be inadvertently activated by components of the breathing system when the system is in certain positions.

Low O_2 warning devices

Low O_2 warning devices are very important on veterinary anaesthetic machines as it is not always possible to monitor gas delivery continuously. Ideally, falling O_2 supplies should curtail N_2O (and CO_2) flow and simultaneously sound an alarm. (As with all safety devices, this alarm should be gas driven and not require batteries or an electrical supply.) The warning system present on a machine is tested by switching on both O_2 and N_2O sources, opening the flowmeter control knobs to give nominal flow rates of 2 and 4 l/min, respectively, and then closing the O_2 cylinder (or other O_2 source). The N_2O and O_2 flow indicators should fall simultaneously and an alarm sound (either intermittently or, preferably, continuously). It is important to establish whether N_2O flow continues through the common gas outlet while the alarm sounds or is vented elsewhere; if, as on old or defective machines, the former is the case, the operator must respond immediately whenever the alarm is heard. On some machines, N_2O flows through the flowmeter and activates a whistle, but is exhausted safely upstream from the common gas outlet.

Emergency air-intake valve

This opens when gas flow from the machine ceases and allows animals to breathe room air until flow is restored. Valve action should be audible, indicating the patient's inspiratory effort. The presence of this device is confirmed by attaching a pipe to the common gas outlet and applying suction.

Overpressure valve

Excessive pressures downstream from the common gas outlet open this valve and sound an alarm. The device is useful for testing breathing systems for leaks; its presence is confirmed by occluding the common gas outlet while pressing the O_2 bypass valve. Overpressure and emergency air-intake valves are often constructed as a single attachment.

Miscellaneous accessories

Useful accessories with anaesthetic machines include:

- Stainless steel work trays
- An eye-level monitor shelf
- Cabinets for equipment
- Circuit hooks
- Large-diameter castor wheels with brakes (desirable on hospital-based machines)
- An adjustable plinth.

Types of anaesthetic machines

Purpose-built machines for small animals

These often have circle breathing systems specially built on. The machines, but not the breathing systems, are suitable for birds, small mammals and companion animals. However, they often lack the warning and fail-safe devices required in human anaesthesia.

Ex-human hospital machines

Usually, these are sophisticated and more likely to have the safety features listed above. They are less expensive than purpose-built small animal models although service arrangements may be difficult to negotiate and components may be obsolete.

Unspecified or improvized equipment

Safe anaesthesia is possible with an assembly of compatible basic components as long as the specifications of each component are known, they function, and they are connected correctly. Components may be salvaged from old machines or bought as new. Combinations of basic components mounted on a portable chassis are available. In machines for unspecified use, flowmeter and vaporizer performance must cover the needs of the species to be anaesthetized. Compactness is useful where space is limited and mobility not required.

Vaporizer in circuit machines

These are circle breathing systems with one or more low-resistance vaporizers positioned within the breathing system, e.g. Stephens' or Komesaroff models or the Mini-Kom (Kruuse). Their operation requires some practice but, once mastered, the systems are safe and easy to use, and because low O_2 flow rates are used they are very economical to operate. The Komesaroff anaesthetic machine consists of an O_2 cylinder, a pressure-reducing valve and a flowmeter attached to a circle breathing system, which incorporates two in-circuit vaporizers for halothane and methoxyflurane. The system is portable (weighing about 15 kg) and its design combines the advantages of inhalation anaesthesia while minimizing atmospheric pollution. The Stephens' anaesthetic machine is similar in design but incorporates a single in-circuit vaporizer and requires a non-integral O_2 supply and pressure regulator. The system is compact and readily adapted for use with halothane, methoxyflurane or isoflurane. The system's efficiency reduces costs when expensive anaesthetics, e.g. isoflurane, are used.

Checking machines before use

The anaesthetic machine should receive a major check at the beginning of each working day and a minor check after each use. To ensure no parts of the test are omitted a list should be attached to the machine:

1. Ensure flow control valves are turned off
2. Ensure cylinders are closed and fitted securely on the hanger yolk
3. Press the O_2 flush valve until no gas flows from the common gas outlet
4. Check that flowmeters and pressure gauges are at zero
5. Open the O_2 cylinder valve (slowly, anticlockwise) and observe the registered pressure. Open then close the O_2 flowmeter control valve to ensure smooth function. Press the O_2 flush valve. (On machines that carry a second O_2 cylinder, the tested cylinder should be closed first and the test repeated on the second cylinder)
6. Label the cylinders either 'in use' or 'full' depending on registered pressure
7. Replace cylinders with little remaining gas
8. Open the O_2 cylinder that is in use and set the O_2 flowmeter control knob at 2 l/min. Examine the status of the N_2O cylinders as in step 5. Label the N_2O cylinders
9. Set the N_2O flow control knob at 4 l/min then turn off the O_2 supply; ensure low O_2 warning device operates (see above)
10. Check the vaporizer (as above)
11. Check overpressure and emergency air-intake valves (as above).

(This routine may need to be modified if the anaesthetic machine is connected to a central gas supply.)

Shutting down the anaesthetic machine

On completion of surgery, the cylinders should be checked for content and relabelled. (If present, the N_2O probe should be removed from the wall socket and the pipe neatly coiled.) The O_2 flowmeter control knob should be opened to produce a flow rate of 2 l/min. The N_2O cylinder valve(s) should then be closed and the N_2O flowmeter turned on until all flow of the gas ceases, when it should be closed again. If O_2 supply pipes are present, they should be disconnected, the O_2 cylinders closed and the O_2 flush valve activated until no pressure registers on the pressure gauge. Machine surfaces should then be wiped with antiseptic.

ANAESTHETIC BREATHING SYSTEMS

Anaesthetic breathing systems connect the anaesthetic machine to the connector for the endotracheal tube (ETT) or mask, and they convey anaesthetic vapour to the patient. They are used during both injectable and inhalational anaesthesia to carry O_2 and to allow intermittent lung inflation. Improper selection of a system, its misuse or circuit malfunction may jeopardize patient safety. Because each circuit has advantages (and disadvantages) in different circumstances, a range should be available to cover all potential clinical situations.

Factors influencing selection of a breathing system

Resistance

Anaesthetized animals hypoventilate when there is increased resistance to inspiratory and expiratory flow, although animals that are lightly anaesthetized may overcome this at the cost of increased work of breathing. Resistance stems from circuit geometry (valves, absorbent canisters, constrictions and hose tortuosity) and hose length. The most important contributor to resistance is hose radius; halving the radius increases resistance to gas flow 16-fold. Selection of a breathing system is normally based on the patient's bodyweight because larger (heavier) animals are able to overcome resistance (lightweight animals are also less able to cope with mechanical dead space). However, the limitations of this criterion must be appreciated; a fit dog weighing 5 kg may tolerate resistance that would compromise an obese, older myasthenic animal weighing 20 kg.

Species	Respiratory rate* (breaths/min)	Tidal volume* (ml/kg)	Minute volume* (ml/kg/min)	Oxygen consumption† (ml/kg/min)
Dogs (> 30 kg)	15–20	12–15	150–250	5.8
(< 30 kg)	20–30	16–20	200–300	6.2
Cats	20–30	7–9	180–380	7.3

*Figure 4.4: Respiratory variables in companion animals. *During surgery, factors like pain, pyrexia and light versus deep anaesthesia will affect these values. †Oxygen consumption depends on factors related to metabolic rate: age, temperature, thyroid status, drugs, muscle tone and response to surgery.*

Controlled versus spontaneous ventilation

Controlled ventilation overcomes most of the problems of resistance to spontaneous breathing and reduces the work of breathing. It is mandatory during thoracotomy, when animals hypoventilate, and during the use of neuromuscular blocking agents. The gas flow requirements of the Magill and Lack breathing systems become uneconomically high during IPPV.

Rebreathing versus non-rebreathing

Rebreathing is the re-inhalation of expired breath. Expired gas is warmer, more moist and higher in CO_2 but lower in O_2 and anaesthetic vapour than fresh (inspired) gas from the machine. Total rebreathing results in undesirable accumulation of CO_2. Partial rebreathing describes re-inspiration of breath from which CO_2 has been removed. This is advantageous (heat and water vapour are retained) and safe, providing O_2 and anaesthetic are replenished. Partial rebreathing is useful in animals at risk from hypothermia and those with certain types of tracheobronchial disease. Circle and to-and-fro systems that allow partial rebreathing are described as rebreathing systems.

Fresh gas flow requirements

In rebreathing systems, gas flow from the machine replaces anaesthetic and O_2 taken up by the patient; flow requirements are based on the animal's O_2 consumption. In non-rebreathing systems, fresh gas is needed to elute CO_2 from the system; flow requirements are based on multiples of minute ventilatory volume (Vm). As these are considerably greater than O_2 consumption (Figure 4.4), non-rebreathing systems are uneconomical in large animals, during prolonged procedures or when carrier gas and vapour economy is important, e.g. anaesthesia with isoflurane.

Inclusion of N_2O

The use of N_2O in rebreathing systems is potentially hazardous when using 'low-flow' or closed systems. Uptake of O_2 and N_2O from the system occurs at different rates and may leave hypoxic gas mixtures. This is identified by measuring inspired O_2 concentrations. Dohoo et al. (1982) showed that flow rates of 30 ml/kg/min O_2 and 60 ml/kg/min N_2O allow the safe use of N_2O in rebreathing systems for dogs. These high flow rates limit partial rebreathing

and increase pollution and wastage of volatile agents and so reduce efficiency.

Mechanical dead space

Mechanical or apparatus dead space accommodates gas, which is re-inspired at every breath but which does not participate in gas exchange. Acting as an extension of the animal's anatomical dead space, it is recognized as the volume between the incisor arcade (rostral limit of anatomical dead space) and that part of the breathing system where inspired and expired gas streams divide (Figure 4.5). It reduces the portion of inspired fresh gas reaching alveoli and, in the absence of increased minute ventilation, causes hypoventilation.

Circuit drag

Heavy hoses, valves and absorbent canisters create drag and facilitate inadvertent extubation or circuit disconnection when animals move or are moved. Lightweight plastic hoses without drag (or rigidity) are desirable in small subjects, e.g. birds. Valves and multiple hoses adjacent to patients contribute to drag; coaxial (tube within a tube) systems have neither, so are useful in very small animals.

Ease of maintenance and sterilization

Disposable lightweight plastic versions of some systems are ideal for animals with infectious diseases. The ease of sterilization depends on the system's complexity: circle systems are difficult to sterilize. Sterilization procedures are beyond the scope of this article.

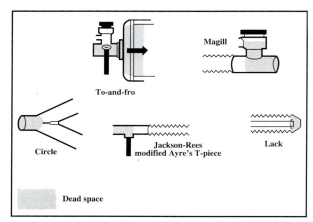

Figure 4.5: Mechanical dead space.

Reproduced from In Practice (1995) 17, pp. 229–237, with permission.

Advantages
Low gas flow requirements
Low volatile agent consumption rate
'Closed' or 'low flow' options
Expired moisture and heat conserved
Ventilation altered (spontaneous to controlled)
    without changing system performance or
    efficiency
Low explosion risk (when explosive gases are used)
Less pollution than other anaesthetic systems

Disadvantages
High resistance to breathing
Nitrous oxide cannot be safely used in
    rebreathing systems at low flows
Expensive to purchase
Regular replacement of soda lime required
Denitrogenation required
Inspired gas content undetermined
Slow to change level of anaesthesia
Cumbersome
Cannot be used with trichlorethylene*

*Figure 4.6: Advantages and disadvantages of rebreathing systems. *No longer available as an anaesthetic. Sevoflurane, a volatile agent currently undergoing clinical evaluation in animals, is unstable in, and absorbed by, soda lime.*

Valve position

Repeated operation of pressure-relief valves located by the head, e.g. to control ventilation, disrupts surgery and may compromise sterility. Coaxial systems reduce this problem.

Ease of scavenging

A scavenging hose attached at pressure-relief valves close to the patient contributes to drag.

REBREATHING SYSTEMS

In circle and to-and-fro systems, soda lime, or bara-lime in the USA, removes CO_2 from expired gas. Advantages and disadvantages of rebreathing systems are shown in Figure 4.6. Some features of rebreathing system operation described in the figure require explanation:

Closed and low flow systems

Rebreathing systems are used in one of two ways. In closed systems, gas inflow precisely replaces anaesthetic and O_2 taken up by the patient (approximately 5–10 ml/kg/min is required). Under these conditions the pressure-relief valve is shut and the system described as closed. Oxygen consumption depends on factors related to metabolic rate, but typical values are given in Figure 4.4. In low flow systems, O_2 delivery exceeds basal requirements (>10 ml/kg/min), with surplus gas

leaking through the partly opened pressure-relief valve. This is the easiest system to operate and therefore the most common. Figure 4.7 shows the advantages and disadvantages of closed and low flow systems.

Nitrous oxide cannot be safely used in rebreathing systems unless inspired O_2 or patient arterial O_2 tensions are monitored or high flows are used.

Denitrogenation

At the onset of anaesthesia, patients expire considerable volumes of nitrogen, which may lower circuit O_2 to hypoxic levels unless purged through the pressure-relief valve (denitrogenation). Hypoxic gas mixtures are likely when N_2O and/or closed systems are used. Denitrogenation is achieved using high flow rates for the first 10–15 minutes of anaesthesia. Alternatively, the reservoir bag should be emptied every 3 minutes for the first 15 minutes and every 30 minutes thereafter.

Anaesthetic concentration

The rate of change of gas concentration in rebreathing systems is inversely proportional to the volume of the system and directly related to the rate of gas inflow. Usually, circle systems have greater volumes than to-and-fro circuits, so rapid increases in concentration (required, for example, when animals become lightly anaesthetized) rely on greater inflow rates and vaporizer settings. Flowmeter and vaporizer performance must meet this requirement.

Advantages
Optimum fresh gas economy
Low pollution and explosion risk
Maximum preservation of heat and moisture
Minimum waste of inhaled anaesthetic
Self-regulating anaesthesia in spontaneously
    breathing subjects when vaporizers are
    incorporated in the breathing system (VIC)

Disadvantages
Constant attention to system required
Accurate flowmeters 0–1000 ml/min required
Denitrogenation mandatory
Nitrous oxide inclusion is imprudent unless
    oximetry performed
Slow response to changing inspired oxygen
    concentration
Use possible only in subjects with oxygen
    consumption lying in a range of vaporizer
    function
High output vaporizers required (VOC) or high
    output low resistance vaporizers (VIC)
Risk of overdose during intermittent positive-
    pressure ventilation when VIC

Figure 4.7: Advantages and disadvantages of closed versus 'low flow' systems.

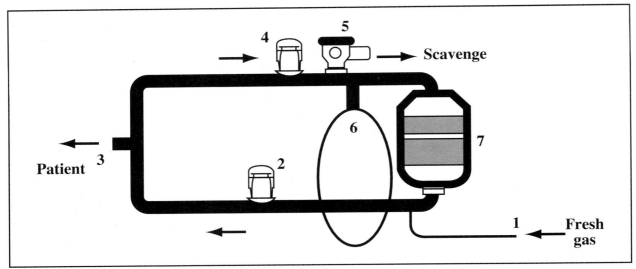

Figure 4.8: *Circle anaesthetic breathing system.*

Reproduced from In Practice *(1995)* **17**, *pp. 229–237, with permission.*

Circle system

Circle systems (Figure 4.8) have valves that permit the movement of gas in one direction. There are seven circuit components: fresh gas inflow (1), inspiratory and expiratory unidirectional valves (2 and 4), the patient 'Y' connector (3), a pressure-relief valve (5), a reservoir bag (6) and an absorbent canister (7). Some circuits have manometers that are useful but not vital. The relative positioning of the components influences efficiency mainly when circle systems are used in a low flow manner.

Fresh gas inflow

This pipe connects the circuit with the common gas outlet on the anaesthetic machine. Its location upstream of the inspiratory valve and downstream from the canister allows best control of inspired gas composition.

Unidirectional valves

These are light transparent discs that rest on the edge of annular valve seats, enclosed within a gas-tight transparent dome. Painted indicators on the discs accentuate their movement. Units are easily disassembled for cleaning and drying.

'Y' connector

This connects inspiratory and expiratory limbs with ETT connectors or masks. In paediatric systems it has a septum that divides inspiratory and expiratory flows, reducing mechanical dead space.

Pressure-relief valve

This is an adjustable unidirectional valve venting at pressures from 1–50 mmHg. It is opened to release surplus gas from low flow systems and during denitrogenation. It is closed when bag compression is imposed for lung inflation. In old systems the valve was sited at the 'Y' connector, which made operation difficult. Pressure-relief valves should be shrouded for attachment to scavenging hoses.

Reservoir (rebreathing) bag

This is normally sited between the expiratory valve and absorber; it allows IPPV and assists in the monitoring of respiratory rate and tidal volume (Vt). The bag's volume should be 3–6 times that of the animal's Vt. Oversized bags increase circuit volume, diminish perceptibility of respiration and are harder to compress manually. Inadequately sized bags collapse during large breaths and over distend during expiration. For small animal use, 2, 4 and 6 litre capacity bags are required.

Absorbent canister

Siting the canister on the expiratory limb downstream from the pressure-relief valve allows CO_2 to be expelled before it reacts with, and consumes, soda lime. In this position, dust aspiration from the absorber granules is unlikely, although heat conservation in the breathing system is poorer.

The filled canister contains approximately 50% absorbent granules and 50% air space. Efficient absorption requires the air space volume between the granules to be greater than the Vt and so the minimum working soda lime volume required is 2 x Vt. Greater volumes than this are needed because the absorbent is progressively inactivated during use. Large canisters may confer increased resistance to breathing, but require less frequent changing.

For optimum absorption efficiency, the canister width:height ratio should be 1:1 or greater. Gas flows more slowly through large-diameter canisters, and resistance caused by turbulent flow is reduced.

Canisters for circle systems should have two compartments. When absorbent in one compartment becomes exhausted, it should be discarded. After refilling, the canister should be replaced in the reverse direction. Expired gas then passes through the remaining partially used absorbent, exhausting this completely before reaching the newly filled compartment. Circle system canisters may have a switch that allows gases to bypass the absorbent. This is used after controlled ventilation when low arterial CO_2 tensions may prevent resumption of spontaneous breathing. Switching the absorbent off allows circuit CO_2 levels to rise without curtailing O_2 and anaesthetic delivery. Inadvertent operation of circle systems with absorbent switched off (excluded) may result in fatal hypercapnia. Absorbent canisters should be easy to open, fill, reseal and replace. They should also have a window so that the colour of the absorbent and the extent of its filling can be checked.

Canisters for human use are suitable for dogs weighing over 15 kg. Mechanical dead space does not increase in the course of time but absorbent exhaustion occurs more acutely than with to-and-fro systems, and replacement may become necessary at inconvenient times during surgery. Small animal systems require about 1.5 litre canisters accepting 1.35 kg of absorbent.

Hoses
Corrugated hosing prevents kinking but generates turbulent gas flow and therefore increases resistance. Smooth-walled hose with external ribbing is preferable. Hoses for human use (22 mm diameter) are suitable for companion animals.

Advantages
Circle systems are very efficient and most suited to dogs weighing over 15 kg. They are more convenient to use than to-and-fro systems. Efficiency becomes particularly high when circle systems are used in a closed fashion (see Figure 4.7). The Komesaroff and Stephens' anaesthetic machines are designed for closed use and have been employed in dogs as small as 2 kg. The level of anaesthesia in animals connected to systems with VIC is to some extent self-regulating; as animals become more lightly anaesthetized their alveolar ventilation increases, which augments vaporizer output and so anaesthesia deepens. Relatively inexpensive lightweight plastic systems are now available. One range is disposable.

Disadvantages
Circle systems are complex, cumbersome and difficult to sterilize. Circuits described as paediatric and adult human (small animal) differ in hose length and radius and in the volume of absorbent canisters. Despite availability, circle systems for small dogs and cats are less popular in the UK than elsewhere because of resistance caused by absorbent and valves, and because dead space in the 'Y' connector is alleged to be excessive. Circle systems designed for human use should not be used in dogs weighing less than 15 kg, although they are useful and efficient in larger dogs. When circle systems are run with VIC, overdosage risk increases when ventilation is controlled. When this is required, animals must be closely monitored and vaporizer output curtailed.

To-and-fro (Water's) system
In this system, gas oscillates through absorbent granules in the Water's canister, which in companion animals is used in a horizontal position (Figure 4.9). To-and-fro and circle systems are compared in Figure 4.10. Desirable features of to-and-fro circuits include:

Fresh gas inflow
Situating gas inflow next to the ETT connector reduces mechanical dead space and allows optimal control over anaesthesia; dialled concentrations of anaesthetic are preferentially inspired.

Filter
A metal gauze screen sited at the patient end of the canister limits inhalation of alkali dust produced by agitation or inferior-grade absorbent.

Scavenging shroud
Old to-and-fro systems may not have a scavenging shroud fixed to the pressure-relief valve; this makes effective scavenging difficult.

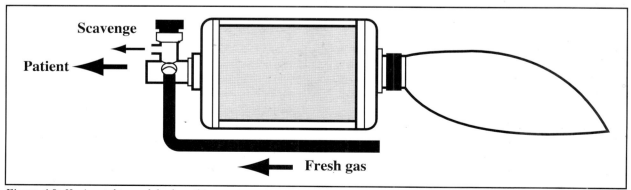

Figure 4.9: *Horizontal to-and-fro breathing system.*

Reproduced from In Practice *(1995)* **17**, *pp. 229–237, with permission.*

Circle
Advantages
High gas efficiency
Mechanical dead space remains unchanged with use
Bronchiolitis unlikely
Low circuit inertia
Ventilation readily controlled
Disadvantages
Expensive
Complex, cumbersome and difficult to sterilize
To-and-fro
Advantages
High gas efficiency
Bidirectional gas flow improves carbon dioxide scrubbing efficiency
Greater heat conservation (hyperthermia is possible in high ambient temperatures)
Lower resistance to breathing than with circle systems (no valves and lower overall circuit length)
Low circuit volume: denitrogenation achieved rapidly; rapid changes in gas concentration
Simple, robust construction
Portable; easily moved from room to room, and in field
Easily sterilized
Inexpensive
Disadvantages
Valve position is inconvenient for positive-pressure ventilation
Mechanical dead space increases during surgery as absorbent is exhausted
'Channelling' of gas over absorbent occurs in poorly packed horizontal Water's canisters
Bronchiolitis; aspiration of alkali dust from canister may cause chemical lung injury
Considerable drag: system has much inertia and is inconvenient during head surgery

Figure 4.10: Comparison of circle and to-and-fro systems.

Canister

Dimension requirements are the same as those for circle systems. Modern horizontal canisters are made from transparent perspex, allowing the colour of the soda lime and filling adequacy to be checked. The latter is important; in horizontal canisters that are improperly filled, expired gas 'channels', i.e. it takes the low resistance path over the absorbent granules so that CO_2 is not absorbed. For dogs weighing over 10 kg it is said that canisters designed for humans, containing 0.5 kg absorbent (650 ml volume), are satisfactory.

Rebreathing bag

See reservoir bags above.

Advantages

Simplicity and durability make to-and-fro systems ideal in animals with infectious airway disease, as they are readily sterilized.

Disadvantages

Considerable circuit drag renders the system cumbersome; extubation is possible when inadequately anaesthetized animals move (although a lightweight plastic system is now available). The proximity of the pressure-relief valve is awkward when IPPV is required during head, neck or dental surgery. Mechanical dead space increases with time. Chemical bronchiolitis and hyperthermia are well known problems. Channelling occurs in the horizontal to-and-fro system.

NON-REBREATHING SYSTEMS

Non-rebreathing (sometimes known as 'semi-closed' in the UK) systems do not use CO_2 absorption and rely on high gas flow rates (based on multiples of minute volume (Vm)) to flush expired CO_2 from the circuit so that it cannot be rebreathed at the next breath. Advantages and disadvantages of non-rebreathing systems are listed in Figure 4.11.

The Magill system

The Magill system consists of a reservoir bag (volume 3–6 x Vt) and a corrugated hose that ends at an expiratory (Heidbrink) valve (Figure 4.12). The expiratory hose volume must exceed the Vt of the animal otherwise rebreathing occurs.

Advantages
Low resistance; ideal for small animals and birds
Simple construction
Inexpensive
Soda lime not required
Inspired gas content similar to that 'dialled' at anaesthetic machine
Denitrogenation not required
Rapid change in level of anaesthesia
Can be used with trichlorethylene and sevoflurane
Disadvantages
High gas flow requirements
High volatile agent consumption rate
High running costs
Expired moisture and heat usually lost
Ventilatory modes affect system performance
Different types of non-rebreathing circuits behave differently and have different flow requirements

Figure 4.11: Advantages and disadvantages of non-rebreathing systems.

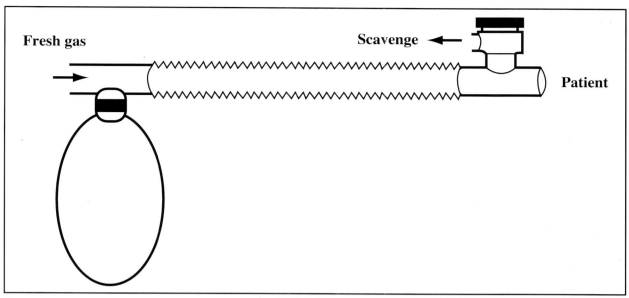

Figure 4.12: *Magill breathing system.*

Reproduced from In Practice *(1995)* **17**, *pp. 229–237, with permission.*

Gas flow

Rebreathing is prevented when gas flow rate equals or exceeds patient Vm (see Figure 4.4). When N_2O is used, its flow rate is included within this value. For example, to supply 66% N_2O to a dog of 15 kg body weight (with a Vm of 3 litres), flow rates of 1 l/min O_2 and 2 l/min N_2O are required. Similarly, 1.5 l/min each of O_2 and N_2O would provide the same dog with a 50% mixture.

Advantages

The Magill system is an efficient general purpose circuit for most companion animal cases up to perhaps 60 kg bodyweight. Gas flow rates required for these and larger animals may exceed flowmeter capability, and reduce economy. The circuit is readily maintained and sterilized.

Disadvantages

Mechanical dead space, inertia and considerable expiratory resistance preclude the usefulness of the Magill system in cats and in dogs with bodyweights <5 kg. The location of the Heidbrink valve is inconvenient for scavenging and operation, especially during surgery on the head. The system should not be used for prolonged positive-pressure ventilation because alveolar gas is rebreathed, causing hypercapnia. Higher gas flow rates and an altered ventilatory pattern permit IPPV without rebreathing, but this cannot be recommended when alternative systems are readily available.

The Lack system

This coaxial system was originally designed for use in humans in an attempt to overcome the inconvenient valve location in Magill circuits. In the Lack system (Figure 4.13) a reservoir bag connects to an outer inspiratory limb; this surrounds an inner expiratory tube that ends at the expiratory valve, which is positioned at the machine connector.

Gas flow

Despite theoretical considerations, the behaviour of the Lack and Magill systems are different; the Lack system was found to be slightly more efficient than the Magill system in dogs (Waterman, 1986). A fresh gas flow rate of 120 ml/kg/min prevented rebreathing in dogs connected to a Lack system, but rebreathing occurred when the same animals were placed on a Magill circuit. There is an inverse relation between bodyweight and the fresh gas flow rate required to prevent rebreathing. Gas flow rates of 193 ml/kg/min were safe for most dogs weighing between 10 kg and 15 kg, and 122 ml/kg/min for dogs over 15 kg. Expiratory resistance in the Lack system is also lower than that of the Magill system, and so the former may be safer in small animals.

Advantages

The circuit is lightweight and exerts less drag than the Magill system. Valve position facilitates operation and scavenging. The system is 1.5 m long, allowing positioning of the anaesthetic machine away from surgery. Lack systems can be used in place of the Magill system; they are more efficient. The expiratory resistance in the Lack system is considerably lower than that in the Magill (and the Bain (Mapleson D)) circuit (Humphrey, 1983). In large dogs, gas flow rates of 200 ml/kg/min in the Magill system and 120 ml/kg/min for the Lack system prevent rebreathing. The advantages of coaxial systems over non-coaxial systems are listed in Figure 4.14.

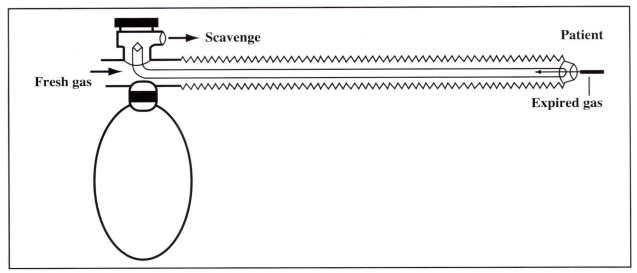

Figure 4.13: Lack breathing system.

Reproduced from In Practice *(1995)* **17**, *pp. 229–237, with permission.*

Simple design

Lightweight plastic construction and absence of valves at the patient end minimizes drag

Valve and reservoir bag position at the machine end allows easy adjustment, imposition of controlled and assisted ventilation and scavenging

System length allows intermittent positive-pressure ventilation to be performed some distance from the animal

Small volume reservoir bag on some versions of the Bain system allows easy recognition of breathing movements

Simple construction favours cleaning and sterilization

In the Bain system, inspired gases (inner limb) are said to be warmed by expired gases in the outer expiratory tube

Figure 4.14: Advantages of coaxial breathing systems.

Disadvantages

Older versions had high expiratory resistance and the inner hose could become broken or disconnected, causing considerable rebreathing. The system is stiff and inconvenient to use in very small animals. Ventilation should not be controlled with this system.

The parallel Lack system

Problems of coaxial geometry (disconnection, fracture or kinking of the inner limb) are avoided when the inspiratory and expiratory limbs are juxtaposed (Figure 4.15) as in the parallel Lack system. The system behaves like a Magill attachment, although the additional bulk created by two hoses increases drag, so conferring little advantage in anaesthesia of very small animals.

Ayre's T-piece

Gas flow

Four T-piece configurations are possible, based on the volume of the expiratory limb. In the most effective type, expiratory limb volume exceeds the patient's Vt and has no reservoir bag nor expiratory valves (Figure 4.16A).

Gas flow rates for T-piece systems must exceed double the Vm otherwise expired gas is rebreathed ($2 \times Vm$). Rapid respiratory rates with short expiratory pauses may require even higher ($3 \times Vm$) flow rates.

Advantages

Minimal mechanical dead space and resistance make the T-piece ideal for cats, small dogs (bodyweight < 5 kg), neonates and birds. It is simple, inexpensive and easy to sterilize. Modest drag occurs because two hoses are present. The system is scavenged with appropriate connectors.

Disadvantages

Ventilation is controlled by occluding the distal end of the expiratory limb, but gas flow must be increased otherwise the duration of inspiration is prolonged and limits adequate ventilation.

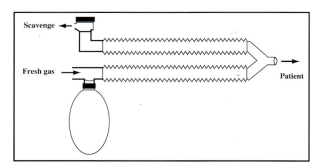

Figure 4.15: Parallel Lack breathing system.

Reproduced from In Practice *(1995)* **17**, *pp. 229–237, with permission.*

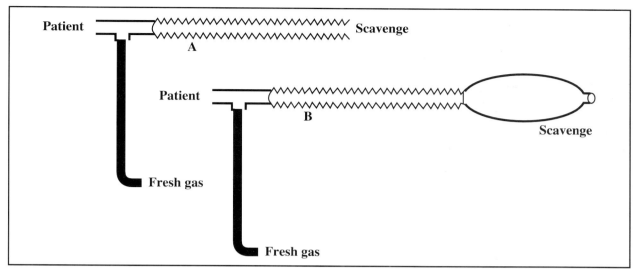

Figure 4.16: Ayre's T-piece and 8th Jackson-Rees modified Ayre's T-piece.

Reproduced from In Practice (1995) *17*, pp. 229–237, with permission.

Ayre's T-Piece with Jackson-Rees' modification

This breathing system is an Ayre's T-piece with an open-ended reservoir bag on the expiratory limb (Figure 4.16B).

Gas flow rate

Flow rates of 2.5–3 x Vm are needed to prevent re-breathing.

Advantages

The bag facilitates IPPV, and bag movement acts as a useful respiratory monitor. Ventilation is controlled by occluding the bag's end, allowing distension, then squeezing the contents into the patient's lungs. The end is then released. The system has the advantage of a T-piece, so is used in similar circumstances. Imposing IPPV does not require increased flow rates.

Disadvantages

Scavenging the system may be complicated; connectors tend to twist and cause rapid over distension of the bag.

The Bain system

The Bain system is a coaxial T-piece with an inner inspiratory limb surrounded by an outer expiratory hose. The expiratory limb ends in:

- A reservoir bag and expiratory valve, Mapleson D (Figure 4.17A), or
- An open-ended tube, Mapleson E (Figure 4.17B), or
- An open-ended bag, Mapleson F (Figure 4.17C).

Valveless Bain systems are preferred in spontaneously breathing dogs, cats, birds and small mammals, while the Mapleson D version can been used in large dogs. Cullen (1989) points out that the Vt of a kitten weighing

1 kg is 10 ml, which makes the mechanical dead space of both Bain and Lack systems unacceptably large.

Gas flow rate

The system probably requires marginally higher flow rates than corresponding T-piece systems, although reports on its performance vary. Manley and McDonell (1979a,b) recommended flow rates between 100 and 130 ml/kg/min in spontaneously breathing dogs and concluded that gas flow rates of 100 ml/kg/min are required when IPPV is imposed using a Vt of 20 ml/kg and respiration rates of 20 per minute. In reviewing coaxial systems, Cullen (1989) recommends a minimum fresh gas flow rate of 200 ml/kg/min in spontaneously breathing dogs and increases this when respiration rate exceeds 15 per minute. He suggests that high flow rates should always be used in coaxial systems when the respiratory rate increases (Cullen, 1989).

Advantages

The (valveless) Mapleson E or F versions are recommended for cats and very small dogs because of low expiratory resistance. Ventilation is controlled by occluding the expiratory limb in 'E' systems. In 'D' systems, the expiratory valve is closed then the bag squeezed. In Mapleson F versions the reservoir bag is used like that in a Jackson-Rees modification. The circuit is useful for IPPV in small dogs and cats, especially when access to the patient is limited. The length of the system (1.8 m) allows the anaesthetic machine to be positioned away from the site of surgery, improving access to the patient. Spontaneous ventilation is satisfactory in dogs weighing more than 10 kg. The system has low drag and mechanical dead space and is easily maintained and sterilized. It is claimed warm expired gas raises the temperature of gas flowing in the inner limb, conserving the patient's temperature.

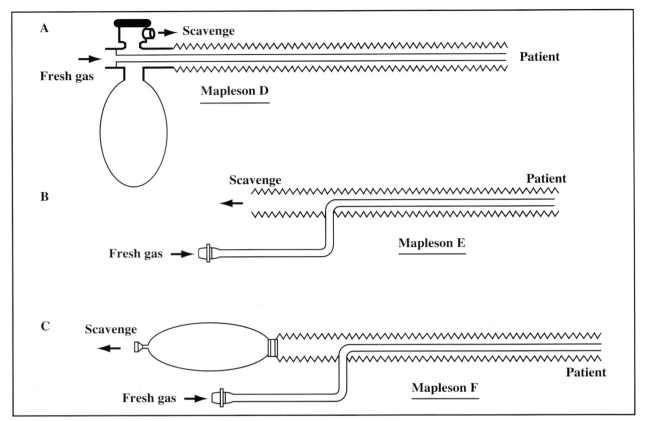

Figure 4.17: *Three coaxial T-piece (Bain) systems.*

Reproduced from In Practice (1995) *17*, pp. 229–237, with permission.

Disadvantages

Expiratory resistance with high flows reduces the system's usefulness in spontaneously breathing cats and small dogs weighing less than 10 kg. Conversely, tube diameters may impose too great a resistance for gas movement in very large dogs breathing spontaneously (Cullen, 1989). A third complication occurs at high flow rates when the inspiratory gas stream entrains CO_2-rich gas from the expiratory reservoir, causing rebreathing. Another complication follows disconnection, kinking or twisting of the inner tube. When this occurs the entire circuit volume becomes mechanical dead space, and severe hypercapnia ensues. The outer limb is made of translucent plastic and the inner limb is coloured (blue or green) so that abnormalities of the inspiratory limb are more obvious. Rebreathing problems caused by disconnection of the inner limb prompted development of a parallel Bain system. However, the integrity of the inspiratory limb is easily tested by occluding its end with a 5 ml syringe plunger; when gas is flowing, the flowmeter indicator falls and/or the overpressure valve is heard.

The relative efficiency of coaxial systems has not been compared in animals. In man, the fresh gas flow rate required to prevent rebreathing in the Bain system is three times greater than that needed in the Lack system. Cullen (1989) suggests that the Lack circuit has less dead space and is more efficient than the Bain system, but that it is less versatile. The Bain system can be used without a valve and in this configuration has lower expiratory resistance.

Disposable anaesthetic breathing systems

A complete range of breathing systems is avai-lable for single use in human patients. Constructed entirely of plastic, these are lighter and less expensive, though less robust, than traditional circuits made of carbonized rubber and stainless steel. They can be safely re-used in animals, but must be discarded when leaks develop (usually around the neck of the reservoir or rebreathing bag) and after use on animals with infective respiratory or systemic disease. Disposable circle and to-and-fro systems cannot be re-used once soda lime is expended, although resourceful users have found ways to replenish exhausted absorbent.

Anaesthetic breathing system safety check

Before use, anaesthetic breathing systems must be examined and tested for leaks. Examination ensures that all components are present and in the appropriate position. Pressure-relief valves are checked for smooth operation, from fully closed to fully open. In rebreathing systems, soda lime is checked for freshness. Testing for leaks is achieved by connecting the breathing system to the common gas outlet, closing all valves (where present) and other ports where gas may escape and connecting a manometer to the patient connector. The system is then filled with O_2 to produce a pressure of 18–22 cmH$_2$O, which it should hold for at least 2 minutes. An occlusion test should be performed on the inner inspiratory limb of the Bain system, while the operation of unidirectional valves should be checked in circle systems.

MECHANICAL VENTILATORS

The lungs can be inflated by the application of positive pressure to the subject's airway (IPPV) or by periodically reducing the pressure around the thoracic cage (negative-pressure ventilation). Negative-pressure ventilation occurs in iron lung type ventilators and has no application in veterinary anaesthesia. Positive pressure ventilation can be imposed by manual or mechanical methods. The advantages and disadvantages of the latter are listed in Figure 4.18. In veterinary practice, a ventilator may be needed:

- For short-term ventilation (1–4 hours) associated with general anaesthesia
- For long-term management of respiratory disease or thoracic trauma
- For short-duration intensive respiratory care (<24 hours).

Requirements
A description of all the ventilator types available for use in animals is beyond the scope of this chapter. Ultimately the choice depends on the machine being:

- Compact, portable, robust and easy to operate
- Economical to purchase, use and maintain
- Electrically safe, isolated, suppressed and explosion proof
- Capable of use with air, O_2 mixtures and all anaesthetics
- Capable of allowing straightforward control and measurement of inspired O_2 concentration (FiO_2)
- Capable of humidifying inspired gas
- Capable of nebulizing drugs
- Capable of rapid disassembly for easy sterilization
- Capable of using disposable hoses
- Fitted with bacterial filters
- Capable of use with non-rebreathing or rebreathing anaesthetic breathing systems
- Capable of rapid conversion for paediatric use.

Mechanical ventilators should have:

- Adjustable flow rates

Advantages
Accurate control of respiratory variables *
Constant arterial gas tensions create stable plasma pH and potassium levels
Regular rhythm depresses ventilation, provides narcosis and improves operating conditions
Constant tidal volume (volume preset) allows compliance measurement
Mechanical ventilator frees anaesthetist for other duties
Special ventilatory modes may be imposed

Disadvantages
Unnoticed disconnection/cuff deflation fatal in 'paralysed' cases†
Mechanical failure possible
Lung trauma more likely if inappropriate variables are set
Purchase and maintenance costs may be high
Some mechanical ventilators may be unsuitable for all patient sizes
Ventilators may become fomites i.e. harbour transmissible respiratory pathogens

Figure 4.18: *Advantages and disadvantages of mechanical ventilation.*

*Examples include tidal volume, respiratory rate, peak inspiratory pressure and I:E ratios.
†Prevention may be possible with low pressure alarms.

- Maximum inspiratory flow rates of 80 l/min allowing:
  Variable inspiratory times of 0.5–3.9 seconds
  Frequencies of 5–50/min
- A Vt range of 50–1500 ml
- A variable I:E ratio (1:1–1:3.5)
- The capability to control all the above simultaneously (altering one variable should not affect others)
- The ability to maintain output even when leaks develop.

Ventilators should be capable of providing:

- 'Sighs'
- Inflation hold (plateau)
- Different airway pressure wave forms
- Low expiratory resistance and positive-end expiratory pressure.

They should be equipped with a pressure-relief valve, and devices to do the following:

- Allow continuous monitoring of airway pressure (P) and of expired volume (V)
- Indicate low pressure and/or circuit disconnection and high pressure and/or pressure overload
- Indicate low expired Vm and low FiO_2

- Display flow rate waveform (*PV* curve)
- Indicate power failure
- Allow rapid manual takeover.

In most types of ventilator, lung inflation is achieved either by the application of a pressure to the upper airway (pressure generation) or by the introduction of a preset volume of gas (flow generation). Constant-pressure devices produce exponential changes in airway pressure and, within limits, compensate for leaks. The output of constant-pressure generators must be periodically adjusted to compensate for changing lung compliance, which often falls during anaesthesia. In constant-flow generators, airway pressure and lung volume increase in a linear fashion, because of constant flow. However, there is no compensation for leaks.

With settings at minimum values, human devices intended for adults are able to ventilate the lungs of dogs weighing more than 20 kg. The lungs of small dogs and cats are more compliant than larger animals, and must be inflated at high respiratory rates and with low tidal volumes. Purpose-built paediatric ventilators, or adult ventilators modified for children, may be suitable. Some modern adult ventilators may be rapidly adjusted to control ventilation in human infants; this normally involves the straightforward exchange of the cuvette and bellows, after a few screws have been slackened or removed. Similarly, Manley ventilators can be rapidly adapted for use in small subjects by inserting a low-flow restrictor that curtails gas flow from the bellows more severely than does the adult version. It should be noted that the cuvettes and flow restrictors necessary for conversion are not integral parts of the ventilator; veterinary practitioners purchasing this equipment must ensure that the vendor supplies these separate components.

In very small dogs and cats, it may be necessary to adapt paediatric ventilators to prevent over expansion of lungs. This can be accomplished by:

- Deliberately incorporating a 'leak' in the inspiratory limb
- Creating a parallel resistance
- Creating a parallel compliance, i.e. a distensible bag.

Alternatively, a laboratory animal ventilator may be used (see below).

Sources

Purpose-built small animal ventilators
Some purpose-built small animal anaesthetic machines incorporate mechanical ventilators. These are not inexpensive and often lack the warning and failsafe devices required in medical anaesthesia. However, they are straightforward in operation and generally robust.

Human ventilators
Medical mechanical ventilators may be designed for use in intensive care or in the operating room. These categories are not rigid, as modern intensive care devices are also capable of delivering anaesthetic vapours. However, intensive care devices tend to be more complicated (and more expensive), being capable of a range of ventilatory modes and functions. Ventilators used in anaesthesia are smaller, more robust, portable, easier to operate and less expensive than those used in intensive care.

Ventilators from human hospitals
Second-hand ventilators are available from human hospitals or the health service and are usually good value for money. They are sophisticated and likely to have the desirable safety features listed above. Components may, however, be difficult to obtain. Machines that are second-hand should be carefully checked and overhauled by trained technicians before purchase.

New medical ventilators
These are expensive complicated devices and tend to be difficult to operate because of their ability to reproduce complex breathing patterns. Most of these patterns are unnecessary in veterinary anaesthesia and so the purchase of such equipment is unwarranted.

Purpose-built laboratory animal ventilators
Although most ventilators can be converted for use in children, care is still needed when they are used in puppies, small cats, birds and small mammals. Many laboratory suppliers produce mechanical ventilators for use in laboratory animals, e.g. rabbits and guinea pigs, which are suitable for use in small patients. They are relatively inexpensive, robust and simple to operate.

Mechanical ventilators
The classification of medical ventilators is beyond the scope of this chapter. Ventilators commonly used in veterinary anaesthesia may be described either as 'bag squeezers' or as 'minute volume' dividers.

Bag squeezers or bag-in-bottle ventilators
These are the simplest form of ventilator, in which the bag, or bellows, is attached to the bag mount of a circle breathing system. The bellows are filled with a mixture of fresh anaesthetic gases and expired breath from the breathing system. The bellows are then compressed either by electrically powered compressors or rotary blowers, or by exposure to high pressure delivered from a separate 'driving gas' (O_2 or air) supply. When the bellows are compressed, gas is expelled into the breathing system and the lungs are thus inflated. Excessive gas flowing into the system is vented from the bellows through a pressure-relief valve that is open only between breaths. The bellows must be designed to

prevent inward gas leaks, i.e. driving gas must not contaminate the delivered gas mixture. Most purpose-built small animal ventilators (e.g. Drager SAV, Hallowell EMC2000 and Mallard 2400) are bellows ventilators. Older ventilators (e.g. Metomatic SA) may have suspended bellows that descend during expiration. Such an arrangement does not allow easy detection of inadvertent disconnection of the patient breathing system because the bellows continue to go up and down in phase with ventilator operation. Modern ventilators tend to be equipped with bellows that ascend on expiration; with this arrangement the bellows stop moving as soon as inadvertent disconnection occurs.

Minute volume dividers

These are driven by the gases that are ultimately delivered to the patient's lungs, i.e. the volume of gas supplied per minute to the device (in l/min) is the patient's Vm. As Vm is the product of Vt and frequency, only one variable can be altered once the flow rate is set; the other variable changes inversely.

Three types of small inexpensive miniature Vm dividers (which operate similarly) have been evaluated for use in dogs: the Minivent, Microvent and Automatic Vent. These devices are positioned at the patient end of the corrugated tubing of the standard Magill attachment after removal of the Heidbrink expiratory valve. Gas flowing into the breathing system causes the reservoir bag to distend and pressure within it to rise (for best results the bag must be new and non-compliant, or stiff). Before inspiration begins, gas flow into the lungs is prevented by a bi-stable valve that is held shut by a nearby magnet. As gas volume in the bag rises, a pressure is reached that overcomes the attractive force between magnet and valve, causing the latter to snap open. Gas is discharged into the subject's lungs owing to elastic energy stored within the bag. As the lungs inflate, the pressure in the bag falls below that needed to keep the magnet and valve separate, so the latter closes. The devices have one or two controls that alter the pressure level at which the bag initiates inspiration.

The Manley Pulmovent is a more complicated minute volume divider. Incoming fresh gas enters a set of bellows, which are restrained by springs. Pressure within the bellows rises as they inflate. Once a pre-set volume is reached, the cycling mechanism trips a valve that allows the pressure in the bellows to inflate the subject's lungs. However, not all this pressure is applied to the airway because a simple screw-in flow restrictor is positioned proximal to the patient and, in addition, there is a pressure-relief valve, which opens at about 7 kPa. Thus a near constant pressure is generated, although it is applied via a flow rate control.

The ADS 1000 is a minute volume divider marketed in the USA for use in small animal patients. It is not designed for connection to an anaesthetic breathing system. Presumably the source of the anaesthetic gas mixture that supplies this ventilator must be capable of delivering intermittently very high flows. At present, there are few published data to support the clinical use of this ventilator.

Hoses

Up to 20% of the tidal volume set can be lost by compression of gas within the ventilator and through expansion of corrugated hoses, and so does not enter the lungs. In non-breathing circuits this may contribute to an increase in total dead space. Problems can be avoided by using low-compliance hoses and/or measuring delivered volume at the endotracheal tube connector.

Safety check

Before use, the ventilator and its controls should be checked for normal operation. The patient port should be occluded to examine operation of the pressure-relief valve. The disconnect alarm, if present, should be operational. Finally, an alternative means of lung ventilation should be available in the event of ventilator malfunction.

SCAVENGING SYSTEMS

Contamination of the operating and recovery room air by waste anaesthetic gases and vapours can be limited in several ways. Scavenging refers to the removal of expired waste gas from the expiratory valves, pressure-relief valves or expiratory limbs of breathing systems and ventilators to a site distant from the working environment. Gas scavenging systems are of two types:

Passive

In passive systems, expired gases are moved by the combined effects of gas flowing into the breathing system from the anaesthetic machine, expiratory effort of the patient and elastic recoil in reservoir or rebreathing bags. Passive systems are simple but their function can be affected by prevailing winds at the exit port. Furthermore, they must not involve excessively long scavenging hose, otherwise resistance to expiration occurs. Passive systems either empty to the atmosphere through ducts in walls, or into a canister of activated charcoal attached to the anaesthetic machine. Activated charcoal does not adsorb N_2O and inefficiently deals with gas rich in trichloroethylene. The life of a single canister is inversely proportional to the concentration of gases passing through it and ranges from 3–6 hours. The exhaustion of an activated charcoal canister is indicated by increased weight.

Active

In active systems, gas is moved by negative pressures generated by an extractor fan or a hospital vacuum system from a shrouded expiratory valve to an air brake receiver (ABR) or scavenger interface. Excessive negative pressures may empty the reservoir bag and make circuits of low flow rate impracticable. However, the ABR prevents the scavenger system from exerting excessive negative pressure on the breathing system and prevents build up of excess pressure if the evacuation system fails (in which case gases are vented to the atmosphere from the ABR). The ABR also allows several systems to be scavenged without affecting the performance of the extraction unit. The need for high flow scavenging is reduced by including a reservoir bag in the system. This accommodates expired gases and evens out fluctuations during the respiratory cycle.

In the event that passive systems become occluded or active systems fail, scavenging systems should incorporate a pressure-relief valve that opens at low pressures, e.g. 5-10 cmH$_2$O.

ENDOTRACHEAL TUBES

Cuffed ETTs:

- Reduce the risk of saliva, regurgitated stomach contents or irrigation fluids being inhaled
- Allow effective imposition of IPPV
- Reduce contamination from waste gas.

Different patterns of ETTs have different advantages in differing circumstances.

Magill pattern tubes

Both oral and nasal Magill pattern ETTs are available. Oral tubes are designed for orotracheal intubation and have thicker walls than the nasal tubes. Oral tubes may be either plain (uncuffed) or cuffed. The cuff is inflated by means of an inflation pipe, which runs as an external moulding. When inflated properly, the cuff produces an airtight seal between the tracheal wall and the tube, which ensures inspired gases pass through the lumen of the tube. However, cuffs inflated to pressures exceeding the perfusion pressure of the capillaries in the tracheal mucosa (about 25-30 mmHg) cause pressure (ischaemic) necrosis of the tracheal mucosa and subsequent tracheal cicatrization. Overinflation can also cause respiratory obstruction when the wall of the tube is compressed into its lumen. The pipe that inflates the cuff may be open ended or fitted with a moulded stopper. The most useful pipe ends in a valve, which accepts the male luer nozzle of an inflating syringe and conveniently closes when the latter is removed.

On all cuffed tubes, the turgidity of a pilot balloon connected to the cuff reflects the degree of cuff inflation. However, this does not indicate an airtight seal, and balloons connected to low pressure-high volume cuffs (see below) may feel soft when the cuff contains considerable volumes of gas. Pre-insertion inflation of the cuff will indicate the approximate volume of gas required to produce a good fit. However, the best way of ensuring that cuff pressure is the lowest required for an airtight airway involves use of an in-circuit manometer. With the breathing system closed, the reservoir bag is compressed until an in-circuit pressure of 18-22 cmH$_2$O is achieved. The cuff is then inflated until 'hissing' ceases. If a manometer is unavailable, the lungs are held in a slightly inflated state and the cuff similarly inflated. Anaesthetic gas mixtures containing N$_2$O may cause cuffs that are inflated with air to expand. This can be avoided by inflating cuffs with gases from the anaesthetic machine. Alternatively, cuff pressures can be monitored using a simple manometer attached to the cuff-inflation pipe, and altered when necessary.

Murphy pattern tubes

These are similar in most ways to the Magill pattern but have a 'Murphy's eye', an oval hole positioned on the bevel facing the opening of the distal tube. This allows gas flow to continue should the distal opening of the tube become inadvertently positioned against the wall of the airway.

Streamlined tubes

The cuff-inflation pipe is embedded within the wall of the ETT, which allows relatively large-diameter tubes to be used in small airways. This configuration means that the tube cannot be cut short (to minimize mechanical dead space).

Armoured, spiral-embedded or flexometallic tubes

These tubes are usually made of silicone rubber and have a steel wire or nylon coil embedded in the wall; the spiral resists kinking and collapse when extreme neck flexion is imposed, as in head or neck surgery. This design has created unique problems. Obstruction and kinking is possible at either end of the tube where it is not reinforced by coils, and the flaccid bevel can invaginate into the tube if pushed against the tracheal wall. Kinking may occur at the proximal (circuit) end if the connector or catheter mount does not overlap the spiral. During boiling or autoclaving, repeated high temperatures soften nylon spirals; when the cuff is inflated, the tube wall beneath the cuff bulges inward, causing obstruction. Furthermore, the steel wire spirals have resulted in the tube lumen remaining occluded after being crushed, precluding ventilation. Flexometallic tubes are considerably more expensive than the standard tubes.

The human trachea is relatively small, and so medical ETTs are only available in sizes up to 11 mm internal diameter. Larger tubes, which are necessary in medium and giant breeds of dogs, must be obtained from a manufacturer of veterinary equipment.

Materials

Endotracheal tubes are available in a variety of materials, which determines their properties, clinical usefulness and longevity. Red rubber tubes are relatively irritant, imperfect for prolonged intubation and firm; their curvature is predetermined. In contrast, plastic (PVC) tubes are non-irritant, soften after a period *in vivo* and mould to body contours at 37°C. Disposable plastic tubes designed for human use may be re-used in animals. The methods of cleaning and sterilization also depend on the material of construction. Red rubber tubes soften with time, frequent use and the necessary cleaning and sterilizing processes. Some materials retain detergents and sterilants more tenaciously than others and a more disciplined approach to their cleaning is required. For example, plastic products that have undergone irradiation are said to react with ethylene dioxide, to produce a tissue irritant, ethylene chlorohydrin.

Cuff profile

The inflated cuffs of red rubber tubes adopt a spherical contour while those of plastic tubes adopt a rectangular outline. Because of this, the area of contact between red rubber tube cuffs and the tracheal mucosa is less than that achieved with plastic tubes. Furthermore, a thin band of relatively high pressure is produced with spherical cuffs, which is more likely to cause mucosal trauma.

Low pressure-high volume cuffs

Low pressure-high volume cuffs with square cuff profiles have much reduced the incidence of iatrogenic tracheal stenosis in human patients. They can be difficult to introduce unless the cuffs are fully evacuated by suction.

Problems with tube size

Using undersized tubes (in terms of diameter) is an effective way to increase airway resistance and the work of breathing, accelerate alveolar collapse and transudation and cause hypoventilation in spontaneously breathing animals. In those breeds where the use of undersized ETTs is unavoidable, e.g. English bulldogs, or in dogs with laryngeal or pharyngeal masses, ventilatory assistance must be provided from the outset.

The main problem in using tubes of inadequate length is tracheal extubation, which occurs with the slightest head movement. Casual re-insertion of the tube will, on most occasions, cause oesophageal intubation. Overly long ETTs create excessive mechanical dead space, which extends rostrally from the level of the incisor arcade to the point of the anaesthetic breathing system where inspiratory and expiratory gas streams divide. This is minimized by choosing an appropriately sized tube: in the conscious standing animal one end of the tube is held at the level of the incisors and is bent to follow the natural airway. The tip of a suitably sized tube ends at the spine of the scapula. If the tip extends beyond the 5th or 6th intercostal space, the tube is too long and may enter a mainstem bronchus if the full length is advanced. Although some mechanical dead space is well tolerated by healthy animals, excessive volumes may compromise those animals susceptible to hypoventilation and respiratory acidosis. In these, surplus tube should be removed with scissors, or ventilation assisted using gas volumes equal to the normal Vt and additional mechanical dead space.

Before use, ETTs must be rinsed of potentially irritant sterilizing solutions. The lumen should be checked for patency (this is especially important in small diameter tubes). The cuff should be inflated and left for 10 minutes before use to ensure its inflation is symmetrical and sustained.

LARYNGOSCOPES

Laryngoscopes are used to hold the root of the tongue and thus improve tracheal examination of the glottis and intubation. They are particularly useful in cats, and in animals with either extensive pharyngeal soft tissue, e.g. Staffordshire Bull Terriers, or small airways, e.g. English Bulldog. They are useful whenever pharyngeal or upper airway disease threatens airway patency, and in Chow-Chows, whose darkly pigmented mucous membranes complicate identification of the rima glottidis.

Patterns

The laryngoscope consists of a handle, which contains the battery power source, and a blade, which mounts the light. It should be noted that the hinge that connects the blade to the handle is not of a standard design, and some handles and blades are incompatible. One edge of the blade is bent at approximately 90 degrees to form the web, which itself curves 90 degrees outwards or inwards to form the flange. The relative dimensions of these components vary and form the basis of a bewildering array of patterns. In the Macintosh pattern, the tongue, web and flange form a reverse 'Z' while in the Miller pattern, they form a reverse 'C'. An important feature of the blade is its straightness or degree of curvature. The Macintosh pattern features a curved blade while the Miller and Wisconsin blades are straight; a curved design is slightly more useful. Most laryngoscope patterns are available in adult and paediatric versions, and blades are available for right- and left-handed operators. An 8 cm Macintosh blade is suitable for cats, and dogs weighing less than 5 kg, while (adult) blade lengths of 12 cm and 20 cm are suitable for most other dog breeds. The Michaels blade is a human paediatric version that is well suited to cats.

Before use, laryngoscopes must be clean and produce adequate illumination. The greatest risk to patients, however, comes from over-aggressive application and not from the laryngoscope itself.

MASKS

The conical shape of the Halls mask accommodates many breeds of dog and is available in a range of sizes. However, these create excessive dead space for cats and brachycephalic breeds of dog and, because they are made of black latex rubber, preclude examination of mucous membrane colour and the position of the mouth and the nostrils. Commercially available cup-shaped masks fitted with a rubber diaphragm circumvent problems of inadequate visibility, but are made of hard plastic and, if used aggressively, can cause facial injury. Furthermore, they add considerable mechanical dead space to the breathing system and so should only be used for induction, rather than the maintenance of anaesthesia.

Before use, masks should be checked to ensure they fit firmly with the chosen anaesthetic breathing system. After use they should be washed in warm soapy water and rinsed. Sterilization is necessary after use in animals with infectious respiratory diseases.

CHAMBERS

Commercially available clear perspex chambers are to be found in several sizes and are most useful for inducing anaesthesia in animals intolerant of physical restraint. The chamber induction technique is satisfactory for fractious small dogs and cats, puppies and toy breeds, as well as large birds and exotic species. Induction chambers should be large, yet contain slots on the inner walls to accommodate clear partitioning walls. The partitioning walls make it possible to create subcompartments that cater for patient size (the smaller the chamber, the more rapid the rate of induction). The lid of the chamber should be capable of being fastened down rapidly, e.g. by toggle levers, and incorporate ports for fresh gas inflow, and an exhaust shroud that connects to a scavenge duct. The edge of the lid should be recessed so that it fits snugly, and should be lined with neoprene, or some other compressible material, to improve gas proofing. Suitably sized chambers can also serve as an O_2 cage for the small animal, and as an incubator and/or O_2 cage for newly delivered whelps. When used for inducing anaesthesia, removal of the patient after induction inevitably causes release of anaesthetic vapour into the room.

Thus, chamber inductions should be used only when deemed necessary.

SUCTION

The presence of a vacuum-generating (suction) device on an anaesthetic machine facilitates the removal of oropharyngeal or endobronchial secretions. In large hospitals, the vacuum source is central, and a vacuum line installed as part of the piped air supply; this is unfeasible in most veterinary practices. However, many ex-health service anaesthetic machines possess an integral suction device, in which a variable vacuum is generated by the passage of an adjustable jet of medical gas over a small aperture. The vacuum thus created draws fluid along a suitable collection pipe into a reservoir. Despite their low cost, safety, simplicity and effectiveness, such devices rapidly consume medical gas. Portable suction devices operating upon an electrically driven reciprocating pump mechanism are available, but are expensive to purchase, although cheap to run. It must be possible to adjust the vacuum generated by all suction devices.

NEBULIZERS AND HUMIDIFIERS

The humidification of inspired gas preserves mucociliary function and limits evaporative heat losses from the respiratory tree, so is desirable in animals with tracheobronchial disease and/or those predisposed to hypothermia. In any process of humidification, the size of the water droplets is most important. Droplets of 20 µm diameter tend to precipitate out in cool parts of the delivery hoses; those of 5 µm pool in the trachea or upper respiratory tract while those of 1 µm reach the alveoli. Devices producing the latter may cause water over load, leading to water intoxication.

Heat–moisture exchangers

The simplest humidification technique involves artificial noses or heat–moisture exchangers. These consist of an adapter attached between the anaesthetic breathing system and the ETT connector. They contain a fine wire mesh on which expired moisture condenses. This moisture then evaporates and is re-inspired at the next breath. These devices are simple, but even those designed for use in children tend to clog and may impose excessive resistance to spontaneous breathing in very small animals. They also contribute to mechanical dead space and can act as effective fomites in animals with infectious respiratory disease. They operate best when the ambient temperature is low but require constant observation.

Humidifiers

Humidification of inspired gas can also be achieved by bubbling dry gases through warm water. The efficiency of this is increased by first passing the gas through sintered glass, which increases the number and reduces the size of gas bubbles formed. Moisture produced in this way, however, tends to condense out in cooler parts of the delivery system.

Nebulizers

Nebulizers are another form of humidifier. In gas-driven nebulizers, a flow of high pressure gas across an orifice causes water to be drawn up and then broken into a spray of droplets in the high pressure stream. In mechanically driven nebulizers, water is dripped either on to a spinning disc (which splits the drop into many droplets before dispersal) or on to a surface that is vibrated at 1–2 MHz frequency by ultrasound. Ultrasonic nebulizers, although expensive, can be adjusted to alter the size of the droplets, and are the most efficient devices. Both devices can be used to create aerosols of water-soluble drug solutions.

REFERENCES AND FURTHER READING

Bain JA and Spoerel WE (1972) A streamlined anaesthetic system. *Canadian Anaesthetists Society Journal* **19**, 426–435

Cullen LK (1989) Coaxial anaesthetic circuits in small animals. *Journal of Small Animal Practice* **30**, 294–297

Dohoo SE, McDonell WN and Dohoo TR (1982) A comparison of fresh gas flows during anaesthesia with nitrous oxide in the dog. *Journal of the American Animal Hospital Association* **18**, 900–904

Humphrey D (1983) A new anaesthetic breathing system combining Mapleson A, D and E principles. *Anaesthesia* **38**, 361–372

Manley SV and McDonell WN (1979a) A new circuit for small animal anesthesia: the Bain coaxial circuit. *Journal of the American Animal Hospital Association* **15**, 61–65

Manley SV and McDonell WN (1979b) Clinical evaluation of the Bain breathing circuit in small animal anesthesia. *Journal of the American Animal Hospital Association* **15**, 67–72

Waterman AE (1986) Clinical evaluation of the Lack coaxial breathing circuit in small animal anaesthesia. *Journal of Small Animal Practice* **27**, 591–598

CHAPTER FIVE

Patient Monitoring

Craig Johnson

INTRODUCTION

All patients should be monitored continuously during anaesthesia. The aim of monitoring is to gather information about the physiological state of the patient so that this can be used as an aid when making decisions about the management of the anaesthetic (Figure 5.1). Appropriate monitoring should allow the anaesthetic technique to be tailored to meet the needs of the patient and the surgeon, by detecting changes at the earliest opportunity and thus allowing early intervention. Careful monitoring should enable the detection of problems before they become severe, so that they can be treated appropriately and crises can be avoided.

Routine anaesthetic monitoring starts with watching, listening to, and touching, the patient. This includes inspection of respiratory function and the colour of mucous membranes, capillary refill time, listening to the sound of breathing and palpation of the peripheral pulse. Attention should be paid to the whole of the patient's environment. In certain instances it may be appropriate to augment this basic monitoring with mechanical aids, which give additional information and allow a more precise picture of the patient's status. This in turn allows closer control over the course of the anaesthetic. The disadvantage of mechanical monitoring devices is that they in turn must be monitored to ensure that the information they are giving is accurate. Unexpected readings should be verified by examination of the patient before they are acted upon.

MONITORS

Many aids to patient monitoring are available. These range from simple devices, such as oesophageal stethoscopes and heart rate meters, to more complex and costly devices such as cardiac output computers. The monitors included here have been chosen to give an overview of what is readily available, concentrating on equipment that is likely to be of use to the small animal practitioner.

Variable (units)	Dog	Cat
Heart rate (beats per minute)	50–100	145–200
Respiratory rate (breaths per minute)	10–20	15–25
Temperature (°C)	37.5–39.2	37.8–39.2
Arterial haemoglobin saturation (%)	>95%	>95%
pH	7.27–7.43	7.25–7.33
$PaCO_2$ (mmHg (kPa))	28–49 (3.7–6.4)	35–49 (4.6–6.4)
PaO_2 (mmHg (kPa))	>100 (1.3)	>100 (1.3)
Bicarbonate (mmol/l)	20–24	18–22
Base excess (mmol/l)	-6–0.5	-6– -3
Arterial blood pressure (mmHg (kPa))		
Systolic	120–140 (15.8–18.4)	??120–140 (15.8–18.4)
Diastolic	80–100 (10.5–1.3)	??80–100 (10.5–1.3)
Mean	100–110 (1.3–14.5)	??100–110 (1.3–14.5)

Figure 5.1: Normal values for physiological variables in the dog and cat. There is some debate concerning these values.

Oesophageal stethoscopes

The oesophageal stethoscope is an economical and useful aid to perioperative monitoring. It consists of a tube with a closed rounded end and a cuff just behind the end, which is connected to the central lumen by a series of holes in the tube. The oesophageal stethoscope functions in the same way as a conventional stethoscope diaphragm and can be connected to a stethoscope earpiece or to a dedicated amplifier with a speaker or headphones. During anaesthesia, the oesophageal stethoscope is lubricated and placed down the oesophagus to the level of the base of the heart. The depth to which it should be inserted can be estimated by measuring from the tip of the patient's nose to the middle of the patient's chest via the caudal border of the mandible and the manubrium. Once placed, the stethoscope's position should be adjusted until heart and breath sounds are loudest.

The oesophageal stethoscope allows the heart and respiratory rates to be counted during anaesthesia without the need to disturb even extensive draping of the patient. In addition, the volume and character of the sounds can give qualitative information about cardiac and respiratory function. The information requires interpretation in the same way as does conventional chest auscultation, and so the value of the information provided by the oesophageal stethoscope increases as the operator becomes more skilled in its use. For this reason it should be used on a regular basis on as many cases as possible to develop a sense of normal variability. This allows the detection of problems at an early stage. The oesophageal stethoscope does not give direct information about tidal or stroke volumes and so its use should always be accompanied by other means of assessment such as palpation of a peripheral pulse and observation of the reservoir bag.

Devices for measuring temperature

A reduction in the patient's temperature can have profound physiological effects. Metabolism is a temperature-dependent process and governs both the rate of recovery from most of the drugs used during anaesthesia and also the rate of oxygen (O_2) utilization that must be supported by the cardiorespiratory system. Anaesthesia-induced hypothermia causes shivering in the recovery period, which may substantially increase oxygen demand at a time when supply is reduced.

Traditional mercury thermometers are not suitable for continuous use during anaesthesia, but there are a large variety of inexpensive devices available that give a constant reading. These usually have probes that are suitable for rectal, oesophageal or nasal use, but can also be obtained with flat probes suited to measurement of temperature at the extremities.

The anaesthetist is usually concerned with the maintenance of core temperature. This can be measured at a variety of sites, but consideration must be given to the surgical site where there will be increased heat loss. This can distort the core area and give misleading results if an adjacent site is used to monitor temperature. For example, rectal temperature usually gives a good indication of core temperature, but during prolonged abdominal surgery, the rectum can be cooled by exposure to the environment and will no longer be a good indicator of core temperature.

The most useful sites for measurement of core temperature are the rectum and the nasopharynx. The latter is one of the closest sites to true core temperature in patients breathing through an endotracheal tube (ETT). The temperature probe should be inserted into the ventral nasal meatus to the level of the medial canthus of the eye.

If core and surface temperatures are measured simultaneously an indication of peripheral perfusion can be gained. This will not give absolute values, but can be used to follow trends in cardiovascular function. An increase in the difference between core and surface temperature indicates that peripheral perfusion is decreasing and may be an early indication of reduced cardiac output.

The electrocardiogram

The electrocardiogram (ECG) gives an indication of the electrical activity of the heart. It is recorded by a number of electrodes (usually three), which are attached to the patient with clips, sticky patches or transcutaneous needles. Electrode gel or surgical spirit is often applied to the electrodes to ensure good electrical contact. As with all electrical monitors, the patient leads must be isolated from the mains supply. This is usually achieved using optical isolators in the preamplifier of the monitoring unit.

The electrodes are classically placed on three limbs (both front limbs and the left hindlimb) to give a standard lead configuration, but during anaesthesia this may not be possible owing to the position of the patient or interference with the surgical field, and so a base/apex configuration is often used. This places one electrode dorsal to the heart (near the base) and one ventral to the heart (near the apex); the third electrode is placed at any distant point on the patient. This will give an ECG that is suitable for diagnosing arrhythmias, but it should be remembered that the detailed morphology of normal sinus rhythm may differ from that given in texts.

The ECG can give information about cardiac arrhythmias and about the myocardial environment. It should be remembered that the ECG gives no information about the mechanical function of the heart and should not be relied upon as a sole monitor of cardiovascular function. Indeed in some circumstances a heart can maintain a normal ECG for several minutes after the cessation of mechanical activity.

Cardiac arrhythmias can only be accurately diagnosed and treated when an ECG is available (see Chapter 14). Changes in the shape of the ECG can also indicate alterations in the myocardial environment such as hypoxia, hypercapnia, hyperkalaemia, acidosis and hypercalcaemia. Many of these changes indicate that the overall condition of the patient is deteriorating and, if diagnosed at an early stage, can be managed appropriately.

Problems

Most of the problems with ECGs relate to electrical interference or the failure of the monitor to detect a signal due to poor electrical contact or the inadvertent dislodging of the leads. Artefactual waveforms rarely mimic the actual ECG and so are easy to spot. The type of artefact can usually be diagnosed with similar ease. Common ECG artefacts are illustrated in Figure 5.2.

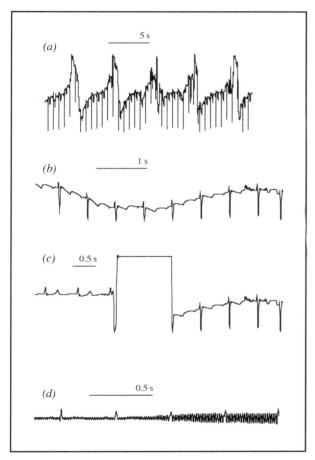

Figure 5.2: *Examples of various artefacts recorded during perioperative electrocardiographic monitoring. (a) The ground electrode of the electrocardiogram (ECG) has become dislodged. The baseline wanders upwards across the display area until the waveform moves out of range. It is then recentred by the monitor but continues to move upwards. (b) Slow movement of the baseline due to patient movement. In this case the baseline continued to rise and fall with chest excursions during respiration. (c) Loss of signal due to lead disconnection. Here one of the leads was repositioned resulting in a change in ECG shape. (d) Mains interference leading to the obliteration of the ECG by 50–60 Hz noise picked up from equipment close to the patient. In this case the interference was due to the animal being placed on an electric heating pad.*

Usefulness

The ECG is a useful monitor in that it provides information that cannot be gained in any other way. However it should not be relied upon as an indicator of cardiovascular function and should always be used in conjunction with other patient monitoring. The ECG is most useful in situations where the development of cardiac arrhythmias or alterations in myocardial environment are likely to develop in the perioperative period. As the electrocardiograph is easy to connect to a patient it can easily become part of routine monitoring.

The pulse oximeter

The pulse oximeter consists of a probe connected to a small computer. By shining light of two different wavelengths (red and infrared) through a tissue and measuring their relative transmissions, it is possible to calculate the relative concentrations of oxygenated and deoxygenated haemoglobin in the tissue. The transmission of light changes with the cardiac cycle and so by comparing the relative magnitude of the change at the two wavelengths it is possible to measure the O_2 saturation of haemoglobin in the blood in the arteries (responsible for this change). This value is referred to as the SpO_2 and is usually quoted as a percentage. Traditionally, the oxygen saturation of blood measured using a bench oximeter is referred to as the SaO_2; SpO_2 is used to indicate the method of measurement used. In addition to providing a measure of SpO_2, pulse oximeters display pulse rate and so are a useful monitor of both cardiovascular and respiratory function.

Pulse oximeters are very easy to use and can quickly generate readings from most animals encountered in practice. When there are problems, these are usually due to the construction or placement of the probe rather than the software, although it should be remembered that many pulse oximeters were developed for use in human patients and there may be problems from the large range of pulse rates encountered in veterinary anaesthesia. There are now a large variety of probes on the market, many of which have been developed for veterinary use (Figure 5.3). A machine with a variety of probe types will be more flexible than a machine with just one, but the potential usefulness of each of the probes available should be considered as some may be primarily for human use. For example, finger probes can be very difficult to use in small animals whereas probes designed for other areas, e.g. ear lobes, or for use in infants can be applied to veterinary patients comparatively easily. Different operators get good results with different probes, and when considering the purchase of a pulse oximeter it is wise to try out several before deciding on a particular machine. Probes for oesophageal or rectal use operate on reflectance of light, rather than transmission. They are convenient to position but are difficult to get consistent results from.

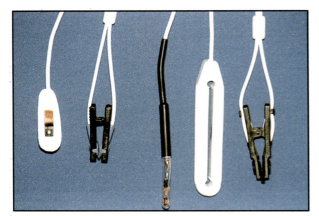

Figure 5.3: *A selection of pulse oximeter probes are available which are suitable for use at various sites. From left to right: surface probe; clip probe; oesophageal/rectal probe; tongue probe; clip probe.*

Photo courtesy of Thames Medical.

Problems

It is not uncommon for a pulse oximeter to fail to get a reliable reading from some sites in some patients. With practice and careful probe placement it is possible to get good results from most veterinary patients. The following can cause a pulse oximeter to fail to give a reading:

Lack of perfusion: The pulse oximeter takes its signal from the arterial blood as the blood perfuses the area of the probe. If there is little or no perfusion then the device will be unable to detect a signal and will not give a reading. Lack of a signal can indicate that the probe has been placed in an area that naturally receives little blood, such as the tip of the pinna, or that there is a generalized lack of tissue perfusion. Particular care should be taken with clip probes as the pressure of the probe can reduce perfusion to the underlying tissues and can cause the probe to lose its signal after a period of time. This often occurs when the probe is located on the tongue. To reduce this problem, the probe should be placed on a different part of the tongue every 10 to 15 minutes.

Inability to locate a signal due to poor perfusion is commonly encountered when anaesthetic techniques including α_2-adrenoceptor agonists are used. These drugs produce vasoconstriction mediated via receptors in blood vessels and hypotension mediated via spinal receptors. The resultant reduction in cardiac output and consequent poor peripheral perfusion can prevent the detection of an adequate signal at the probe site. Other causes of shutdown of peripheral perfusion, such as cold or the use of vasoconstrictors, may result in the loss of signal from the pulse oximeter.

Pigment or fur: Probes often cannot get signals from heavily pigmented or furred areas. In most animals an area of unpigmented tongue or a white digit can be found from which a signal can be obtained. If a digit or other area of skin is to be used, the signal can be greatly improved by clipping the hair where the probe is to be attached.

Ambient light: Pulse oximeters produce red and infrared light from light emitting diodes (LEDs). Bright light falling on the preplaced probe can overwhelm the light from the LEDs and so prevent the light sensor from getting an accurate reading. This problem can be easily solved by shading the probe with a drape or piece of card.

Movement: Movement of the probe over the tissue from which a signal is being measured will result in artefactual changes in the transmission of light, which will obscure the signal. This is a particular problem in conscious animals or those recovering from anaesthesia. If a pulse oximeter is to be used into the recovery period, it is advisable to choose a site which is less likely to suffer from movement artefact and to secure the probe firmly in position without undue pressure. For example, the tongue is often used for perioperative pulse oximetry, but is less useful in the recovery period as animals may lick or chew at it, stopping the probe from recording a good signal and even damaging it. In these cases it is better to secure the probe to a digit with a light bandage. This will allow the pulse oximeter to function well into the recovery period.

Haemoglobin abnormalities: Pulse oximeters are unable to cope with abnormal haemoglobins such as methaemoglobin and carboxyhaemoglobin. The presence of these in the blood can lead to erroneous readings. In patients where the presence of one of these haemoglobins is suspected, pulse oximetry should not be regarded as a reliable indicator of SpO_2. The effects of admixture of artificial blood substitutes on pulse oximetry have yet to be evaluated in animals.

Sites for probe placement

There are many possible locations for the pulse oximeter probe. The best site in a given circumstance will depend upon the type of probe, the size and type of patient and the preferences of the clinician. Figure 5.4 lists some possible sites.

Problems

The pulse oximeter is non-invasive and so carries very little risk of complications. The infrared light will heat the tissues through which it shines, and very minor burns have been seen in some patients after prolonged probe use. These are usually seen as an area of reddening where the probe was attached, which fades after the probe is removed.

Significance of information

The pulse oximeter provides two important pieces of information – pulse rate and SpO_2 at the probe site. The

Site	Type of probe	Placement of probe
Tongue	Clip or tongue	Place as far back on tongue as possible. Blood supply can be occluded as tongue is pulled out of mouth. It sometimes helps to replace tongue with attached probe into mouth
Symphysis of mandible	Clip	Useful in cats. Place probe between canines to shine through tissues behind mandible
Gastrocnemius tendon	Clip	Cats and small or thin dogs. Place probe over tissues between tendon and tibia
Digit	Clip	Useful on white digits. Clip fur and place probe from side to side across digit
Oesophagus	Rectal	Place as oesophageal stethoscope
Rectum	Rectal	Ensure that probe is adjacent to rectal wall and not obscured by faeces
Superficial artery	Flat	Clip fur and place over metatarsal artery
Prepuce	Clip	Place across fold of skin between penis and body wall
Vulva	Clip	Place clip across one wall of the vulva
Scrotum	Clip	Place in area between testicle and body wall
Pinna	Clip	Useful in rabbits. Place probe across pinna from inside to out as far down as possible

Figure 5.4: *Sites for attachment of pulse oximeter probes.*

arterial blood at the probe site is almost always representative of the arterial blood as a whole because of the mixing that occurs as the blood passes through the heart. Several important inferences can be drawn from this information.

Perfusion: The presence of a signal indicates that the tissues under the probe are being perfused by arterial blood. This implies that the heart is effectively pumping blood around the body. Some pulse oximeters have a waveform display or signal strength indicator, which can be used as a crude indication of increasing or decreasing perfusion. This indicator should be treated with caution as the signal strength can be affected by factors other than tissue perfusion. In addition, some pulse oximeters automatically amplify the signal so that it is scaled to the size of the waveform display. This renders the display useless as an indicator of perfusion. Even when using units that do not scale the signal, alterations in signal strength should only be used to alert the anaesthetist to possible alterations in perfusion. They should not be relied upon as the sole indicator of peripheral perfusion.

Pulse rate: The pulse rate indicated by the pulse oximeter is an indication of the rate of effective stroke volumes and not of the rate of electrical activity of the heart. This information can be used in conjunction with an ECG to detect pulse deficits. It should be remembered that small differences in the rate shown by the ECG and the pulse oximeter may be due to differences in the rate-calculating algorithms used by the two devices and are not necessarily a cause for concern.

A change in pulse rate implies an alteration in cardiovascular function, which is usually brought about by changes in activity of the autonomic nervous system. A rising pulse rate (tachycardia) is often an indication of inadequate anaesthesia or hypovolaemia, and a falling pulse rate (bradycardia) is often an indication of overdose of anaesthetic agents or of overhydration. This information should be interpreted in the light of the clinical situation. Measurement of central venous pressure (CVP) or arterial blood pressure can be helpful in differentiating between the causes of bradycardia and tachycardia.

Saturation: The saturation of the arterial blood gives an indication of the amount of oxygen carried in the blood as a percentage of the total carrying capacity of that blood. An alteration in packed cell volume (PCV) can cause a change in the total carrying capacity of the blood that will not be detected by the pulse oximeter. The PCV should be borne in mind when interpreting arterial O_2 saturation, e.g. there is less reserve O_2 carrying capacity in anaemic patients and a smaller fall in saturation than would normally be of concern may result in inadequate delivery of O_2 to tissues.

Because O_2 saturation is a linear measure of the carrying capacity of the blood (unlike partial pressure of

O_2 in arterial blood, PaO_2), a given reduction of saturation anywhere across the spectrum will reduce the O_2 carried in the blood to the same extent. For example, assuming a haemoglobin concentration of 15 g/dl, a decrease in saturation of 5% will result in a reduction in O_2 content of about 0.85 ml/dl regardless of whether the decrease was from 95–90% or from 85–80%.

Normal arterial blood saturation as measured by the pulse oximeter is considered to be between 95% and 100%. A reading of <90% is usually considered to indicate hypoxaemia. Cyanosis of the mucous membranes will not usually be noticed until arterial saturation reaches 70%. A normal reading implies that the patient is breathing a sufficient volume of gas containing an adequate partial pressure of O_2, that the O_2 is able to diffuse across the alveolar membrane and that the oxygenated blood is being pumped from the lungs to the tissues. In the absence of a monitoring error, falling saturation can indicate any of the following:

·   A hypoxic gas mixture is being breathed
·   There is insufficient minute volume (Vm) to oxygenate the blood
·   There is an increased shunt fraction (proportion of blood which passes through the lungs without becoming oxygenated)
·   There is an impairment of alveolar diffusion
·   There is insufficient cardiac output to deliver the blood to the tissues (usually accompanied by loss of signal).

Because the supply of O_2 to the peripheral blood can be interrupted at any stage in the process, it is wise to investigate each possibility until the cause is isolated.

A pulse oximeter reading of <90% represents an immediate threat to the patient because it relates to the blood that is currently perfusing the tissues. For this reason it should be investigated as a priority and appropriate action taken as soon as possible.

Usefulness

A pulse oximeter is a very useful device in routine surgical patients. It can be rapidly attached and is non-invasive, yet provides valuable information about cardiovascular function and oxygenation of the arterial blood. It is especially useful in patients with respiratory insufficiency or where a procedure which is likely to compromise oxygenation, such as bronchoscopy or bronchoalveolar lavage, is to be carried out. With an appropriate probe, a pulse oximeter is also very useful during the recovery period where it can provide a relatively early indication of respiratory depression or obstruction. It is useful in patients receiving supplemental O_2 therapy, and it can be used to optimize O_2 delivery and to help ensure that the blood remains well oxygenated as the inspired O_2 concentration is reduced.

ANALYSIS OF RESPIRATORY GASES

The composition of the gas breathed in and out by an anaesthetized patient can provide valuable information about the patient's cardiovascular and respiratory systems as well as the extent of anaesthesia. Traditionally, physiological gases such as O_2 and carbon dioxide (CO_2) together with nitrous oxide (N_2O) and volatile anaesthetic agents have been measured by separate monitors, although machines are now available that monitor all of these gases. Several different methods are used to analyse respiratory gases and the following are intended as examples. Measurement is made either on the gas stream as it flows into the ETT (main stream) or by removing a continuous sample of gas for analysis inside the monitor (side stream).

Measurement

Carbon dioxide

Analysis of CO_2 is usually based on its ability to absorb infrared light. Peak absorption occurs at a wavelength of 4.28 μm, and at this wavelength there is little interference from other gases such as N_2O. Continuous monitoring of the CO_2 concentration in the gas produces a readout which is usually displayed as a waveform (Figure 5.5). From the waveform, the end-tidal and inspiratory CO_2 tensions and the respiratory rate can be measured, and these are usually displayed in numerical fashion.

Oxygen

Several oxygen measuring devices make use of light absorption by this gas. Analysis of O_2 may also make use of the paramagnetic property of this gas. Unlike most other gases (e.g. nitrogen), which are weakly repelled by magnetic fields, O_2 is attracted by them. If a glass dumbbell containing nitrogen is suspended in a chamber by a filament and placed in a magnetic field it will rotate on the filament. This arrangement will come to rest when the tension in the filament equals the force developed by the magnetic field on the gas in the two spheres of the dumbbell. When O_2 is added to the gas in the chamber it will be attracted to the magnetic field and tend to displace the spheres. This will alter the forces on the filament and the dumbbell will rotate to find a new equilibrium. A beam of light is reflected from a mirror placed on the dumbbell, and the position of the reflected beam can be read off a scale that can be calibrated in per cent O_2 in the gas in the chamber. Over the respiratory cycle the percentage of O_2 can be measured, and inspired and expired O_2 displayed. The percentage of O_2 extracted from the inspired gas is also often displayed.

Nitrous oxide

The concentration of nitrous oxide is usually measured by absorption of infrared light in a similar manner to that of CO_2. The wavelength of infrared light used is 3.9 μm.

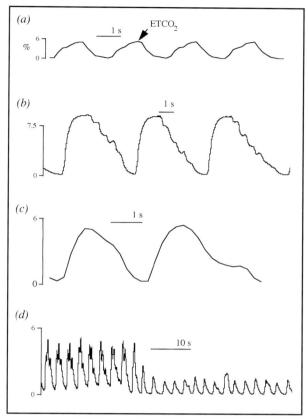

Figure 5.5: *Examples of end-tidal carbon dioxide (ETCO₂) traces recorded during the perioperative period. (a) Normal waveform showing return to 0 with each inspiration and plateau as alveolar gas is expired. The peak of each cycle is taken as end-tidal CO₂ (marked by arrow). (b) In this recording fluctuations can be seen in the waveform during the expiratory pause. These are in time with the heart beat and are due to gas moving in and out of the chest as the heart contracts and relaxes. (c) Abnormal waveform showing hypoventilation. The tidal volume is reduced and no alveolar plateau is reached at the end of expiration. It would be expected that true end-tidal CO₂ would be higher than the peak of this recording. (d) Sudden decrease in end-tidal CO₂ due to reduction of cardiac output. This recording was taken during ligation of a patent ductus arteriosus. The reduction in cardiac output was due to tamponade caused by bleeding into the pericardial sac from a torn pulmonary artery.*

Volatile anaesthetic agents

Traditional anaesthetic agent monitors have also utilized the absorption principle of infrared light, but this has been associated with problems such as interference from changing N_2O concentrations in the gas. A particular problem in veterinary anaesthesia has been interference from methane, which occurs in the expired gas of herbivores such as horses and ruminants. A newer technique that is not affected by other gases passes a stream of gas over a piezo-electric crystal. When a voltage is applied to the crystal, the crystal oscillates and the frequency of this oscillation is altered by the concentration of volatile agent in the gas stream. Anaesthetic agent monitors usually display the minimum and maximum agent concentration through

the respiratory cycle. Which of these values is from inspired gas and which is from end-tidal gas will vary with the course of the anaesthetic. When the patient is taking up anaesthetic agent at the start of anaesthesia, the greatest value will be from inspired gas, but at the end of anaesthesia when the agent has been removed from the inspired gas the greatest value will be from expired gas. The monitor will be unable to differentiate the two unless it also measures another gas such as CO_2.

Significance of information

Carbon dioxide

Inspired CO_2 is important as it is a sensitive indicator of rebreathing and is used to ensure that the fresh gas flow delivered to a non-breathing system is adequate. It can also warn of a malfunction of the breathing system such as the failure of a unidirectional flow valve in a circle breathing system or soda-lime exhaustion. It should, however, be noted that some breathing systems such as the Bain and Ayre's T-piece can allow a small amount of rebreathing under normal operating circumstances. The absence of CO_2 in the expired air may indicate that the anaesthetic system is disconnected from the ETT, that the tube is incorrectly placed (usually in the oesophagus) or that there is no effective gas exchange taking place in the lungs.

The gas contained in the upper airway at the end of expiration was in the alveoli at the start of expiration. Because alveolar gas is equilibrated with arterial blood, end-tidal gas concentrations reflect arterial gas concentrations. End-tidal CO_2 concentration is closely related to arterial CO_2 tension unless there is respiratory dysfunction such as the presence of excessive shunt or dead space. End-tidal CO_2 concentration is related to the balance between CO_2 production (metabolic rate) and CO_2 removal (alveolar Vm). Changes under anaesthesia usually relate to Vm and give a good indication of hypoventilation or hyperventilation. This information can be useful in helping to assess adequacy of anaesthesia. A sudden fall in end-tidal CO_2 concentration can indicate a sudden disturbance in pulmonary perfusion such as cardiac arrest or pulmonary embolism. Complete loss of the end-tidal CO_2 waveform can indicate apnoea or the disconnection of the patient from the breathing system. More subtle alterations in respiratory function can be detected as alterations in the shape of the waveform (see Figure 5.5). With non-rebreathing circuits, the constant flow of fresh gas close to the endotracheal tube causes mixing of expired gas and fresh gas, making end-tidal observations unreliable with this type of breathing system.

The respiratory rate of the patient is usually derived from the CO_2 waveform and can be combined with the concentration of end-tidal CO_2 to give an indication of the patient's respiratory function. Rapid respiratory rates can be associated with an increased Vm due to surgical stimulation. In this case the concentration of end-tidal CO_2 will be low and the shape of the waveform will be normal. Anaesthetic agent overdose can also lead to a rapid respiratory rate, but in this case it is accompanied by a reduced tidal volume (Vt), and the resultant Vm will be decreased with an increase in end-tidal CO_2 concentration. Under these circumstances the apparent concentration of end-tidal CO_2 displayed by the monitor can be low if Vt is insufficient to allow true alveolar gas to reach the gas sampling port during expiration. When this is the case the shape of the waveform will be abnormal with no true plateau. True decreased end-tidal CO_2 concentration can be differentiated from this situation by squeezing the rebreathing bag to produce a large Vt. If Vm is high, the concentration of end-tidal CO_2 for this breath will be low, but if there is respiratory depression the concentration for this breath will be much higher than for the patient's usual breaths and will bear a closer relation to $PaCO_2$.

Oxygen
The measurement of inspired O_2 concentration is useful as an assurance that the patient is not breathing a hypoxic gas mixture. This can be especially useful when using a rebreathing system as it can allow the safe use of N_2O. The measurement of inspired O_2 concentration combined with blood gas analysis or pulse oximetry can also be useful in assessing the severity of pulmonary dysfunction. When used with pulse oximetry, the minimum concentration of inspired O_2 required to produce an SpO_2 of >95% can easily be determined and changes used as an indicator of worsening or improving respiratory function. When used with blood gas analysis, the difference in alveolar/arterial O_2 tension can be calculated using a derivation of the alveolar air equation:

$$PAO_2 = PIO_2 - (1.1 \times PaCO_2)$$

where PAO_2 is alveolar PO_2, PIO_2 is inspired PO_2 and $PaCO_2$ is arterial PO_2.

PAO_2 is then used in a second equation:

$$P(A-a)O_2 = PAO_2 - PaO_2$$

In normal animals this value should be <15 mmHg (2 kPa), but it becomes larger if lung function deteriorates.

Nitrous oxide
The measurement of N_2O concentration is useful at the end of anaesthesia, when it can be used to monitor the decreasing expired concentration of N_2O when the patient is breathing 100% O_2. If the patient is not disconnected until the expired N_2O concentration has substantially decreased then there is no risk of diffusion hypoxia in the early postoperative period.

Volatile anaesthetic agents
The inspired and expired concentration of volatile anaesthetic agent is largely used as a teaching and research tool. The concentration of end-tidal anaesthetic agent is related to the effect of the agent at a steady state and is used in the definition of minimum alveolar concentration (MAC). When used in the clinical setting it is unwise to rely on an agent monitor to judge adequacy of anaesthesia as there is large variability between patients. Agent monitoring can be useful to alert the anaesthetist to other problems especially when using a rebreathing system. For example, if the patient requires much less anaesthetic agent than expected, this may indicate the presence of another problem such as hypothermia or a severe acid/base disorder. Conversely, if much more agent is required than expected this may indicate that perioperative analgesia is inadequate.

Usefulness
Respiratory gas analysis is most useful in patients undergoing major surgery, especially if intermittent positive-pressure ventilation is used as part of the anaesthetic technique. Gas monitors are non-invasive and very easy to attach to patients and can easily form part of a routine monitoring system in theatres where they are available.

ARTERIAL BLOOD PRESSURE

Arterial blood pressure is one of the most useful measures of cardiovascular function available to the anaesthetist. Unfortunately it cannot be appreciated without monitoring equipment of some kind. There are two methods of measuring blood pressure which are widely used in clinical practice – direct and indirect.

Direct blood pressure measurement
This technique involves the placement of a cannula into a peripheral artery. In the dog, the dorsal metatarsal artery and femoral artery on the hindlimb or the palmar artery on the forelimb are the most common sites for cannula placement. The middle auricular artery can be used in breeds that have large ears, e.g. Basset Hound. In the cat, the femoral artery is the most common site. The cannula is connected to a pressure transducer via a column of heparinized saline. The transducer can be a flexible membrane fluid/air interface (e.g. the Pressureveil, Figure 5.6) connected to a Bourdon pressure gauge, or an electronic strain gauge connected to an electronic monitoring device. The transducer is zeroed at the level of the right atrium. Both methods give a continuous reading of blood pressure.

The Pressureveil measures mean blood pressure, but cannot respond to the change in pressure over the cardiac cycle rapidly enough to give an indication of systolic or diastolic pressure. A strain gauge transducer responds instantly to changes in pressure and

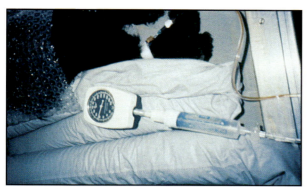

Figure 5.6: Direct arterial blood pressure measurement using a Pressureveil system connected to the dorsal metatarsal artery of a dog. Note that the saline/air interface should be placed at the level of the right atrium.

should be connected to the cannula using narrow non-compliant tubing to prevent distortion of the signal due to damping or resonance (ringing). Systolic and diastolic pressures are taken as the cyclic maximum and minimum pressures respectively, and mean pressure is calculated using the area under the curve (integral) of the waveform. Interpretation of the systolic and diastolic pressure is complicated by the frequency response characteristics of the catheter/transducer system and the location of the catheter. Nevertheless, trends in these pressures are useful clinical tools.

Indirect blood pressure measurement

There are several variations of this technique all of which are based on the occlusion of blood flow to an extremity by the inflation of a cuff tourniquet. Any of the limbs or the tail can be used. Pulsatile flow of blood is detected either by pulsatile pressure changes in the cuff itself (oscillometric) or by the placement of a flow transducer over an artery distal to the cuff. The transducer is usually an ultrasound probe and either detects flow of red cells through the artery (Doppler) or movement of the arterial wall (Arteriosonde). Indirect blood pressure monitors give intermittent readings of blood pressure.

The cuff is inflated until all flow through the artery ceases and then deflated slowly until the first flow is detected. The pressure at which blood flow recommences is taken as systolic blood pressure. As the cuff is further deflated, diastolic and mean blood pressure are measured. Oscillotonometric devices record mean blood pressure as the pressure at which the pulses in the cuff are maximal and diastolic pressure as the pressure below which they disappear. When using a flow transducer, diastolic pressure is taken at the point when blood flow occurs throughout the cardiac cycle, and mean pressure is calculated as diastolic pressure plus one third of the difference between systolic pressure and diastolic pressure:

$$\text{Mean pressure} = \text{Diastolic pressure} + \left(\frac{\text{Systolic pressure - diastolic pressure}}{3} \right)$$

Problems

The problems with direct blood pressure measurement are mostly those of arterial cannulation. There is potential for accidental displacement of the catheter and subsequent haematoma formation. Pressure should always be applied to an artery for 5 minutes after failed attempted cannulation or removal of a cannula, to allow the wall to seal through thrombus formation. In addition the accidental intra-arterial injection of drugs through an arterial catheter can be disastrous. Agents such as thiopentone can crystallize out of solution after arterial injection and can block the arterioles leading from the artery causing ischaemia and necrosis of the area served by that vessel.

Indirect arterial blood pressure measurement has few complications, but can give inaccurate results if attention to detail is not paid when performing this procedure. The width of the occlusive cuff used affects the result. In general, the wider the cuff the lower will be the values obtained. The ideal cuff width is usually quoted as 40% of the circumference of the limb to which it is applied, but this is a compromise as the ideal width also varies with the pressure range being measured. With automatic techniques attention should also be paid to the correct rotation of the cuff compared to the artery. Most cuffs have a mark which should be placed directly over the artery. Indirect blood pressure measurements become more difficult in very small animals and when the patient is hypotensive. When using a manual method the quality of the sounds should give an indication that the technique is working properly. Mechanical methods tend to fail by giving results which are less and less accurate. When using such a method the correct function of the monitor can be checked by counting the pulse rate and comparing this to the pulse rate given by the monitor. The stability of the results over several estimations can also be used as an indicator of correct function.

Significance of information

Arterial blood pressure monitoring gives information about the ability of the heart to pump blood around the body and the fluid balance of the patient. Blood flow to the major organs of the body is autoregulated across a range of mean blood pressures from about 60 mmHg (8 kPa) to about 120 mmHg (16 kPa). When blood pressure falls below this range, blood flow to major organs is compromised and there may be serious long- and short-term consequences. Such a reduction in organ flow will result in the accumulation of lactic acid in the tissues and the development of acidosis. Long-term consequences of reduced organ blood flow can be seen due to ischaemic damage to tissues that have undergone periods of inadequate O_2 delivery. The most common consequence of these in the dog is renal failure, the onset of which may be precipitated or hastened by such a period of reduced renal blood flow.

Changes in blood pressure over time can be used

in conjunction with heart rate to help diagnose the development of inadequate anaesthesia, anaesthetic agent overdose, hypovolaemia and overhydration (Figure 5.7).

When monitoring arterial blood pressure using a direct method with an electronic monitor, much information can be gained from the shape of the trace in addition to the absolute values of systolic, diastolic and mean pressures. The rate of rise of the waveform in the early systolic period is the best clinical indicator of ventricular contractility. The degree of curvature in the diastolic part of the waveform gives an indication of the presence of hypovolaemia (Figure 5.8).

Usefulness

Arterial blood pressure monitoring is not a technique that is widely used on all cases. This is because all the techniques available to monitor blood pressure require a degree of time and effort to set up and take measurements. Blood pressure gives a direct indication of the adequacy of cardiovascular function, which can respond very rapidly to changing situations. As such, it is extremely useful in patients with significant cardiovascular disease and patients undergoing major surgery. Like any technique, it becomes easier and also quicker and more accurate with practice, and so if a blood pressure monitoring device is purchased, it should be used on a regular basis. Staff will then learn both how to set up and use the system and the significance of the information obtained. With increased familiarity, blood pressure monitors can be used on a wider population of patients and should become routine monitoring equipment.

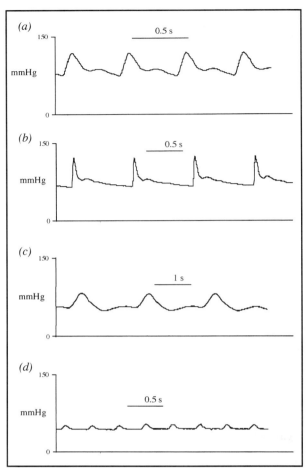

Figure 5.8: Recordings of arterial blood pressure taken using an electronic pressure transducer connected to an arterial cannula. (a) Normal arterial blood pressure. Note brisk increase in the early systolic period and 'springy' baseline in the diastolic period. (b) The large pulse pressure and flat baseline indicate hypovolaemia. This dog has lost considerable blood from an arterial bleed during thoracic surgery. (c) The slow rate of rise in the early systolic period indicates myocardial depression in this case due to relative halothane overdose. (d) Combined hypovolaemia and myocardial depression. This is the same case as in Figure 5.8b. When this recording was made, the ongoing blood loss was compromising oxygen delivery due to falling packed cell volume and reduced perfusion.

CENTRAL VENOUS PRESSURE

Central venous pressure (CVP) is taken as the pressure in the great veins within the thoracic cavity. In common with arterial pressure, CVP is measured with reference to a zero point, taken to be the level of the right atrium. This is approximated by the level of the manubrium in lateral recumbency and the scapulohumeral joint in patients on their backs. In order to measure CVP, a cannula must be inserted into the jugular vein so that its tip lies beyond the thoracic inlet. This is connected to a pressure transducer usually in the form of a saline manometer (Figure 5.9).

Central venous pressure is the first cardiovascular

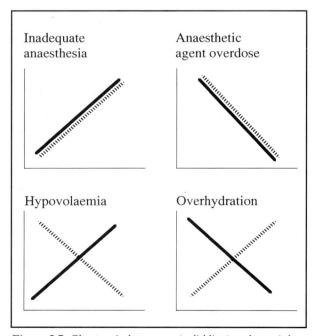

Figure 5.7: Changes in heart rate (solid line) and arterial blood pressure (dashed line), which occur over time.

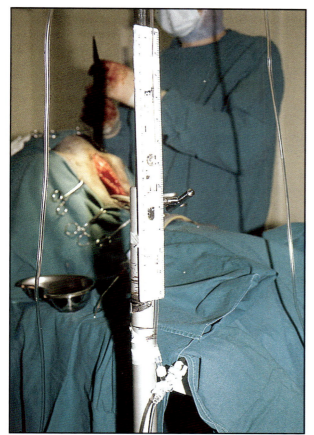

Figure 5.9: *Measurement of central venous pressure (CVP) from a Dobermann during ventral cervical intervertebral disk fenestration. Note that the 10 cm mark is used as a zero (CVP can be negative) and placed at the level of the right atrium.*

variable to alter in response to changes in fluid balance and as such gives a good indication of the hydration status of the animal and of the ability of the heart to pump blood. The normal range in the dog and cat is large, making single readings of limited value, but a small change over time can be interpreted as an alteration in cardiovascular function. A low (or falling) CVP occurs when the central venous reservoir is depleted, and so indicates hypovolaemia. A high (or increasing) CVP occurs when the central venous reservoir is well filled, and so can indicate hypervolaemia or cardiogenic–cardiovascular insufficiency. Central venous pressure can be a valuable aid in differentiating low arterial blood pressure due to hypovolaemia from low arterial blood pressure due to heart failure.

URINE OUTPUT

Urine output is measured over a period of time by collecting urine from the bladder. This is usually performed in a semi-continuous manner in patients with an indwelling urinary catheter and a closed collection system. Careful attention should be paid to sterile technique when setting up and managing such a system, and the patient should normally be receiving antibiosis to prevent nosocomial infection. The collection system and bladder are both emptied and the urine that accumulates measured over a known period (usually 30 minutes to 1 hour). A reduction in urine production to below 1 ml/kg/h indicates that renal perfusion is reduced or that the patient is dehydrated and is conserving water by resorption of glomerular filtrate. Both circumstances indicate hypovolaemia or cardiovascular collapse and can lead to the development of acute renal failure if not remedied.

Urine output is usually only measured when a urinary catheter is placed for other reasons. In such animals it can be used as a reasonable medium-term indicator that arterial blood pressure is sufficient to maintain renal perfusion. It is also invaluable in the treatment of acute renal failure where the renewed production of urine gives evidence of response to treatment.

BLOOD GAS ANALYSIS

Blood gas analysers measure the pH of the blood and the tension of O_2 and CO_2 and can also calculate other variables such as plasma bicarbonate concentration, total plasma CO_2, haemoglobin saturation and base excess. More modern machines can often perform additional measurements such as concentration of sodium, potassium, chloride and ionized calcium, and haematocrit. Traditional blood gas monitors have electrodes that are placed in contact with the blood and rely on the setting up of an electrical half cell to perform their measurements. These machines are expensive and require frequent skilled maintenance in order to remain functioning accurately. Recently, however, blood gas analysers using newer technology, such as disposable modules, have become available. These are cheap to buy and require little or no maintenance. Despite the higher sample costs of these units they have brought blood gas analysis within the reach of the general practitioner.

The blood gas machine utilizes samples of heparinized blood. The blood samples should be withdrawn anaerobically and analysed promptly so that the measured values reflect the actual gas tensions in the blood and not ones that have been altered by contact with room air. Blood gas analysis can be performed on any blood sample, but it is usual to use arterial blood wherever possible. Arterial blood is preferred because it can provide information about the ability of the lungs to oxygenate the blood and also because it is mixed and so can be taken from any artery. Venous blood can only provide information about the tissues that are drained by the vein from which the sample is taken.

Significance of information
The results of blood gas analysis can provide invaluable information about the oxygenation and acid/base

status of the patient. The detailed interpretation of blood gas measurements can be complex as all the results are interrelated.

Problems

Ordinarily, blood gas analysis requires a sample of arterial blood. Taking an arterial blood sample is relatively easy, but complications such as haematoma or bruise formation at the site of sampling can occur without careful attention to technique. In particular, pressure should be applied to the site for several minutes after sample collection to allow the vessel to seal. If it is likely that multiple samples will be required from a case then the placement of an arterial cannula should be considered.

Usefulness

Blood gas analysis is useful in the management of critical patients and those presenting for major surgery. Accurate assessment of the ability of the lungs to oxygenate the blood and the acid/base status of the animal is invaluable in the evaluation of a case. Specific treatment can be planned from the results of initial blood gas analysis and the response to this treatment can be monitored by taking further blood gas samples.

RESPIRATORY AND CARDIAC 'BLEEP' MONITORS

Many monitors are available that detect the presence of an electrocardiograph or movement of respiratory gases, and that bleep with respiration or with an ECG complex. In the past these monitors have found a place in many practices, but they should be treated with extreme caution as they provide very little information about the physiological state of the patient and it is dangerous to rely on them. The respiratory monitors usually respond to a change in temperature at the end of the ETT. This provides information about the rate of respiration, but nothing about the Vt. In addition, it is possible for these monitors to continue to bleep in time with the heart rate in patients that have undergone respiratory arrest. The cardiac monitors respond to the ECG and so give no information about the mechanical function of the heart. In addition, they can respond to some arrhythmias as 'normal' complexes and give no information about the kind of arrhythmia present when an irregularity is detected.

ANAESTHETIC RECORDS

In order to get the best out of monitoring equipment it is advisable to keep a written record of every anaesthetic procedure. Anaesthetic records are useful for four main reasons:

- They allow trends in patient variables to be noticed at an early stage. For example, a sudden change in heart rate from 100 beats per minute to 60 beats per minute should be obvious to anyone monitoring an anaesthetic. If this same change occurs over 10 or 20 minutes then it is much less obvious but will be immediately visible if the heart rate is recorded every 5 minutes. Such detection of trends will allow the anaesthetic to be adjusted to compensate for this slowing heart rate sooner than would otherwise be the case
- An archive of anaesthetic records will enable similar situations that occur in a number of cases to be directly compared to each other. For example, if a change is made in routine anaesthetic protocols and occasional instances of hypoventilation occur, then the records from several cases can be inspected and can give a detailed picture of the circumstances surrounding this complication. This may highlight the reason for the problem, which can then be rectified
- They can concentrate the mind of inexperienced personnel and improve their standard of patient monitoring. In this case the improvement in anaesthetic monitoring comes through paying more attention to the patient and the record itself is of secondary importance
- It is increasingly common for courts to become involved in disputes involving the management of veterinary patients. In cases where the anaesthetic management of a case needs to be defended, an anaesthetic record is of enormous worth both as a reminder of the details of the individual case and as evidence of the general standard of care given by the veterinary practice. To be admissible as evidence, an anaesthetic record must be contemporaneous i.e. it must have been made at the same time that the anaesthetic was given.

ELECTRICAL SAFETY

When any electrical equipment is connected to a patient there is a risk of injury to the patient from leakage of electrical current. This risk can be minimized by ensuring that the equipment used is of a medical standard and is electrically isolated from the patient. It is also important to ensure that the equipment is regularly serviced so that faults which may lead to a leakage of current through the patient do not go undetected. Leakage of electrical current can lead to burns developing at the contact or earthing point of the patient and can lead to cardiac arrest if sufficient current passes across the heart. In the UK, electrical monitoring equipment that makes an electrical connection to the patient is categorized into two safety standards: CF is used for equipment that has a direct intracardiac connection and must have a leakage current of <50 µA, even if a single fault develops, and B or BF is only suitable for non-cardiac or surface connection and must have a leakage current of < 500 µA, even if a single fault develops. In the USA, the leakage current for an ECG that uses surface electrodes should not exceed 300µA. These standards are not obligatory for equipment used in veterinary medicine, but it is sensible to ensure that any equipment purchased conforms to the appropriate safety standard.

WHICH MONITOR TO BUY

As more ambitious surgical procedures on high-risk patients are undertaken in veterinary practice, the need for adequate patient monitoring increases. When considering which anaesthetic monitors to buy it is important to bear in mind the case load as well as the expertise of the staff operating the monitor. It is useful if an overall idea of the ideal or desired monitoring set-up can be gained before the first monitor is purchased so that possibilities can be assessed both in terms of their immediate usefulness and how they will fit in to a broader picture. An ideal monitoring device or combination of devices will provide information appropriate to the expected complications of the patients encountered and will be used often enough for the staff to become familiar with its function and skilled at interpreting the information given.

CHOOSING A MONITOR FOR A CASE

When selecting a monitor for a particular case, the selection will be made from those available within the practice. It is not always appropriate to attach every monitor to every patient as this may lead to prolonged anaesthetic times for minor surgical procedures and can actually reduce the monitoring efficiency of inexperienced staff. At the same time it should be remembered that for the best to be gained from a monitor, it should be familiar to staff and it should be used on a regular basis.

FURTHER READING

Edwards NJ (1987) *Bolton's Handbook of Canine and Feline Electrocardiography, 2nd Edition.* WB Saunders, Philadelphia
Moyle JTB (1994) *Pulse Oximetry.* BMJ Publishing Group, London
O'Flaherty D (1994) *Capnography.* BMJ Publishing Group, London
Parbook GD, Davis PD and Parbrook EO (1990) *Basic Physics and Measurement in Anaesthesia.* Butterworth-Heinemann, Oxford

CHAPTER SIX

Analgesia

Avril E. Waterman-Pearson

INTRODUCTION

Pain is a universal experience and, although everybody knows what it feels like, it is very much more difficult to define. Humans can express and describe the sensations they experience, and these descriptions are well accepted. Assessment in animals is much more difficult. One must rely on the observation of overt signs and the correct interpretation of these signs, for it is only when pain is recognized that steps can be taken to alleviate it.

ADVANTAGES AND DISADVANTAGES OF PAIN

The ability to feel pain has clear survival advantages: limiting the extent of an injury, encouraging rest and healing of the injured area and ensuring that the individual learns to avoid noxious stimuli in the future. Ongoing pain, however, has no benefit and many disadvantages. Ongoing pain:

- Is distressing for the animal; postoperatively, dogs and cats in pain are dull and depressed and do not recover as well as might be expected
- Provokes an enhanced stress response and increases catabolism causing delayed wound healing
- Depresses food intake
- Results in impaired respiration. Especially after upper abdominal or thoracic surgery, animals are more prone to pulmonary atelectasis, hypoxia, hypercapnia and the retention of mucus and sputum, due to a reluctance to cough. This increases the risk of pneumonia
- Can lead to self-mutilation
- Causes sensitization of the central nervous system (CNS).

The reasons for the relative neglect of analgesia by veterinarians may be because:

- Pain in animals is difficult to recognize
- There are misconceptions about the use of analgesic drugs, especially opioids
- There is a limited number of licensed products available for use
- There are reservations about the potential side effects of analgesics.

Analgesic drugs are often withheld because the clinician is not absolutely sure that the animal is experiencing pain, and yet that same clinician may administer antibiotics without proving the presence of bacterial contamination or infection. Precisely because pain is difficult to assess, a liberal attitude to the use of analgesic drugs should be maintained; overtreatment may occur, but the adverse consequences of this are minimal compared with the distress caused by withholding pain relief. It is sometimes suggested that analgesics should be withheld so that the protective function of pain is maintained. However, provided that effective measures are taken to immobilize or protect damaged tissues, and competent surgical techniques are employed, the abolition of pain rarely causes problems. It is hard to concede that leaving a patient without pain relief can ever be advantageous.

ASSESSING PAIN IN DOGS AND CATS

Humans can express and define the sensations they are experiencing and can localize the site of the pain. In animals one must rely on the observation of behavioural cues and their correct interpretation. The judgement of pain in animals is bound to be based on personal experiences and, although such an anthropomorphic approach is potentially dangerous, it is reasonable as a first line of approach. Animals probably have no psychological expectation of pain, and so the confounding influence of anticipation is removed. Animals are generally less demonstrative about their pain than humans, not least because for those animals that are hunted there is a survival advantage in not displaying abnormal behaviours overtly as this would attract the attention of predators.

Changed responsiveness to human contact is often a first indicator that the animal is in discomfort. Aggression and avoidance of human contact may increase, or conversely some animals may seek excessive human reassurance. Acute postoperative pain provokes signs of guarding and vocalization, especially if the painful area is manipulated. Lack of vocalization, however, should not be interpreted as lack of pain.

Moderate discomfort often leads to attempts to bite or scratch the area, while deafferentation pain (e.g. following peripheral nerve or spinal cord injury) can give rise to self-mutilation. Increased restlessness is often a feature of postoperative discomfort, especially if the source of the pain is visceral, while extreme somatic pain leads to reluctance to move. This may be a reflection of the poor localization of visceral pain as opposed to pain of orthopaedic origin.

More chronic localized sources of pain such as limb injuries give rise to stiffness, difficulty in walking or rising, changes in gait and obvious avoidance responses if the affected area is manipulated. Chronic visceral pain is less easy to quantify – low-grade discomfort tends to reduce the animal's general well being and demeanour, while increasing pain levels lead to abnormal postures and guarding or straining.

Disturbances to the normal sleep pattern, with a dog sleeping less, is also an indicator of discomfort. Thoracic pain makes dogs and cats reluctant to lie down or sleep despite obvious exhaustion. Reduced grooming and eating behaviour are often manifestations of more chronic pain.

Cats in pain are less vocal and demonstrative than dogs and tend to be less active: they sit unresponsive and hunched in sternal rather than in curled lateral recumbency. The most severe pain may cause cats to vocalize spontaneously, although more usually growling or hissing is reserved for pain provoked by manipulation of the wound site. Aggression and resentment of handling is a common manifestation of pain in cats. Self-mutilation is rare but may be provoked by intense neurogenic pain.

A SCORING SYSTEM FOR PAIN

A useful way of learning how to assess pain is to use a simple scoring system. A four point numerical rating scale can be used:

· 0 – No pain, no overt signs of discomfort, no resentment to firm pressure
· 1 – Some pain, no overt signs of discomfort, resentment to firm pressure
· 2 – Moderate pain, some overt signs of discomfort, made worse by firm pressure
· 3 – Severe pain, overt signs of persistent discomfort, made worse by firm pressure.

Postoperatively, scoring should be carried out at 1 and 4 hours, and the scores should be recorded. The aim should be to keep scores in the 0 or 1 category at all times.

This scoring system combines visual appraisal of spontaneous behavioural signs indicative of pain with a qualitative assessment of response to palpation of the affected area. If the animal is in pain, palpation can produce an exaggerated behavioural response such as aggression, vocalization or avoidance. Such an interactive method of assessing pain, which includes handling the animal, allows a far more accurate assessment of the severity of the discomfort than can be ascertained from mere observation.

MECHANISMS OF PROCESSING NOCICEPTIVE INFORMATION

The 'pain pathway' can be split into three principal components:

· Peripheral tissue nociceptors detect the stimulus and permit transmission of the nociceptive signal via primary afferent nerve fibres to the spinal cord or cranial nerve nuclei. There are four types of peripheral nociceptors: high- and low-threshold mechanoreceptors, thermoreceptors and polymodal nociceptors, while visceral receptors are activated by dilation or ischaemia. Nociceptive signals are conveyed by primary afferent axons (slowly conducting unmyelinated C-fibres or small myelinated Aδ nerve fibres).
· Signal processing occurs in the spinal cord or brainstem before transmission to supraspinal structures. The primary afferent axons enter the spinal cord via the dorsal root into the dorsal horn and terminate mostly in lamina I (Aδ nerve fibres) or lamina II (C-fibres). There are two classes of nociceptive neurons within the dorsal horn:
  – Wide dynamic range neurons which respond mainly to innocuous stimuli, unless the stimulus level is great (i.e. noxious), when the frequency of their discharge is increased
  – Nociceptive specific neurons which respond exclusively to noxious stimulation.
  Pain behaviours correlate better with firing in wide dynamic range neurons than in nociceptive specific neurons
· After further processing at supraspinal sites, the signal induces the conscious perception of pain.

There are, in addition, various intrinsic segmental, spinal and supraspinal endogenous mechanisms for inhibiting the transmission of the nociceptive signals which are mediated by endogenous neurotransmitter systems (opioid, serotonergic, cholinergic, adrenergic).

CNS sensitization

The appreciation of pain does not simply involve a moment by moment analysis of afferent noxious input relayed by a hard-wired transmission system, but is more a dynamic process that is influenced by past experiences. The system has great plasticity, and is able to change over time according to experience. This concept is not new. In 1883, Sturge proposed that peripheral injury triggered a change in the excitability of the CNS so that normal inputs evoked exaggerated responses leading to pain hypersensitivity, and in 1913, Crile made similar observations.

Clinical pain can be classified as inflammatory or neuropathic and is distinguished from physiological pain by the presence of pathological hypersensitivity. Inflammatory pain relates to peripheral tissue damage, and neuropathic pain relates to a damaged CNS. Both are characterized by changes in sensitivity, such that stimuli that are not normally perceived as painful become painful (allodynia) and an exaggerated responsiveness to a given noxious stimulus (hyperalgesia) develops and spreads to uninjured tissue (secondary hyperalgesia).

This sensitization can occur at either or both peripheral and central levels:

- Peripheral sensitization develops because of an increase in the sensitivity of nociceptors as a result of exposure to a 'soup' of inflammatory mediators (bradykinin, prostaglandins, leucotrienes, 5-hydroxytryptamine (5-HT), histamine, substance P, thromboxanes, platelet activating factor) released by tissue injury. These inflammatory changes may also induce normally unresponsive ('sleeping') nociceptors to become active. The net result is an increase in firing rate of afferent nerve fibres
- Central sensitization develops as a result of changes in the spinal cord. An activity-dependent increase in excitability of dorsal horn neurons develops which outlasts the nociceptive afferent inputs (Woolf, 1983). This produces secondary hyperalgesia, i.e. there is a spread of hypersensitivity to uninjured tissue. 'Central hypersensitivity' results in a modified response to subsequent afferent inputs, which lasts between 10 and 200 times the duration of the initiating stimulus (Woolf and Chong, 1993). There are several receptors involved in the mediation of these changes in the spinal cord, one of the most significant clinically being the N-methyl-D-aspartate (NMDA) subtype of the glutamate receptor.

Central sensitization is responsible for some of the changes in the zone of primary hyperalgesia, but all of the changes in the zone of secondary hyperalgesia.

Peripheral sensitization differs from central sensitization because it enables low intensity stimuli to produce noxious signals by activating sensitized nociceptors and primary afferents, whereas central sensitization represents an abnormal interpretation of information from low-threshold sensory fibres, their input now interpreted as pain.

The clinical implications of this hypersensitivity are that:

- Once pain is established, analgesic drugs, for a given dose, are much less effective, i.e. pain is more difficult to control
- The pain is perceived to be greater by the animal.

Thus, the evidence is overwhelming that pain should be prevented rather than merely treated. By preventing the surgical afferent barrage from entering the spinal cord, these changes in spinal nociceptive processing can be prevented and, thus, the severity of postoperative pain can be markedly decreased. The concept of 'pre-emptive analgesia' is the administration of analgesics preoperatively to reduce the severity of postoperative pain.

It has been shown experimentally in rats (Woolf and Wall, 1986) and clinically in dogs (Lascelles et al., 1997) that preinjury treatment with opioids prevents or markedly decreases the development of central hypersensitivity, but these treatments are far less effective if administered after the injury is initiated. Local analgesics (Coderre et al., 1990) have a similar protective effect, both experimentally and clinically, e.g. phantom limb pain after amputation in humans (Bach et al., 1988).

STRATEGIES FOR CONTROLLING PAIN

At this point it is important to make a distinction between the prevention of sensitization of the CNS and the alleviation of postoperative pain. Pre-emptive analgesia may block the development of sensitization, but it cannot eliminate postoperative pain; additional measures are still required to ensure a comfortable recovery. The aim of pre-emptive analgesia is solely to reduce the severity and duration of postoperative pain and to minimize the chances of a persistent pain state becoming established.

Effective analgesia depends on giving the correct combination of drugs in effective doses by the most appropriate route, i.e. balanced analgesia. Since individuals vary in their response to surgery, the adequacy of pain alleviation can only be determined by continual assessment of the animals and adjustment of the treatment protocol as necessary. Effective pain control is not achieved by waiting until the animal shows overt signs of pain before giving another dose of analgesic. The aim must always be to provide a completely pain-free postoperative period, and this is best achieved by having a planned protocol of drug(s) administration beginning preoperatively and continuing intra- and postoperatively, using a rational combination of two or three of the main types of analgesic drugs.

The optimum form of pain therapy should be continuous pre-emptive analgesia, continuously preventing the establishment of sensitization. The administration of opioids or local anaesthetic drugs blocks central sensitization while non-steroidal anti-inflammatory drugs (NSAIDs) reduce the severity of the peripheral inflammatory response.

Clinically, the aim should be to provide balanced analgesia using a combination of an opioid and an NSAID. Their combined use is more effective than using either drug alone.

ANALGESIC AGENTS

Local anaesthetic agents

Local anaesthetics can produce complete pain relief by blocking all sensory input from the affected area. It is a reasonable view that the risk of CNS sensitization after surgery is such that some form of regional anaes-thesia should always form part of any anaesthetic regimen, but in practice the site of injury/surgery will determine the feasibility of using regional anaesthesia to control pain. While certain sites lend themselves to the use of local blocks (intercostal blocks after thoractomy, mandibular nerve block after mandibulectomy), other sites can be more difficult to desensitize. Local anaesthetics may also be employed topically, e.g. on the mucosa following nasal or rectal surgery; EMLA (Eutectic Mixture of Local Anaesthet-ics) cream is most effective in reducing the pain associated with venepuncture in restless cats. Brachial plexus blocks are technically difficult to master, but provide excellent pain prevention for major surgery of the forelimb and should be mandatory before forelimb amputation to minimize the risk of possible phantom limb pain. Similarly, extradural (epidural) analgesia is highly recommended as an adjunct to hindlimb sur-gery and is essential if amputation is contemplated. Local anaesthetics produce analgesia when given in small doses intravenously, but are potent proconvulsants and can induce marked myocardial depression and cardiac dysrhythmias when administered by this route.

The local anaesthetic drug chosen for postopera-tive pain relief should ideally have a long duration of action and, therefore, bupivacaine (onset 15 minutes, duration of action 4–6 hours) or ropivacaine are the drugs of choice, although they are not licensed for veterinary use. Lignocaine, which is licensed, may be used during surgery for a more immediate effect.

Safe maximum doses are: 4 mg/kg lignocaine or 1–2 mg/kg bupivacaine. These doses should be diluted to the volume required to facilitate the application of the block.

Opioids

All opioids are chemically related and in the UK most are controlled drugs under the Misuse of Drugs Act, 1971, which governs their purchase, storage and use. Opioids are similarly controlled in the USA by the Controlled Substances Act, 1970. Most countries have comparable legislation for regulating the use of opioids.

All opioids have a similar mode of action, although their activity at the various opioid receptors varies. Currently, four opioid receptors have been cloned: OP1(δ), OP2(κ) OP3 (μ) and the orphan opioid receptor (ORL1). The latter seems to be linked to the endo-genous peptide nociceptin, which seems to have anta-gonist properties. Most opioids used clinically are selective for the μ receptor and mimic the effects of endogenous opioids in the CNS and possibly peripher-ally in inflamed tissue. There are two types of opioid drug used clinically: full agonists and partial agonists. Full μ-agonists, such as morphine, have a predictable profile of activity, a high ceiling of effect and provide the most reliable degree of pain relief postoperatively. Although partial μ-agonists (or κ-agonists) can be very effective, they are less reliable against a wide range of types of pain, have a poor dose/response relationship and, should they fail to be effective, increasing the dose is not likely to increase the degree of analgesia; chang-ing to another opioid can then prove difficult.

The major effects of opioids are:

- Analgesia
- Sedation in low doses
- Euphoria/excitement in high doses (especially in cats)
- Respiratory depression. This is potentially one of the most serious side effects in humans, but it is rarely a clinical problem in dogs and cats unless the drugs are combined with other potent respiratory depressants during general anaesthesia. Opioids should be used with caution in animals with respiratory disease, but since thoracic pain can cause impairment of adequate respiratory excursions, their use can be beneficial
- Cough suppression
- Nausea, vomiting and defecation
- Gut sphincter stimulation/constipation. The use of most opioids should be avoided in animals with biliary obstruction or pancreatitis because they cause an increase in tone in the sphincter of Oddi, with the exception of pethidine, which has a spasmolytic action on this sphincter
- Oculomotor nucleus stimulation. High doses tend to cause pupillary dilation in cats, which can make the assessment of neurological status difficult.

Drug absorption is more reliable and, therefore, drug efficacy is better if opioids are administered intramuscularly; however, some animals violently re-sent intramuscular injections, and extensive clinical

Drug	Dogs	Cats
Pethidine	Dose: 3.5–10 mg/kg i.m. or 10–15 mg/kg s.c. L CD Duration: 2.5–3.5 hours	5–10 mg/kg i.m. or 10–15 mg/kg s.c. L CD Duration: 2 hours
Morphine*	Dose: 0.1–0.5 mg/kg i.v., i.m. or s.c. NL CD Duration: 4–6 hours	Dose: 0.1–0.2 mg/kg i.m. or s.c. NL CD Duration: 6–8 hours
Fentanyl	Dose: 0.002–0.005 mg/kg i.v. or i.m. NL Duration: 20–30 minutes	
Methadone	Dose: 0.1–0.25 mg/kg i.v., i.m. or s.c. NL CD Duration: 4–6 hours	
Oxymorphone	Dose: 0.05–0.2 mg/kg i.v., i.m. or s.c. L (USA); CD Duration: 2–4 hours	Dose: 0.05–0.4 mg/kg i.v., i.m. or s.c. L (USA); CD Duration: 2–4 hours
Buprenorphine	Dose: 0.010–0.020 mg/kg i.m. or s.c. L CD Duration: 6–8 hours	Dose: 0.005–0.020 mg/kg i.m. or s.c. NL CD
Butorphanol	Dose: 0.2–0.5 mg/kg i.v., i.m. or s.c. L Duration: 1–2 hours	Dose: 0.2–0.8 mg/kg i.m. or s.c. L2 Duration: 2–4 hours
Pentazocine	Dose: 2–3 mg/kg i.m. NL Duration: 1.5–2 hours	Dose: 2–3 mg/kg i.m. NL Duration: 2–3 hours
Naloxone (antagonist)	Duration: 0.04–1.0 mg/kg i.v., i.m. or s.c. NL	Duration: 0.04–1.0 mg/kg i.v., i.m. or s.c.

Figure 6.1: *Doses and routes of administration of opioid analgesics used in the dog and cat.*

L=licensed; CD=controlled drug; NL=not licensed in the UK. * = Approved for veterinary use in the USA.

experience confirms that the subcutaneous route can be successfully employed in these situations, as long as a higher dose is used.

Doses and routes of administration are shown in Figure 6.1.

Morphine

Morphine is still the analgesic of choice for the most severe pain in dogs and cats and is the benchmark by which other drugs are assessed. It is a pure -agonist and is a potent analgesic and a good sedative, but is not licensed for use in animals in the UK. However, it can cause nausea and vomiting, especially when used preoperatively. Following administration, the onset of action is not rapid, but its duration of action is longer than its plasma half-life would suggest. Morphine is metabolized by conjugation, so its half-life is longer in the cat than in the dog (3 hours versus 60 minutes). Much of the notorious reputation of morphine in cats resulted from its use in gross overdosage, based entirely on the work of Joel and Arndts (1925), who used a dose of 20 mg/kg. It is certainly a safe drug to use in this species.

Papaveretum ('Omnopon')

Papaveretum is a preparation containing all the alkaloids of opium, with 50% morphine content. The presence of the other alkaloids seems to reduce the incidence of nausea and vomiting and improve sedation. Doses are roughly double those for morphine.

Pethidine (Meperidine)

Pethidine is a synthetic compound with approximately 1/10 the potency of morphine. It is a μ-selective agonist, but unlike morphine it is devoid of adverse gastrointestinal effects. The clinical value of pethidine lies in its relative lack of unpleasant side effects and its excellent sedative and spasmolytic properties. Its fast onset of action and its predictability make it a very useful analgesic. It has a relatively short duration of action, although postoperatively this may not be such a drawback. There is no nausea or vomiting and its atropine-like structure gives it spasmolytic properties, which makes it very useful for visceral pain. However, it does induce histamine release if given intravenously, which leads to profound hypotension.

Following anaesthesia and surgery in old dogs, or those with liver disease, its duration of action is prolonged, but it is still very safe. Cats are able to metabolize pethidine normally by demethylation and it has a similar elimination half-life in dogs and cats (30–60 minutes).

Fentanyl

Fentanyl is a pure μ-agonist, 1000 times more potent than morphine. It is not licensed in animals, except in combination with fluanisone. It causes marked bradycardia and respiratory depression in high doses. It has a rapid onset of effect (1–2 minutes) and short duration of action (20–30 minutes). Its main value is as an intraoperative analgesic to control acute intense pain and as a 'rescue analgesic' postoperatively if pain is proving difficult to control.

Methadone

Methadone is a synthetic μ-agonist, equipotent with morphine, but not licensed for use in animals. It produces less sedation than morphine, but has a long duration of action in dogs.

Oxymorphone

Oxymorphone is a semi-synthetic μ-agonist with approximately 10 times the potency of morphine. It is not available in the UK or Europe, but is widely used in the USA. It is said to cause less nausea and vomiting than morphine, but a greater degree of auditory hypersensitivity and bradycardia with a predilection to cause tachypnoea, as it disrupts thermoregulation. Its duration of action is quoted as 2–4 hours.

Buprenorphine

Buprenorphine is an extremely potent analgesic with 30–100 times the potency of morphine, and it is highly lipophilic. It is a partial μ-agonist but also has antagonistic actions. Thus, while low doses are analgesic, higher doses may be less effective. It has a slow onset of action and is not equally effective against different types of pain. These pharmacological properties have clinical implications. First, the dose must be chosen carefully and, second, the slow onset of action means that the drug must be administered up to 45 minutes before the analgesic effect is required. If animals are allowed to recover in pain before the drug is active then it is unlikely to be successful. Because buprenorphine binds avidly to the receptor, it is very difficult to displace, so if the drug is not effective, alternative opioid analgesic agents cannot be used to top up analgesia, nor can conventional antagonists reverse its actions. If severe respiratory depression occurs, doxapram must be given.

Butorphanol

In addition to being a partial μ-agonist, butorphanol is also a κ-agonist. Like buprenorphine, its effect reaches a plateau (or ceiling) as the dose increases. This is certainly the case in the cat, where the optimal dose for visceral analgesia seems to be 0.2 mg/kg. Its efficacy against somatic pain is very poor at doses from 0.2 to 0.8 mg/kg. It has a very short elimination half-life and clinically appears to give only brief (30–40 minutes) analgesia postoperatively, with a relatively high number of 'failures'. Its effectiveness as a sedative and antitussive seem to be better than its analgesic potency (Waterman and Kalthum, 1992).

Pentazocine

Pentazocine is a benzomorphan derivative. It is a partial μ-agonist, and κ-agonist with a potency 1/4 that of morphine. It has a flat dose–response curve and a tendency to produce dysphoria. Analgesia is reasonable postoperatively, with a duration of around 1–2 hours although sedation lasts considerably longer (Waterman and Kalthum, 1992). It has a short elimination half-life in the dog, lasting slightly longer in the cat.

NSAIDs

Most NSAIDs are potent inhibitors of prostaglandin production, so that gastrointestinal, hepatic and renal toxic side effects are seen with high or prolonged dosing. Relative or absolute hypovolaemia (such as often occurs under anaesthesia or perioperatively) and renal disease cause renal prostaglandins to become active in maintaining normal renal haemodynamics. The use of any NSAID that affects the production of prostaglandins is inadvisable in these circumstances. This potential problem precludes their pre-emptive use (with the exception of carprofen, which has a prostaglandin sparing effect). The older drugs in this group are not effective for severe pain, but the newer agents e.g. flunixin, ketoprofen and carprofen, can provide excellent relief of acute postoperative pain (Lascelles et al., 1994a). Doses for use in the cat and dog are shown in Figures 6.2 and 6.3 respectively.

Acetylsalicylic acid (aspirin)

Acetylsalicylic acid is the oldest NSAID, but it is very toxic and can cause gastric irritation, aplastic anaemia and hepatoxicity. In cats, its half-life is so long (40 hours) that cumulation can occur. There are safer compounds available for analgesia.

Phenylbutazone

Phenylbutazone is also cumulative, especially in cats (elimination half-life 18 hours), and there is a high incidence of gastrointestinal and renal toxic side effects with its use.

Flunixin meglumine

Flunixin is an extremely potent analgesic, but can cause severe gastrointestinal and renal damage, especially in animals with pre-existing hypovolaemia. It is equipotent to morphine in providing postoperative pain relief in dogs (Reid and Nolan, 1991), but it is not safe to use preoperatively. It has a shorter half-life in the cat than the dog, but nevertheless should still be used with extreme caution.

Ketoprofen

Ketoprofen is a powerful inhibitor of both cyclo-oxygenase and lipo-oxygenase enzymes and also inhibits bradykinin. It is, therefore, a very effective anti-inflammatory agent and a good analgesic. It provides effective, long duration postoperative analgesia in cats and dogs, but may only be safely used postoperatively because of its cyclo-oxygenase inhibitory properties. A recent study in cats (Slingsby and Waterman-Pearson, 1998) has shown that it provides postoperative analgesia equal in efficacy and of longer duration than pethidine or buprenorphine.

Meloxicam

Meloxicam is marketed mainly for treating chronic skeletal pain in dogs. It is not licensed for use in cats although it provides good postoperative analgesia for around 18–24 hours (Slingsby and Waterman-Pearson, unpublished data). It has also proved clinically effective in the amelioration of the pain associated with severe stomatitis in cats. Its safety margin, however, is unclear in the cat and gastrointestinal side effects are most likely, which may make the therapeutic margin rather narrow. It may also be useful for long-term postoperative analgesia if the dog or cat is eating.

Carprofen

Carprofen differs from other NSAIDs because, despite being a good anti-inflammatory and potent analgesic agent, it has relatively very little effect on prostaglandin production. It seems to be tolerated extremely well in dogs and cats, with few side effects. The main indication for carprofen is as an analgesic, and because it can safely be given preoperatively, its efficacy in the immediate postoperative period is maximized. Its safety and efficacy, which are comparable to pethidine and

Drug	Suggested dose (mg/kg)	Length of treatment	Particular indications
Licensed			
Tolfenamic acid	4.0 s.c. q24h 4.0 orally q24h	Maximum of 2 injections Maximum of 3 days	Analgesia (unlicensed) and adjunct to treatment of upper respiratory tract infections Febrile conditions Not for cats with gastrointestinal, renal or cardiac disease or hypovolaemia
Ketoprofen	2.0 s.c. q24h 1.0 orally q24h	Maximum of 3 days Maximum of 5 days	Analgesia and anti-inflammatory Not for preoperative use Not for cats with gastrointestinal, renal or cardiac disease or hypovolaemia
Carprofen	2.0–4.0 i.v., s.c. q18–24h 4.0 orally q24h	Single dose Tablets for long-term treatment of chronic pain or inflammation (unlicenced use in cats)	As a perioperative analgesic Safe to use preoperatively
Unlicensed			
Meloxicam	0.3 orally on day 1, followed by 0.1 orally q24h	Maximum 4 days Probably well tolerated long-term	Postoperative analgesia Not for preoperative use
Flunixin meglumine	1.0 s.c., i.v. or orally	Single dose	Postoperative analgesia Not for preoperative use Not for cats with gastrointestinal, renal or cardiac disease or hypovolaemia
Acetylsalicylic acid (aspirin)	10 orally q48–72h		Anti-inflammatory Analgesic Prophylactic anti-thromboembolic agent in cats with cardiac disease

Figure 6.2: Non-steroidal anti-inflammatory drugs for use in the cat.

Drugs	Suggested dose (mg/kg)	Length of treatment	Particular indications
Licensed			
Tolfenamic acid	4.0 s.c. q24h 4.0 orally q24h	Maximum of 2 injections Maximum of 3 days	Analgesia, not for preoperative use Anti-inflammatory Gastrointestinal side effects as for all NSAIDs
Ketoprofen	2.0 s.c., i.m. or i.v. q24h 1.0 orally q24h	Maximum of 3 days Maximum of 5 days	Analgesia, not for preoperative use Anti-inflammatory Contraindicated with gastrointestinal, renal or cardiac disease or hypovolaemia (absolute or relative)
Carprofen	4.0 i.v., s.c. q18–24h 4.0 orally q24h	Single dose Tablets for long-term treatment of chronic pain or inflammation	As a perioperative analgesic Safe to use preoperatively
Meloxicam	0.2 s.c. 0.2 orally on day 1, followed by 0.1 orally q24h	Maximum 1 injection Well tolerated long term	Postoperative analgesia For the relief of chronic pain, e.g. osteoarthrosis on a ?long-term basis
Flunixin meglumine	1.0 s.c., slow i.v. or orally	Maximum 1 injection Maximum 3 days orally	Postoperative analgesia Do not use preoperatively or in dogs with gastrointestinal, renal or cardiac disease or hypovolaemia (absolute or relative) Do not use in dogs under 6 weeks of age or elderly animals
Dipyrone (in Buscopan Compositum)	1.0–2.5 ml i.v. or i.m.		Analgesia Spasmolytic (for visceral pain especially)
Unlicensed			
Acetylsalicylic acid (aspirin)	10–25 orally q24–48h		Anti-inflammatory Analgesic

Figure 6.3: *Non-steroidal anti-inflammatory drugs (NSAIDs) for use in the dog.*

morphine (but with a longer duration of action), make it the most versatile drug to use as the basis for a planned analgesic protocol for dogs and cats. Recent work in the dog (Slingsby and Waterman-Pearson, unpublished data) has shown that it use in combination with pethidine produces enhanced analgesia compared with when either drug is used alone.

It may be used orally to provide fairly long-term postoperative pain relief, although cats sometimes find the tablets unpalatable.

Tolfenamic acid

Tolfenamic acid is chemically related to mefenamic acid. It has both analgesic and anti-inflammatory properties. It is not recommended for use in very young or very old animals or in those with any degree of dehy-

dration or liver, gastrointestinal or renal disease. It seems to offer no advantage over other NSAIDs, and in many respects it seems to be less safe. It is licensed for use in dogs for the treatment of postoperative pain and in cats for the treatment of febrile conditions and upper respiratory disease. In a clinical trial of postoperative analgesic efficacy in the cat, its duration of action was shorter than ketoprofen or carprofen (Slingsby and Waterman-Pearson, unpublished data).

Etodolac

Etodolac is an indole acetic acid derivative that is approved in the USA for use in the dog as an analgesic, anti-inflammatory and antipyrexic. It is said to inhibit cyclooxygenase-2 and therefore produce minimal adverse effects on the gastrointestinal and renal systems.

However, occasionally it produces vomiting and regurgitation. It is used to manage the pain of osteoarthritis in the dog at a dose of 10–15 mg/kg orally and is given once a day. Until it has been fully evaluated, the use of etodolac should be accompanied by the restrictions and cautions that apply to the other NSAIDs.

Miscellaneous drugs

Alpha$_2$-adrenoceptor agonists
Alpha$_2$-adrenoceptor agonists (e.g. medetomidine, xylazine) are analgesic, but they are not often used solely for their analgesic action. If atipamezole is used to reverse their effects, the analgesic effect is also reversed and, thus, pain relief is lost in the postoperative period. These drugs are dangerous if there is any degree of cardiovascular compromise. Very low doses (0.1–0.2 mg/kg xylazine, 2 µg/kg medetomidine) may be worth considering to control visceral pain or opioid-unresponsive pain in dogs with spinal cord damage.

Ketamine
Ketamine, an NMDA antagonist, can play a part in reducing postoperative pain. Since it acts on the NMDA receptor it may both prevent and reverse the development of CNS sensitization. It is a good analgesic against ischaemic and somatic pain, although it has a relatively short duration of action. High doses provide longer analgesia, but will induce dissociative anaesthesia. A dose of 1–2 mg/kg i.m. provides good analgesia in cats, and should certainly be considered for the initial management of a difficult trauma case.

Benzodiazepines
The involvement of benzodiazepines in the modulation of pain mechanisms remains controversial. Benzodiazepines (diazepam or midazolam) enhance the inhibitory actions of GABA by modulating GABAergic neurotransmission through the GABA$_A$/benzodiazepine receptor complex. Extradural and intrathecally administered midazolam produces postoperative analgesia after thoracic and limb surgery in humans, but is less effective in alleviating visceral pain. Clinically, combinations of midazolam or diazepam with opiates are reported to enhance opiate-mediated analgesia in humans.

Volatile and gaseous agents

Methoxyflurane: This is an excellent analgesic at subanaesthetic doses, which in the past made it an ideal choice for orthopaedic surgery, where its slow elimination kinetics provided many hours of postoperative analgesia. It is no longer available in the UK.

Nitrous oxide: This has good analgesic properties, but these only persist for as long as it is administered. Its use, however, certainly helps reduce intraoperative nociception.

Sevoflurane: This new volatile agent has also been shown to have some analgesic properties when used in combination with intrathecal fentanyl.

ROUTES OF DRUG ADMINISTRATION

Most analgesics are given by the intramuscular, intravenous or subcutaneous routes to control acute postoperative pain, or orally for more chronic pain. However, alternative routes can sometimes offer advantages.

Extradural approach
Extradural analgesic drug administration is only logical if the effects of the drug are more localized and more intense than when it is given systemically. The advantage to using local anaesthetics by this route is indisputable; whether there are such obvious benefits from using other analgesics in this way is less clear.

Drugs given by this route act directly on the spinal cord by diffusing through the dura mater to neuronal tissue, and also via the dural cuffs. Systemic absorption may also occur, especially if drugs are highly lipophilic.

Local anaesthetics
Local anaesthetics are routinely given extradurally and offer maximal block of sensory input. This technique is recommended for all major surgery of the hindlimb, perineal surgery and some abdominal surgery. Lignocaine (1–2%) or bupivacaine (0.25%) should be used at a rate of about 0.1–2 ml/kg or 0.5 ml/10 cm crown–rump length administered via the lumbosacral space.

Opioids
Opioids may be administered extradurally to provide analgesia in both dogs and cats. The advantage of their use by this route is that analgesia is prolonged without motor impairment. Morphine has proved to be the most useful drug, but pethidine is also effective. Highly lipophilic drugs such as fentanyl are far less effective. Morphine is given at half the dose recommended for systemic use, and made up to a total volume of 0.125 ml/kg for pelvic surgery, or 0.25 ml/kg for surgery of the abdomen. Onset of action is 20–60 minutes and given thus, it provides 16–24 hours' analgesia. Side effects include pruritus, some respiratory depression and urinary retention. These side effects seem to be reversible with systemic administration of naloxone, which does not seem to significantly reverse the analgesia produced.

Combinations of morphine and lidocaine can be used for surgery, offering the advantage of an immediate sensory block with prolonged analgesia without long-term motor impairment.

Alpha$_2$-agonists
Alpha$_2$-agonists have been used extradurally in large animals to provide long-term analgesia, but their cardio-

vascular side effects are such that their routine use extra-durally cannot yet be recommended in cats or dogs. They may, however, have some potential in combination with opioids or local anaesthetics when much lower doses can be employed, thus reducing their dangerous side effects.

Ketamine and NSAIDs
Ketamine and NSAIDs have also been shown to be analgesic when given extradurally, but there are also reports of neurotoxicity when they are given by this route (Pascoe, 1997).

Transdermal approach
The transdermal approach provides a simple method of continuous parenteral drug administration. To overcome the skin barrier to transdermal transport, drugs need to be of small molecular weight, lipophilic, uncharged and potent. Clinically, in animals, only fentanyl has been used in this way. Absorption is slow and the fentanyl patches have to be applied 12–24 hours before surgery to provide background postoperative pain relief. There are practical problems with maintaining patches in place in dogs, and there is tremendous variation in the plasma concentrations of fentanyl that are achieved. While this technique may offer a background level of analgesia, rapid and reliable changes to the delivery rate are not possible and so it is not versatile enough to control acute peaks of postoperative pain, and additional parenteral doses of other drugs are needed, making the logic of their use questionable.

The use of fentanyl patches to control chronic pain may theoretically offer some advantages to repeated injections or the prolonged use of NSAIDs. Side effects include reduced appetite, respiratory depression and bradycardia. Increases in body temperature can markedly enhance absorption, making overdosage possible. There is, in addition, the risk of both deliberate and inadvertent human misuse of these patches, with potentially lethal results. It is difficult to envisage the widespread use of this technique in veterinary practice in the UK.

Iontophoresis is an enhanced mode of transdermal drug administration using an electrical current to ionize drugs. The advantage of this over simple occlusive patches is obvious; there will be rapid achievement of a steady state and an ability to vary the rate of drug administration, allowing far greater flexibility in the control of acute pain.

Intranasal approach
Intranasal administration of opioids, using a metered spray, may offer advantages in needle-shy animals or ones where venous access is not possible. Butorphanol, pethidine and fentanyl have all been used in this way in humans; absorption is very rapid and bioavailability is good. Metered doses of 10–25 µg/kg of fentanyl have proved to be safe in lambs (Waterman-Pearson and Thornton, unpublished data).

FACTORS AFFECTING THE SEVERITY OF POSTSURGICAL PAIN

Patient considerations
In general, young animals of all species have a more limited repertoire of behavioural signs with which to register their distress and so tend to exhibit similar overt signs whether they are in pain, hot, cold or hungry. Older animals, however, seem to tolerate postoperative discomfort more stoically. Recent evidence from lambs suggests that neonates have a lower pain threshold than older animals (Thornton and Waterman-Pearson, unpublished data). Very young kittens and puppies have immature kidney and liver function, making the metabolism and excretion of drugs limited compared with adults. They also become hypothermic very easily, which further decreases the rate of elimination of drugs. Drugs that are generally rapidly metabolized, such as pethidine, should therefore be used, and the dosing intervals should be increased to prevent cumulation.

Elderly animals also need to be treated with care. They are likely to be thin and have reduced hepatic and renal reserves. These ageing changes will lead to a smaller volume of distribution for drugs and a slower rate of elimination. Again, drug doses and dosing intervals may need to be adjusted accordingly.

Certain breeds seem to be more susceptible to pain, or at least exhibit more overt signs. Notably the Greyhound family, some toy breeds and Staffordshire Bull Terriers often seem to suffer great distress after relatively minor surgery, whereas Labradors, for example, seem much more stoical.

Surgery
A major factor influencing the severity of pain is the nature of the surgical interference. The severity of tissue damage, amount of inflammation, degree of tension and/or movement of surrounding muscles, strength of contraction of smooth muscles or degree of distension of hollow organs all influence the severity of postoperative pain. In addition, if there is damage to, or pressure on, nerves (which may be iatrogenic in origin, e.g. too tight bandaging), or tissue ischaemia, postoperative discomfort will be increased. It is axiomatic, therefore, that there should be no unnecessary disruption of tissues. Exposed tissues should be kept vital and covered in warm saline-soaked swabs. Tourniquets can cause intense noxious stimulation and marked hyperalgesia within 20 minutes in conscious animals. If they are used under anaesthesia this should be borne in mind. Skin sutures that are too tight can also cause intense irritation.

SPECIFIC RECOMMENDATIONS

Trauma
Following trauma, dogs and cats may be difficult to handle, and provision of analgesia with a drug that has

some sedative properties can be beneficial. In order to allow frequent re-evaluation of the case, a short-acting drug such as pethidine or butorphanol should be chosen initially. Animals with head injuries need to be monitored very carefully, as any respiratory depression will lead to an increased $PaCO_2$, cerebral vasodilation and an increase in intracranial pressure. Fractious cats may be given low doses of ketamine in combination with midazolam (see Chapter 7).

Ophthalmic surgery

Ocular pain can be most distressing, and animals will attempt to rub and scratch their eyes if relief is not provided. The mediation of the pain associated with intraocular surgery is such that it is best controlled by a combination of topical local anaesthesia and an NSAID, although the sedative properties of pethidine can also be beneficial. Following ocular surgery, a rise in intraocular pressure can be disastrous, and therefore drugs that may cause retching or vomiting must be avoided; the administration of low doses of a sedative such as acepromazine postoperatively can also promote a quiet pain-free recovery (see Chapter 12).

Aural surgery

This can be very painful and if the animal starts to shake its head, a vicious circle of increasing pain provoking more head shaking can easily be set up. A potent opioid, given as part of the premedication and topped up postoperatively should provide good pain relief. In addition, a single dose of an NSAID such as carprofen should be given at the start of surgery and, if possible, topical anaesthesia with EMLA cream should also be provided at this stage.

Dental extractions

In the case of dental extractions, opioids are not very effective. In these cases postoperative analgesia should be provided by the use of an NSAID such as carprofen or ketoprofen. Mandibular and/or maxillary nerve blocks may also be used (see Chapter 13).

Orthopaedic surgery

Orthopaedic procedures, especially those involving joints, or long bone fractures with over-riding of the fracture and muscle spasm, are extremely painful. The source of the pain is difficult to localize, but muscle damage as much as periosteal disruption may be responsible for any distress. The analgesic protocol should include a potent opioid (morphine) given preoperatively, to provide cover during the surgery, which should then be topped up in the postoperative period for 12 hours or so. In addition, an NSAID should also be administered perioperatively to give longer-term pain relief (carprofen or ketoprofen).

Limb amputation is extremely painful, although there is no way of knowing whether animals, like humans, suffer from phantom limb pains. Animals should certainly be given the benefit of the doubt and analgesia provided before, during and after surgery, utilizing potent opioids, NSAIDS and a local block (extradural or brachial plexus block) if possible.

Spinal surgery leads to marked discomfort postoperatively, the source of the pain being largely the extensive muscle disruption caused, although haemorrhage around the spinal cord can also lead to an increase in pressure on the cord and spinal nerves, which is intensely painful. The severity of the pain with these types of surgery makes the use of potent μ-opioids, usually with an NSAID, mandatory. The addition of a benzodiazepine in low doses may also prove beneficial. Occasionally these patients suffer severe opioid-unresponsive pain postoperatively, especially when there is spinal cord ischaemia. This pain often responds to low doses of α_2-agonists or ketamine.

Thoracic surgery

Thoracic surgery is very painful in humans, but in dogs and cats there is less long-term discomfort once the indwelling chest drain is removed. However, the immediate postoperative period can be very distressing, especially in small dogs and cats. The pain emanates from disruption of the intercostal muscles and the pleural pain associated with the presence of the chest drain. Impairment of respiration, caused by reluctance to expand the thoracic cage, is not such a problem in dogs as it is in humans, although if there has been an extensive repair to the diaphragm, ventilation can be impaired. Postoperative pain control should always include some form of regional block with a long-acting local anaesthetic agent infiltrated intercostally and/or intrapleurally, as well as administration of a balanced combination of an opioid and an NSAID.

Abdominal (visceral) surgery

In small animals, intra-abdominal manipulations cause much less postoperative discomfort than in humans, probably due to the fact that quadrupeds do not have to move their abdominal muscles as much while walking or breathing. Cranial abdominal surgery is more painful because of the necessity to stretch the costal area during manipulations. Perianal and rectal surgery is, likewise, painful, and dogs will often strain incessantly or be reluctant to defecate postoperatively.

For most types of visceral surgery, pethidine rather than morphine is preferred since it does not provoke vomiting, spasm of sphincters or urinary retention, and its spasmolytic effect can be beneficial. Partial μ-/full κ-agonists such as butorphanol can also be effective. Both these drugs will require repeated administration postoperatively.

Other causes of postoperative pain

A distended bladder or a leg swollen by the extravasation of intravenous fluids can cause marked discomfort and postoperative restlessness.

Muscle spasms may provoke marked pain after surgery, and some thought should be given to adding a drug with muscle relaxant properties into the analgesic treatment regimen for cases where this may be a problem. Benzodiazepines are particularly useful here, as their mild sedative properties can be beneficial and they also have some analgesic activity.

Wound care is also of great importance since infection increases inflammation causing increased pain. Good toilet includes proper care of all intravenous or urinary catheters and any invasive monitoring equipment.

Finally, the animal's mental state should not be neglected. Anxiety is a well recognized contributory factor to the severity of pain in humans and, although animals do not worry about the risk of dying under anaesthesia, or the long-term prognosis, there is no doubt that the experience of waking up in a strange place and separation from the owner can cause anxiety and distress.

NON-PHARMACOLOGICAL METHODS OF PAIN RELIEF

All too often the only considerations in the management of pain relief or prevention are pharmacological measures. There are, however, sound nursing measures that can also have a major impact on reducing the level of postoperative pain.

The redeeming feature of acute postoperative pain is that, by and large, its intensity declines quickly with time and, if the patient can sleep, the pain diminishes. The environment should therefore be quiet, and one might even consider giving a low dose of a sedative to encourage sleep if the patient is particularly agitated. Cats, in particular, appreciate a quiet environment postoperatively; a barking dog in the next cage is not conducive to a stress-free recovery!

Giving the animal some attention once every so often is of immeasurable benefit and helps decrease the distress associated with pain and the unfamiliar environment, otherwise a cycle of pain/distress/sleeplessness can develop.

Animals benefit from the provision of a comfortable bed in a warm, though not too hot, environment. They should be offered food and water, if appropriate, fairly early in the postoperative period. Pain and inflammation cause an increase in basal metabolic requirements, and a high level of nutrition will be required to promote healing. Offering food early in the postoperative period not only speeds recovery, but can also have a soothing effect on a restless animal.

DURATION OF ANALGESIC TREATMENT

The length of time that treatment should be continued postoperatively is variable, depending on the degree of trauma and the patient's ability to cope. Experience suggests that pain is profound for at least 2–3 days and so some form of analgesic treatment should be continued for at least 72 hours. Potent opioids may be discontinued after 24 hours, with NSAIDs becoming the mainstay of treatment.

Ideally, the drug chosen for longer-term pain relief should be safe, orally active and palatable and should have a short latency and a long duration of action so that it may be used tactically rather than on a continuous basis. Clearly, at present there is no ideal drug available, although the new NSAIDs are far safer than older agents and may be usefully employed as long as the animal is monitored carefully and re-evaluated frequently to minimize the risk of serious side effects occurring.

REFERENCES AND FURTHER READING

Bach S, Norveng MF and Tjjellden NU (1988) Phantom limb pain in amputees during the first twelve months following amputation after preoperative lumbar epidural blockade. *Pain* **33**, 297–230
Coderre TJ, Vaccarino AL and Melzack R (1990) Central nervous system plasticity in the tonic pain response to subcutaneous formalin injection. *Brain Research* **535**, 155–158
Joel E and Arndts F (1925) Beitrage zur Pharmakologie der Korperstellung der Labyrinth. XIX Mitteilungen. *Morphin. Arch. Gesellschaft (Physiology)* **210**, 280
Lascelles BDX, Butterworth SJ and Waterman AE (1994) Postoperative analgesic and sedative effects of carprofen and pethidine in dogs. *Veterinary Record* **134**, 187–191
Lascelles BDX, Cripps PJ, Mirchandani S and Waterman AE (1995) Carprofen as an analgesic for post-operative pain in cats: dose titration and assessment of efficacy in comparison to pethidine hydrochloride. *Journal of Small Animal Practice* **36**, 535–541
Lascelles BDX, Cripps PJ, Jones A and Waterman A (1997) Postoperative central hypersensitivity and pain: the pre-emptive value of pethidine for ovariohysterectomy. *Pain* **73**, 461–471
Lascelles BDX and Waterman AE (1997) Analgesia in cats. *In Practice* **19**, 203–213
Lascelles BDX, Waterman AE, Cripps PJ, Livingston A and Henderson G (1995) Central sensitization as a result of surgical pain – investigation of the pre-emptive value of pethidine for ovariohysterectomy in the rat. *Pain* **62**, 201–212
Pascoe PJ (1997) Drugs in the epidural space. *Proceedings of the 6th International Congress of Veterinary Anaesthesia.* pp. 53–62
Reid J and Nolan AM (1991) A comparison of the post-operative analgesic and sedative effects of flunixin and papaveretum in the dog. *Journal of Small Animal Practice* **32**, 603–608
Slingsby LS and Waterman-Pearson AE (1998) A comparison of pethidine, buprenorphine and ketoprofen for postoperative analgesia after ovariohysterectomy in the cat. *Veterinary Record* **143**, 185–189
Wall PD and Melzack R (1994) *Textbook of Pain.* Churchill Livingstone, Edinburgh
Wall PD and Woolf CJ (1984) *Journal of Physiology* **356**, 443–458
Waterman AE (1988) Analgesia in the dog and cat. *Advances in Small Animal Practice* **1**, 159–181
Waterman, AE and Kalthum W (1992) The use of opioids in providing postoperative analgesia in the dog: a double blind trial of pethidine, pentazocine, buprenorphine and butorphanol. In: *Animal Pain and its Control (Proceedings of a Symposium, Cornell University July 1990)*, ed. CE Short, pp 466–479. Churchill Livingstone Inc., New York
Woolf CJ (1983) Evidence for a central component of post injury pain hypersensitivity. *Nature (London)* **306**, 686–688
Woolf CJ and Chong M-S (1993) Pre-emptive analgesia treating postoperative pain by preventing the establishment of central sensitisation. *Anesthesia and Analgesia* **77**, 326–343
Woolf CJ and Wall PD (1986) Relative effectiveness of C primary afferent fibres of different origins in evoking a prolonged facilitation of the flexor reflex in the rat. *Journal of Neuroscience* **6**, 1433–1442

CHAPTER SEVEN

Premedication and Sedation

Victoria M. Lukasik

INTRODUCTION

Preanaesthetic drugs are an important component of a complete anaesthetic protocol. They help relieve anxiety and decrease stress before induction of anaesthesia. They also increase patient and staff safety during restraint and facilitate manipulations such as placing intravenous catheters. Preanaesthetic drugs contribute to a smooth induction and recovery from anaesthesia. Specifically, premedication protocols should be designed to:

- Reduce anxiety and calm patients
- Produce mild to moderate sedation
- Provide analgesia before surgery
- Increase muscle relaxation
- Decrease saliva and airway secretions
- Reduce unwanted side effects of subsequent anaesthetic drugs
- Suppress vomiting and regurgitation
- Decrease the amount of drug needed to produce unconsciousness
- Contribute to analgesia postoperatively.

Surgical procedure, anaesthetic duration, anticipated complications, postoperative needs and patient age, size, temperament and physical condition should all be considered when choosing drugs for premedication. Preanaesthetic protocols usually include combinations of anticholinergics, sedatives or tranquillizers, and opioid analgesics.

ANTICHOLINERGICS

Anticholinergics are parasympathetic antagonist drugs that are often included in premedication protocols to decrease salivation and prevent bradycardia. These drugs also cause bronchodilation and a decrease in gastrointestinal secretions and gastrointestinal motor function. The administration of an anticholinergic decreases the undesirable autonomic effects of drugs used to reverse neuromuscular blockade (e.g. neostigmine, edrophonium, physostigmine). Routine use of anticholinergics has decreased over the past few years, but their use is still recommended in combination with drugs anticipated to cause bradycardia or increase salivation.

Anticholinergics are contraindicated in patients with pre-existing tachycardia. This includes patients with sinus tachycardia as well as patients with other tachyarrhythmias.

Atropine sulphate

Effective doses of atropine sulphate in dogs and cats range from 0.02 to 0.04 mg/kg s.c. or i.m. and from 0.01 to 0.02 mg/kg i.v. When given intravenously, atropine may initially cause an increase in vagal tone leading to bradycardia, which is followed by cholinergic blockade and tachycardia. Atropine will cross the blood–brain barrier and the placenta. Atropine overdose leads to stimulation of the central nervous system (CNS) and can precipitate seizures. Although controversial, severe cases of atropine overdose can be treated with physostigmine 0.02 mg/kg i.v., given slowly to effect. Administration of physostigmine should probably be reserved for cases in which patients undergo seizures, experience extreme agitation or are at risk of injuring themselves or others.

Atropine relaxes the iris sphincter muscle, causing the pupil to dilate. This effect is especially prominent in cats. For this reason, atropine is contraindicated in patients with narrow angle glaucoma and synechia. Atropine has been shown to decrease tear formation in dogs. It may be beneficial to protect the patient's eyes with sterile lubricant when atropine is included in preanaesthetic protocols.

Other uses of atropine include:

- Treatment of sinus bradycardia, sinoatrial arrest and incomplete atrioventricular block
- Antidote for overdose of cholinergic drugs like physostigmine
- Antidote for organophosphate poisoning
- Antidote for muscarinic mushroom poisoning
- Treatment of hypersialism
- Treatment of bronchoconstrictive disease.

Atropine is reportedly *compatible* when mixed in syringes and intravenous tubing with:

- Butorphanol
- Buprenorphine
- Diphenhydramine
- Droperidol
- Fentanyl
- Glycopyrrolate
- Pethidine (meperidine)
- Morphine
- Oxymorphone
- Pentazocine.

Atropine is reportedly *incompatible* when mixed in syringes and intravenous tubing with:

- Noradrenaline
- Methohexitone
- Sodium bicarbonate.

Antihistamines, benzodiazepines, pethidine, phenothiazines, procainamide and quinidine may all enhance the activity of atropine. Long-term corticosteroid use can potentiate the adverse effects of atropine, and intraocular pressure may increase. Atropine may enhance the effects of sympathomimetics and may antagonize the effects of metoclopramide.

Glycopyrrolate
Effective doses of glycopyrrolate in dogs and cats range from 0.01 to 0.02 mg/kg s.c. or i.m. and from 0.005 to 0.01 mg/kg i.v. Vagal inhibition lasts 2 to 3 hours, and secretions may be decreased for as long as 7 hours. Glycopyrrolate is a large polar quaternary ammonium molecule that does not readily diffuse across lipid membranes such as the blood–brain barrier and placenta. Because of its quaternary structure, minimal effects on the CNS and fetus would be expected after overdose with glycopyrrolate.

At clinically useful doses, glycopyrrolate is slightly less arrhythmogenic than atropine. The manufacturer of the veterinary product in the USA lists only mydriasis, tachycardia and xerostomia as adverse effects in dogs and cats when glycopyrrolate is used at recommended doses.

Other uses of glycopyrrolate include:

- Treatment of bradyarrhythmias
- Treatment of hypersialism
- As a bronchodilator.

Glycopyrrolate is reportedly *compatible* when mixed in syringes and intravenous tubing with:

- Buprenorphine
- Diphenhydramine
- Droperidol
- Droperidol and fentanyl
- Fentanyl
- Lignocaine (lidocaine)

- Pethidine
- Morphine
- Neostigmine
- Oxymorphone.

Glycopyrrolate is reportedly *incompatible* when mixed in syringes and intravenous tubing with:

- Dexamethasone
- Diazepam
- Methohexitone
- Methylprednisolone
- Pentazocine
- Pentobarbitone
- Sodium bicarbonate
- Thiopentone.

Antihistamines, benzodiazepines, pethidine, phenothiazines, procainamide and quinidine may enhance the effects of glycopyrrolate. Long-term corticosteroid use can potentiate the adverse effects of glycopyrrolate, and intraocular pressure may increase. Glycopyrrolate may enhance the effects of sympathomimetics and may antagonize the effects of metoclopramide.

TRANQUILLIZERS

Tranquillizers and sedatives are used to calm patients and to improve the quality of anaesthesia induction and recovery. They also decrease the amount of induction drug needed to produce unconsciousness. It is important to allow sufficient time for tranquillizers to take full effect before anaesthesia induction otherwise a relative overdose of induction and maintenance drugs may occur. It is best to leave patients in a quiet area for 15 to 30 minutes while tranquillizers are taking effect. Tranquillizers and sedatives commonly used in premedication protocols are the phenothiazines, benzodiazepines and butyrophenones.

Phenothiazines
Acepromazine is the most commonly used phenothiazine in veterinary medicine. Other phenothiazines used on rare occasions include chlorpromazine, promazine, promethazine, trimeprazine and methotrimeprazine.

Acepromazine maleate
Although not consistent with manufacturers' recommendations, effective doses of acepromazine in dogs and cats range from 0.02 to 0.075 mg/kg s.c. or i.m. to a maximum dose of 3 mg, regardless of patient size. Large and giant breed dogs are easily overdosed with acepromazine, and the lower end of the dose range should be used in these patients. The onset of action can be relatively slow, requiring 30 to 60 minutes before peak effects are seen. It is important to allow sufficient time for acepromazine to take full effect before giving anaesthetic induction drugs.

Desirable effects of acepromazine include tranquillization, sedation and decreased adrenaline-induced ventricular arrhythmias. Acepromazine also has antiemetic, antispasmodic and weak antihistaminic properties. Some researchers have reported that acepromazine has anticonvulsant properties. However, conventional thinking in veterinary medicine holds that acepromazine may lower the seizure threshold in epileptic patients and precipitate seizures.

Increasing the dose of acepromazine may not lead to increased sedation, but the incidence of unwanted side-effects increases. If desired levels of sedation do not occur after acepromazine administration, it is better to add another type of tranquilliser in combination with acepromazine than to increase the dose. The tranquillizing effects of acepromazine may be overridden by catecholamines, and acepromazine cannot always be counted upon when used as a sole restraining drug.

Undesirable effects of acepromazine include:

- Alpha-adrenergic blockade – may cause adrenaline reversal
- Hypotension – can be profound
- Hypothermia
- Excessive vagal tone
- Bradycardia
- Potentiation of organophosphate toxicity
- A decrease in packed cell volume – occurs within 30 minutes, and may be as great as 50%
- Ventilatory depression.

If profound hypotension occurs after acepromazine administration, cardiovascular function should be supported by aggressive administration of intravenous fluid. Treatment with vasopressors or catecholamines may be indicated if cardiovascular compromise is severe. *Adrenaline is contraindicated in patients overdosed with acepromazine.* In the presence of α_1-adrenergic blockade, adrenaline administration may lead to unopposed β_2-receptor activity. This effect augments vasodilation, and hypotension may become more severe.

Noradrenaline, phenylephrine and ephedrine are better choices for treating acepromazine overdose because their primary site of action is the α_1-receptor, and they have minimal activity at β_2-receptors. Dobutamine is mainly a β_1-receptor agonist, and dopamine has α_1-receptor, β_1-receptor and dopaminergic effects. Although either drug may be appropriate for treating acepromazine overdose, their short duration of effect requires that dopamine and dobutamine be administered by constant rate infusion.

Acepromazine is contraindicated in hypovolaemic patients and those in shock. Acepromazine should be used cautiously in patients with cardiac dysfunction, decreased cardiac reserve, hepatic dysfunction or general debilitation. Paediatric patients are quite susceptible to the hypotensive effects of acepromazine. In

geriatric patients, very low doses have been associated with prolonged drug effects. Low doses have also resulted in prolonged recoveries in large and giant breed dogs. Acepromazine should be used with caution in these patients.

Acepromazine has no analgesic effects, so patients should be treated with appropriate analgesics to control pain.

Acepromazine is reportedly *compatible* when mixed in syringes and intravenous tubing with:

- Atropine
- Buprenorphine
- Butorphanol
- Ketamine
- Oxymorphone.

Both glycopyrrolate and diazepam are reported to be physically incompatible when mixed with acepromazine in syringes, but glycopyrrolate is commonly combined with acepromazine immediately before administration, with no apparent adverse effects.

Chlorpromazine
Chlorpromazine is used mainly as an anti-emetic, but may be used as a tranquilliser or, in combination with other drugs, as a premedicant. Chlorpromazine is similar to acepromazine with regard to pharmacological activity, but is less potent and has a longer duration of effect. Effective doses in dogs and cats range from 0.05 to 1.1 mg/kg i.m., administered 60 to 90 minutes before anaesthesia induction.

Promazine
Promazine has pharmacological actions similar to acepromazine. Effective doses in dogs and cats range from 2.2 to 4.4 mg/kg i.m.

Promethazine
Promethazine is more commonly used as an antihistamine than as a tranquilliser.

Trimeprazine
Trimeprazine has antihistaminic, sedative, antitussive and antipruritic qualities. It is rarely used in premedication combinations.

Methotrimeprazine
The combination etorphine/methotrimeprazine is commercially available. Each millilitre contains 18 mg of methotrimeprazine and 0.074 mg of etorphine. This combination produces neuroleptanalgesia and hyperglycaemia in dogs; it is not recommended in cats. It can be given intramuscularly or intravenously and provides deep sedation, hypnosis and analgesia that may be adequate for some minimally invasive surgical procedures. Analgesia lasts for 60 to 90 minutes. If general anaesthesia is to follow administration of etorphine/methotrimeprazine, very small doses of an-

aesthetic drugs are needed to produce and maintain unconsciousness. Caution must be exercised to avoid inadvertent anaesthetic overdose.

Adverse effects of etorphine/methotrimeprazine include bradycardia, hypotension and respiratory depression that may be severe enough to cause cyanosis. Supplemental oxygen, intravenous fluids and assisted ventilation may be necessary in patients sedated with etorphine/methotrimeprazine. This drug combination should not be used in geriatric patients or in any patient that may have decreased organ reserve.

Humans are extremely susceptible to the effects of etorphine, and the combined drug should be handled cautiously. Steps should be taken to avoid inadvertent injection, absorption through breaks in the skin or absorption across mucous membranes. Care must also be exercised when disposing of needles and syringes. Naloxone, or another opioid antagonist suitable for use in humans, should be readily available. Staff should be familiar with emergency procedures and prepared to administer aid if an emergency develops.

Benzodiazepines

The benzodiazepines exert their effects by binding to a specific benzodiazepine binding site on the γ-aminobutyric acid (GABA) receptor. These drugs act as anxiolytics, hypnotics and anticonvulsants, and they produce muscle relaxation through their effects on the CNS. *Benzodiazepines have no analgesic activity.* They decrease postoperative restlessness in patients receiving adequate analgesic medication. As preanaesthetics, benzodiazepines are often used in combination with opioid analgesics. More commonly, benzodiazepines are used in combination with the dissociative drugs ketamine and tiletamine to induce general anesthesia. Benzodiazepines help prevent hypertonus and enhance sedation when used with dissociative drugs. The benzodiazepines include diazepam, midazolam and zolazepam. Zolazepam is only commercially available in the USA and then only in combination with tiletamine.

Diazepam

Effective doses of diazepam in dogs range from 0.1 to 0.6 mg/kg i.v. and in cats from 0.05 to 0.4 mg/kg i.v. Diazepam is formulated in a propylene glycol base. This formulation is not water soluble which makes the uptake of diazepam after intramuscular or subcutaneous administration unpredictable and poor at best. Therefore, diazepam should only be given intravenously. An emulsion of diazepam for injection is available in several countries. This preparation obviates some of the problems associated with propylene glycol but may have reduced bioavailability. Because diazepam decreases inhibition, patients given only diazepam may actually become more difficult to handle. Diazepam works well in combination with opioid analgesics, increasing sedation and patient manageability.

Clinical doses of diazepam have very little effect on the cardiac and respiratory systems. High intravenous doses can slightly depress ventilation, blood pressure, left ventricular function and cardiac output. An increase in heart rate may occur after diazepam administration. The toxicity of diazepam is relatively low. In the event of diazepam overdose, the benzodiazepine antagonist, flumazenil, should be administered. In addition, cardiopulmonary function should be supported by administration of intravenous fluids, adequate ventilation and oxygen supplementation.

Diazepam should be given slowly to decrease the incidence of venous thrombosis, and it should not be given intra-arterially. In addition, rapid intravenous injection of diazepam may cause haemolysis and cardiotoxicity secondary to the propylene glycol base. Diazepam has been implicated in causing congenital abnormalities in humans if given during the first trimester of pregnancy. The veterinary significance of this effect is unclear, but caution should be exercised if contemplating using diazepam in a patient during early pregnancy. Diazepam is also used to relieve status epilepticus in dogs and cats.

Diazepam may adsorb to plastic and should not be stored in plastic syringes. It may also adsorb significantly to plastic bags containing solutions for intravenous administration, and to infusion tubing. Diazepam is reportedly not compatible when physically mixed with any other drugs or solutions, but is commonly mixed with ketamine immediately before administration. Do not administer any solution in which a precipitate forms and does not clear.

Midazolam

Effective doses of midazolam in dogs and cats range from 0.07 to 0.22 mg/kg i.m. or i.v. Midazolam is water soluble and is suitable for both intravenous and intramuscular administration. It is twice as potent as diazepam. Midazolam is supplied at pH 3.5. After administration, when pH increases to above 4.0, the chemical configuration of midazolam changes and it becomes lipid soluble. Midazolam is rapidly and almost completely absorbed after intramuscular administration.

Midazolam has very little effect upon cardiovascular function, but may depress ventilation at high doses. Midazolam overdose may be treated by administration of flumazenil, supporting cardiovascular function and ensuring adequate ventilation.

Midazolam is reportedly *compatible* when mixed in syringes and intravenous tubing with:

- Atropine
- Fentanyl
- Glycopyrrolate
- Ketamine
- Morphine.

Zolazepam

Zolazepam can be combined with the dissociative drug tiletamine (see section on ketamine in sedation). In one preparation, zolazepam/tiletamine is supplied as a lyophilized powder in 5 ml vials. Each vial contains 250 mg of tiletamine hydrochloride and 250 mg of zolazepam hydrochloride. After reconstitution with 5 ml of sterile water, each millilitre of solution contains 100 mg/ml of drug (50 mg of tiletamine and 50 mg of zolazepam). Doses for this product are reported in mg/kg of the combined product: the two drugs are considered one product for dosing purposes. Effective doses in dogs range from 6.6 to 9.9 mg/kg i.m. or 2 to 4 mg/kg i.v., and in cats from 6 to 11.9 mg/kg i.m.

The drug combination provides sedation and analgesia that may be adequate for minor diagnostic procedures. When combined with an opioid analgesic it may allow minimally invasive surgical procedures. If the combination is used as a premedication, the dose of subsequent anaesthetics may be greatly reduced.

Adverse effects include tachycardia, especially in dogs, either hypertension or hypotension, respiratory depression (common), apnoea, cyanosis and pulmonary oedema. Oxygen supplementation, assisted ventilation and administration of intravenous fluids may be necessary in patients sedated with zolazepam/tiletamine.

Athetoid movements (constant succession of slow, writhing, involuntary movements of flexion, extension, pronation, etc.) may occur; additional zolazepam/tiletamine should not be given in an attempt to diminish these movements. The eyes usually remain open after heavy sedation with the drug combination and should be protected with a sterile eye lubricant.

Zolazepam/tiletamine is contraindicated in patients with pancreatic disease, severe cardiac disease or pulmonary disease. It crosses the placenta and may cause depression of the newborn. Patients given the drugs are predisposed to develop hypothermia, therefore an external heat source should be provided. In addition, the drugs will not abolish pinnal, palpebral, laryngeal or pharyngeal reflexes.

Other undesirable effects include:

- Emesis
- Excessive salivation – decreased by pre-emptive use of an anticholinergic
- Excess tracheal and bronchial secretions – decreased by pre-emptive use of an anticholinergic
- Vocalization
- Erratic or prolonged recovery
- Involuntary muscle twitching
- Muscle rigidity (especially during recovery)
- Pain at the injection site.

In addition to sterile water, zolazepam/tiletamine is commonly reconstituted with xylazine or a combination of xylazine and ketamine, with no apparent physical incompatibility. Solutions that are discoloured or that contain a precipitate should not be used.

BENZODIAZEPINE ANTAGONIST

Flumazenil

The actions of the benzodiazepines can be effectively antagonized by the drug flumazenil. The effective dose of flumazenil in dogs and cats is 0.1 mg/kg i.v. Flumazenil's duration of effect is short (about 60 minutes). It may be necessary to redose with flumazenil when large doses of benzodiazepine need to be reversed. The effects of flumazenil are usually observed after 2 to 5 minutes. Reversal is smooth, and patients usually do not experience tachycardia, hypertension, anxiety or other signs of stress.

Flumazenil is *compatible* when mixed in the same syringe or intravenous tubing with:

- Lactated Ringer's solution
- 0.9% saline solution
- 5% dextrose in water.

BUTYROPHENONES

Droperidol

Droperidol is available in combination with the opioid analgesic fentanyl citrate. Each millilitre of one preparation available in the USA contains 0.4 mg of fentanyl citrate and 20 mg of droperidol. When this combined drug is used for premedication, the effective dose in dogs ranges from 0.05 to 0.1 ml/kg i.m., and in cats from 0.1 to 0.11 ml/kg s.c. Maximal effects occur in 30 to 60 minutes. Caution must be exercised when using this product in cats because undesirable CNS stimulation may occur.

In dogs, droperidol/fentanyl produces profound analgesia of short duration (about 30 minutes) and sedation, which lasts considerably longer. The effects of droperidol/fentanyl may be sufficient to allow minor procedures without the need for additional anaesthetic drugs. Adverse cardiopulmonary effects after administration of droperidol/fentanyl include bradycardia, hypotension and respiratory depression.

Other effects that may be seen after administration of droperidol/fentanyl are:

- Alpha-adrenergic blockade
- Panting
- Aggressiveness up to 48 hours after recovery
- Defecation
- Salivation
- Vomiting (rare).

Pretreating patients with an anticholinergic decreases or eliminates some undesirable side effects. Dogs sedated with droperidol/fentanyl may be easily aroused by auditory stimuli. Reversal of the analgesic and sedative effects of fentanyl can be accomplished by administering naloxone hydrochloride 0.04 mg/kg i.v. The CNS effects of both droperidol and fentanyl can be antagonized with a combination of naloxone 0.04 mg/kg mixed with 4-aminopyridine 0.5 mg/kg, given intravenously.

Droperidol/fentanyl is reportedly compatible when mixed in syringes or intravenous tubing with:

- Glycopyrrolate
- Pethidine.

Fluanisone

Fluanisone can be combined with fentanyl citrate. Each millilitre of one commercial preparation contains 10 mg/ml fluanisone and 0.315 mg/ml of fentanyl citrate. This combined drug is no longer licensed for use in dogs in the United Kingdom. Fluanisone/fentanyl produces deep sedation and excellent analgesia that may be adequate for minimally invasive surgical procedures. Peak drug effects are observed in 15 minutes and analgesia lasts for about 30 minutes. The sedative effects of fluanisone/fentanyl last considerably longer than the analgesic effects. Fluanisone effectively prevents opioid induced vomiting. When fluanisone/fentanyl is used as a preanaesthetic, the amount of drug necessary to induce and maintain general anaesthesia can be greatly reduced.

Adverse effects of fluanisone/fentanyl include:

- Bradycardia – may be treated with an anticholinergic
- Defecation
- Responsiveness to auditory stimuli
- Hypotension
- Respiratory depression.

Fluanisone/fentanyl is contraindicated in patients with respiratory disease, renal disease or hepatic disease. The effects of fentanyl can be effectively antagonized with naloxone, but due to fentanyl's short duration of effect reversal is usually unnecessary.

Azaperone

Azaperone is indicated to control the aggressiveness of weanling and feeder pigs when pigs are mixed together. It is not recommended for use in small animals.

OPIOIDS

The pharmacology of the opioids is also described in Chapter 6. Their analgesic effects may be accompanied by mild sedation, but loss of proprioception or consciousness does not occur unless excessive doses are administered.

Butorphanol, morphine, oxymorphone, fentanyl, buprenorphine and other potent opioids are usually combined with tranquillizers in premedication combinations. Opioids increase sedation and provide analgesia in the preoperative period and intraoperatively, and provide some postoperative analgesia.

Morphine sulphate

Effective doses of morphine in dogs range from 0.1 to 2 mg/kg s.c., i.m. or very slowly i.v. Dogs generally exhibit CNS depression after morphine administration, but on rare occasions may become excited. Morphine has central antitussive effects, may cause pupillary constriction and can stimulate the chemoreceptor trigger zone (CTZ) to cause vomiting. Dogs may become hypothermic after morphine administration, therefore an external heat source should be available. Morphine can cause histamine release from mast cells and should be administered very slowly if given intravenously. Morphine does not seem to adsorb to plastic syringes, tubing or bags.

Morphine is considered a respiratory depressant; dogs may pant heavily after its administration without decreasing arterial carbon dioxide ($PaCO_2$). It may cause bronchoconstriction in dogs when given at moderate to high doses. Its cardiovascular effects in dogs range from bradycardia to tachycardia and include coronary vasoconstriction, increased coronary vascular resistance and decreased systemic arterial blood pressure.

Morphine decreases gastrointestinal motility and secretions, but dogs often defecate immediately after administration. Urination after morphine administration is also common, but bladder hypertonia may occur, resulting in difficult urination.

Other uses of morphine sulphate in dogs include:

- Analgesia
- Treatment of hypermotile diarrhoea
- As an antitussive
- An adjunctive treatment of cardiogenic oedema
- An adjunctive treatment of supraventricular premature beats
- Extradural analgesia – use preservative-free morphine.

Effective doses of morphine in cats range from 0.05 to 0.1 mg/kg s.c. or i.m. Morphine should be used cautiously in cats, because significant CNS stimulation can occur if it is used without a concurrent tranquillizer. Cats can experience hyperthermia after morphine administration, and vomiting may occur. Because the major route of morphine elimination is through hepatic glucuronidation, its half-life may be prolonged in cats compared with dogs.

Morphine is reportedly *compatible* when mixed in syringes or intravenous tubing with:

- Atropine
- Diphenhydramine
- Dobutamine
- Droperidol
- Fentanyl
- Glycopyrrolate
- Metoclopramide.

Morphine is reportedly *incompatible* when mixed in syringes or intravenous tubing with:

- Aminophylline
- Heparin sodium
- Pentobarbitone
- Phenobarbitone
- Sodium bicarbonate
- Thiopentone.

Pethidine hydrochloride (meperidine hydrochloride)

Effective doses of pethidine in dogs range from 2 to 6.5 mg/kg s.c. or i.m and in cats from 2 to 4.4 mg/kg s.c. or i.m. Intravenous use is not recommended. The duration of effect in both dogs and cats is only 1–2 hours.

Pethidine is the only opioid used in veterinary medicine that has vagolytic and negative inotropic properties at clinically useful doses. Pethidine reduces salivation and respiratory secretions and does not cause vomiting or defecation in most patients. It can cause histamine release, particularly when given intravenously.

Pethidine is reportedly *compatible* when mixed in the same syringe or intravenous tubing with:

- Atropine
- Diphenhydramine
- Dobutamine
- Droperidol
- Fentanyl
- Glycopyrrolate
- Metoclopramide
- Xylazine.

Pethidine is reportedly *incompatible* when mixed in the same syringe or intravenous tubing with:

- Aminophylline
- Heparin sodium
- Hydrocortisone
- Methylprednisolone
- Pentobarbitone
- Phenobarbitone
- Thiopentone.

Oxymorphone hydrochloride

Effective doses of oxymorphone in dogs range from 0.05 to 0.2 mg/kg s.c., i.m. or i.v., and in cats from 0.05 to 0.4 mg/kg s.c., i.m. or i.v. Oxymorphone may cause

mild respiratory depression and bradycardia – the latter may be reversed with atropine or glycopyrrolate. Dogs may pant quite heavily after oxymorphone administration without decreasing $PaCO_2$. Histamine release rarely occurs, and there are minimal effects on cardiac output and arterial blood pressure. If used at higher doses in cats, concurrent use of a tranquilliser is recommended to avoid excitement.

Oxymorphone is reportedly *compatible* when mixed in the same syringe or intravenous tubing with:

- Acepromazine
- Atropine
- Glycopyrrolate.

Oxymorphone is reportedly *incompatible* when mixed in syringes or intravenous tubing with:

- Barbiturates
- Diazepam.

Other uses of oxymorphone hydrochloride in dogs and cats include:

- Analgesia
- Sedation
- Anaesthesia induction in geriatric and sick dogs
- Intraoperative analgesia
- Extradural analgesia.

Fentanyl citrate

Fentanyl is available alone or combined with either droperidol or fluanisone. When fentanyl is used in preanaesthetic combinations, effective doses in dogs range from 0.01 to 0.02 mg/kg s.c., i.m. or i.v. (see doses used for analgesia in Chapter 6). Fentanyl has a short duration of effect, about 20 to 30 minutes. Fentanyl may cause profound excitement in cats and is not recommended for use without the concurrent administration of a tranquilliser.

Fentanyl has little effect upon cardiac output and blood pressure at clinically useful doses. Histamine release rarely occurs. Intravenous and intramuscular administration may cause bradycardia that is easily reversed with atropine or glycopyrrolate. Fentanyl usually does not induce vomiting in dogs, but defecation frequently occurs.

Fentanyl is reportedly *compatible* when mixed in the same syringe or intravenous tubing with:

- 5% dextrose in water
- Lactated Ringer's solution
- 0.9% saline
- Glycopyrrolate
- Heparin
- Hydrocortisone
- Potassium chloride
- Sodium bicarbonate.

Other uses of fentanyl in dogs include:

- Analgesia – by constant rate infusion, transdermal patch or multiple injections intravenously
- Anaesthetic induction in sick dogs – often in combination with a benzodiazepine.

Etorphine hydrochloride

Etorphine is an opioid agonist that is up to 1000 times more potent than morphine. It is available in combination with the phenothiazide tranquillizer methotrimeprazine. In this commercial preparation each millilitre contains 0.074 mg of etorphine and 18 mg of methotrimeprazine. This drug combination produces neuroleptanalgesia and hyperglycaemia in dogs. Bradycardia and hypotension may occur after etorphine administration. Etorphine is not recommended for use in cats (see section on methotrimeprazine above).

Etorphine is extremely potent and great caution must be exercised when handling this drug. If accidental self-administration occurs, death may result if a reversal drug is not given immediately. Either nalorphine or diprenorphine is recommended to reverse etorphine in emergency situations.

Butorphanol tartrate

Butorphanol is a synthetic opioid that has both agonist and antagonist properties. Butorphanol will partially reverse exogenous and endogenous opioid agonists and will diminish the analgesia afforded by these compounds. For this reason, this drug should be used cautiously in animals with moderate to severe pain that has been present for more than 24 to 48 hours. Effective doses in dogs range from 0.2 to 0.8 mg/kg s.c., i.m. or i.v, and in cats from 0.2 to 0.4 mg/kg s.c., i.m. or i.v.

The respiratory depressant effects of butorphanol are less than those of morphine and seem to reach a ceiling effect beyond which higher doses do not increase depression. Slight decreases in heart rate and blood pressure can occur after butorphanol administration. However, butorphanol does not seem to cause histamine release. Butorphanol has excellent sedative properties in dogs, but on rare occasions can produce excitement when used alone. At higher doses, butorphanol may cause excitement in cats if a tranquillizer is not also given.

Butorphanol is reportedly *compatible* when mixed in the same syringe or intravenous tubing with:

- Acepromazine
- Atropine
- Diphenhydramine
- Droperidol
- Xylazine.

Butorphanol is reportedly *incompatible* when mixed in the same syringe or intravenous tubing with:

- Pentobarbitone.

Other uses of butorphanol in dogs include:

- As an antitussive – excellent for this purpose
- Analgesia – for acute pain of less than 24 to 48 hours' duration
- As an anti-emetic before cisplatin treatment.

Buprenorphine hydrochloride

Effective doses of buprenorphine in dogs range from 0.01 to 0.02 mg/kg s.c., i.m. or i.v., and in cats from 0.005 to 0.02 mg/kg s.c. or i.m. Onset of action is relatively slow, requiring 20 to 30 minutes, but analgesia may last 8 to 12 hours. Excitement may be seen in cats if buprenorphine is given alone, therefore concurrent administration of a tranquillizer is recommended.

Like butorphanol, this drug partially reverses exogenous and endogenous opioid agonists, and diminishes the analgesia afforded by these compounds. For this reason buprenorphine should be used cautiously in animals with moderate to severe pain that has been present for more than 24 to 48 hours. Buprenorphine has little effect on cardiovascular function. Occasionally, respiratory depression may occur after buprenorphine administration.

Buprenorphine is reportedly *compatible* when mixed in syringes or intravenous tubing with:

- Acepromazine
- Atropine
- Diphenhydramine hydrochloride
- Droperidol
- Glycopyrrolate
- Xylazine.

Buprenorphine is reportedly *incompatible* when mixed in syringes or intravenous tubing with:

- Diazepam.

Other uses of buprenorphine include:

- Analgesia – for acute pain of less than 24 to 48 hours' duration
- Extradural analgesia.

Pentazocine lactate

Pentazocine has poor sedative effects compared with other opioids and is not usually used as a premedicant. Pentazocine can cause dysphoria in cats and is possibly best avoided in this species. Effective doses in dogs range from 0.2 to 3.3 mg/kg i.m.

Undesirable effects associated with pentazocine include:

- Increased salivation
- Respiratory depression
- Hypotension

- Decreased gastrointestinal motility
- Fine muscle tremor
- Emesis
- Swelling at the injection site.

Pentazocine is reportedly *compatible* when mixed in syringes or intravenous tubing with:

- Atropine
- Diphenhydramine
- Droperidol
- Metoclopramide.

Pentazocine is reportedly *incompatible* when mixed in syringes or intravenous tubing with:

- Aminophylline
- Flunixin meglumine
- Glycopyrrolate
- Pentobarbitone
- Phenobarbitone
- Sodium bicarbonate.

OPIOID ANTAGONISTS

The opioid antagonists have no analgesic activity. They will effectively reverse all pharmacological effects of opioid agonist and agonist-antagonist drugs. This includes the reversal of all analgesic effects. If a patient becomes severely depressed after the administration of an opioid agonist, partial reversal with an opioid agonist-antagonist would be more appropriate if analgesia was still desired.

Naloxone hydrochloride
Effective doses of naloxone range from 0.04 to 0.1 mg/kg i.m. or i.v. in both dogs and cats. Its duration of effect is about 30 to 60 minutes. If reversal of etorphine is necessary, naloxone can be used at a dose of 0.6 to 0.8 mg/kg i.v., but the duration of effect is extremely short and renarcotization may occur in 10 to 15 minutes.

Nalorphine hydrochloride
Nalorphine has a longer duration of effect than naloxone. When used to reverse etorphine, nalorphine is dosed at the volume:volume ratio nalorphine:etorphine of 1:10 to 1:20 given slowly intravenously. After intravenous injection, reversal takes place in about 3 minutes. Nalorphine has some opioid agonistic properties; overdosing may prolong immobilization.

Diprenorphine
Diprenorphine effectively reverses the effects of etorphine. In all species, diprenorphine is dosed at 0.272 mg/kg i.v. by slow injection. Dogs given diprenorphine to reverse the effects of combined etorphine hydrochloride and methotrimeprazine may still experience moderate sedation due to the lingering effects of methotrimeprazine. Dogs may renarcotize after 4 to 8 hours, and redosing of diprenorphine may be necessary. Diprenorphine has some opioid agonistic properties; overdosing may prolong immobilization.

ALPHA$_2$-ADRENERGIC AGONISTS

Alpha$_2$-adrenoceptors are prejunctional inhibitory receptors within the sympathetic nervous system and are found in the CNS, gastrointestinal tract, uterus and kidney and on platelets. Alpha$_2$-agonists produce analgesia, sedation, muscle relaxation and anxiolysis. When used as premedicants, they reduce the dose of subsequent intravenous and inhalant anaesthetics by as much as 50%. Special attention is required to prevent inadvertent overdose. The anaesthetic sparing effect is somewhat dose dependent, but patients that seem poorly sedated still require reduced doses of subsequent anaesthetic drugs. The uptake of inhalant anaesthetics may be delayed after administration of α_2-agonists, therefore more time may be necessary to induce general anaesthesia by mask.

Alpha$_2$-agonists may cause bradycardia and decrease cardiac output. Atropine and glycopyrrolate are more effective at preventing bradycardia if given before α_2-agonists than at reversing bradycardia after it develops. Therefore, the pre-emptive administration of an anticholinergic drug may be recommended when using α_2-agonists for premedication or sedation, although this remains controversial (see below).

Hypotension, which can be severe, is often seen after a short period of increased blood pressure that immediately follows drug administration. Supporting cardiovascular function with intravenous fluids is recommended when using α_2-agonists. After the administration of these drugs, peripheral veins may be difficult to visualize. Placing intravenous catheters before sedation is less difficult and allows for easy administration of subsequent intravenous drugs and fluids.

After administration of α_2-agonists, ventilation may become shallow and intermittent. Some patients become cyanotic. Pulmonary oedema has also been associated with the use of α_2-agonists. In addition, because hypothermia is common in patients sedated with α_2-agonists, an external heat source should be available.

Other side effects include vomiting, especially in cats, slight muscle tremor, reduced intestinal motility and increased uterine tone. Alpha$_2$-agonists inhibit insulin release resulting in hyperglycaemia, and decrease antidiuretic hormone causing marked diuresis.

Xylazine hydrochloride

Xylazine is a mixed α_2/α_1-agonist with an $\alpha_2:\alpha_1$ selectivity ratio of 160:1. It was first synthesized in the 1960s as an antihypertensive, but was found to have potent sedative effects in animals. Effective doses in dogs and cats range from 0.2 to 1.1 mg/kg s.c., i.m. or i.v. The concentration of the product should be checked before drawing xylazine into a syringe. The onset of action after subcutaneous or intramuscular administration is approximately 10 to 15 minutes, and after intravenous administration is 3 to 5 minutes. Analgesic effects last for about 15 to 30 minutes, and sedation may persist for 1 to 2 hours. Without reversal with an α_2-antagonist, complete recovery after xylazine administration may take 2 to 4 hours.

Xylazine should be used cautiously in patients with pre-existing cardiac disease and those with ventricular arrhythmias, hypotension, shock, respiratory dysfunction, hepatic or renal insufficiency and pre-existing seizure disorder, or if debilitated. Because the α_2-agonists may increase uterine tone, xylazine should not be used, or used with extreme caution, during pregnancy. Xylazine depresses thermoregulatory mechanisms, and either hypothermia or hyperthermia may occur depending upon ambient temperature. This effect may last beyond the sedative and analgesic effects of xylazine. Patients may be aroused by sharp auditory stimuli, and fractious patients may not be adequately sedated with xylazine alone. Increasing the dose of xylazine does not generally increase the level of sedation but prolongs the duration of effect.

Its effects upon the cardiovascular system include an initial increase in total peripheral resistance with increased blood pressure followed by a longer period of hypotension. Bradycardia may be seen and some patients develop second degree heart block. Cardiac output may be decreased up to 30%. Xylazine has been shown to potentiate the arrhythmogenic effects of adrenaline. Respiratory function is usually not affected with clinically useful doses of xylazine, but brachycephalic dogs may develop dyspnoea. Pulmonary oedema has been reported after xylazine administration in some species.

Decreased gastro-oesophageal sphincter pressure has been reported in dogs after xylazine administration and may increase the likelihood of gastric reflux. Emesis may be induced in cats and to a lesser degree in dogs. Vomiting is usually seen within 3 to 5 minutes after administration. To prevent aspiration, further anaesthetics should not be given until this time period has lapsed. Xylazine also prolongs gastrointestinal transit time in dogs. Acute abdominal distension may occur in large dogs (bodyweight ≥ 25 kg). This may be caused by aerophagia or by parasympatholytic gastrointestinal atony with accumulation of gas. Sedation with xylazine may not be appropriate for upper gastrointestinal radiography in large breed dogs.

The manufacturers warn against using xylazine in conjunction with other potent tranquillizers. Xylazine is commonly used with opioid analgesics in patients that will be given an α_2-antagonist at the conclusion of a procedure.

Xylazine is reportedly *compatible* when mixed in syringes or intravenous tubing with:

· Buprenorphine
· Butorphanol
· Ketamine
· Pethidine
· Several other compounds (do not administer any solution in which a precipitate has formed).

Other uses of xylazine include:

· Sedation
· As an emetic in cats
· Extradural analgesia.

Detomidine hydrochloride

Compared with xylazine, detomidine hydrochloride has a higher specificity for α_2-receptors with an $\alpha_2:\alpha_1$ selectivity ratio of 260:1. Detomidine activates α_1-receptors at higher doses. Detomidine is more potent than xylazine and was developed as a tranquilliser for use in horses and cattle. Effective doses in dogs range from 0.005 to 0.02 mg/kg i.m. or i.v., but its use is not recommended in small animals.

Like other α_2-agonists, detomidine is contraindicated in patients with cardiac arrhythmias, coronary insufficiency, cerebrovascular disease, respiratory disease, hepatic disease or renal disease. Detomidine should be used with extreme caution in patients with traumatic or endotoxic shock, hypotension or dehydration, and those stressed by temperature extremes, fatigue or high altitude. The manufacturer warns against using detomidine with intravenous potentiated sulphonamide antibiotics because fatal arrhythmias may develop.

Medetomidine hydrochloride

Medetomidine is the newest α_2-agonist approved for veterinary use. It is more potent and more effective than other drugs in this class. Medetomidine is highly selective for the α_2-adrenoceptor, having an $\alpha_2:\alpha_1$ selectivity binding ratio of 1620:1. Effective doses in dogs range from 0.01 to 0.04 mg/kg s.c., i.m. or i.v. and in cats from 0.04 to 0.08 mg/kg s.c., i.m. or i.v.

Higher doses do not result in deeper sedation, but prolong the duration of effect. Subcutaneous administration produces less reliable effects than intramuscular or intravenous administration. Fractious or excited patients may not become sedated after the administration of medetomidine. Addition of an opioid or benzodiazepine in combination with medetomidine enhances sedation and analgesia beyond any effects achieved with medetomidine alone. If adequate sedation is not obtained, repeat dosing is not recommended.

Bradycardia is common after medetomidine administration. The pre-emptive use of an anticholinergic is more effective at preventing bradycardia than reversing it, if it develops. Atropine and glycopyrrolate can increase the initial hypertensive effects of medetomidine. Anticholinergic plus medetomidine combinations should be used with caution in patients that may not tolerate hypertension. When medetomidine is administered with ketamine 5 mg/kg i.m. in cats, the sympathomimetic properties of ketamine offset the bradycardic effects of medetomidine.

After medetomidine administration, there is an initial increase in total peripheral resistance and blood pressure followed by a longer period of hypotension. Respiratory depression may occur; some patients become cyanotic and require supplemental oxygen. Hypothermia may occur in some patients, and an external heat source should be available.

Other undesirable effects reported after medetomidine include:

- Vomiting
- Muscle twitching
- Second degree heart block
- Diuresis
- Hyperglycaemia
- Excitement
- Prolonged sedation
- Circulatory failure (this occurs with two times the recommended dose or higher).

The manufacturer warns against using medetomidine in patients that are exercise intolerant, have cardiac disease, respiratory disorders, hepatic disease or renal disease or are in shock. Medetomidine should not be used in debilitated patients or those stressed due to heat, cold, fatigue or altitude.

ALPHA-$_2$ ANTAGONISTS

Yohimbine hydrochloride
Yohimbine is indicated for the reversal of xylazine in dogs and cats. Effective doses in dogs range from 0.1 to 0.11 mg/kg i.v. and the dose in cats is 0.1 mg/kg i.v. Yohimbine may cause transient apprehension, CNS excitement, muscle tremors, salivation, increased respiratory rate and hyperaemic mucous membranes. Yohimbine will reverse any analgesia afforded by xylazine and is contraindicated in patients that are dependent upon α_2-agonists for analgesia. Yohimbine should be used cautiously in patients with seizure disorders and renal dysfunction.

Atipamezole hydrochloride
Atipamezole is indicated for the reversal of medetomidine. Effective doses in dogs and cats range from 0.04 to 0.5 mg/kg i.m. Intravenous administration of atipamezole is not recommended. Atipamezole will reverse sedation and analgesia within 5 to 10 minutes of administration. Appropriate analgesia should be provided for patients that require pain relief. Vomiting, hypersalivation, diarrhoea, tremors and excitement may occur after atipamezole administration.

NON-PROPRIETARY PREANAESTHETIC COMBINATIONS

Many drug combinations have been used to premedicate dogs and cats. The following combinations are those with which the author has personal experience, and the list is not comprehensive. When choosing drug combinations, the surgical procedure, anaesthetic duration, anticipated complications, adverse drug effects, postoperative needs and patient age, size, temperament and physical condition should all be considered. The following protocols are designed to serve as examples, and doses should be adjusted to meet individual patient needs.

When drawing multiple drugs into the same syringe care must be exercised not to contaminate vials. The order of drugs listed in the following combinations is the recommended order for drawing drugs into syringes. If anticholinergics are mixed with other drugs, the anticholinergic should be drawn into the syringe first. If anticholinergics are |used pre-emptively, intramuscular administration 5 minutes before the other drugs are administered is most beneficial.

Phenothiazine combinations
These combinations are generally used in young healthy active patients with enough organ reserve to withstand the hypotensive and other adverse effects of phenothiazines. Unless otherwise noted, combinations listed may be appropriate for both dogs and cats. The addition of glycopyrrolate 0.01 mg/kg s.c., i.m. or i.v. or of atropine 0.04 mg/kg s.c. or i.m. or 0.01 mg/kg i.v. to any of the following protocols may be appropriate in some patients.

Butorphanol and acepromazine
Butorphanol 0.4 mg/kg and acepromazine 0.05 mg/kg mixed in the same syringe and administered subcutaneously or intramuscularly.

Oxymorphone and acepromazine
Oxymorphone 0.05 mg/kg and acepromazine 0.03 mg/kg mixed in the same syringe and administered subcutaneously or intramuscularly.

Morphine and acepromazine (dogs only)

Morphine 0.8 mg/kg and acepromazine 0.05 mg/kg mixed in the same syringe and administered subcutaneously or intramuscularly.

Buprenorphine and acepromazine

Buprenorphine 0.01 mg/kg and acepromazine 0.05 mg/kg mixed in the same syringe and administered intramuscularly.

Benzodiazepine combinations

These combinations are generally used in paediatric and geriatric patients. They are also appropriate choices in patients with physiological compromise or decreased organ reserve. The addition of glycopyrrolate 0.01 mg/kg s.c., i.m. or i.v., or atropine 0.04 mg/kg s.c. or i.m. or 0.01 mg/kg i.v. to any of the following protocols may be appropriate in some patients.

Butorphanol and midazolam or butorphanol and diazepam

- Butorphanol 0.3 mg/kg and midazolam 0.1 mg/kg mixed in the same syringe and administered intramuscularly.
- Butorphanol 0.3 mg/kg i.m. followed 10 to 15 minutes later by diazepam 0.15 mg/kg i.v.
- Butorphanol 0.2 mg/kg slowly i.v. followed by diazepam 0.15 mg/kg i.v.

Fentanyl and midazolam (dogs only) or fentanyl and diazepam (dogs only)

- Fentanyl 0.01 mg/kg slowly i.v. followed by midazolam 0.1 mg/kg i.v.
- Fentanyl 0.01 mg/kg slowly i.v. followed by diazepam 0.15 mg/kg i.v.

Buprenorphine and midazolam or buprenorphine and diazepam

- Buprenorphine 0.01 mg/kg and midazolam 0.1 mg/kg mixed in the same syringe and administered subcutaneously, intramuscularly or intravenously.
- Buprenorphine 0.01 mg/kg i.m. followed 20 to 30 minutes later by diazepam 0.15 mg/kg i.v.
- Buprenorphine 0.01 mg/kg slowly i.v. followed by diazepam 0.15 mg/kg i.v.

Oxymorphone and midazolam or oxymorphone and diazepam

- Oxymorphone 0.05 mg/kg and midazolam 0.1 mg/kg mixed in the same syringe and administered subcutaneously, intramuscularly or intravenously.
- Oxymorphone 0.05 mg/kg i.m. followed 10 to 15 minutes later by diazepam 0.15 mg/kg i.v.
- Oxymorphone 0.03 mg/kg slowly i.v. followed by diazepam 0.15 mg/kg i.v.

Alpha$_2$-agonist combinations

Combinations that include α_2-agonist drugs are generally used in healthy exercise-tolerant patients. The preemptive use of glycopyrrolate 0.01 mg/kg i.m. or atropine 0.04 mg/kg i.m. administered 5 minutes before any of the following protocols may be appropriate in some patients.

Butorphanol and xylazine or butorphanol and medetomidine

- Butorphanol 0.4 mg/kg and xylazine 0.3 mg/kg mixed in the same syringe and administered intramuscularly.
- Butorphanol 0.4 mg/kg and medetomidine 0.04 mg/kg mixed in the same syringe and administered intramuscularly.

Midazolam and xylazine or midazolam and medetomidine

- Midazolam 0.1 mg/kg and xylazine 0.3 mg/kg mixed in the same syringe and administered intramuscularly.
- Midazolam 0.1 mg/kg and medetomidine 0.04 mg/kg mixed in the same syringe and administered intramuscularly.

Medetomidine and ketamine (cats only)

Medetomidine 0.05 mg/kg and ketamine 4 mg/kg mixed in the same syringe and administered intramuscularly.

SEDATION FOR MINOR PROCEDURES, DIAGNOSTICS AND RADIOLOGY

Physical restraint of veterinary patients is accompanied by varying degrees of stress. Some calm patients that do not resist handling can be physically restrained with minimal risk of injury to staff or patient. However, most patients benefit from some type of chemical restraint for procedures that require exact positioning or that are invasive. Drugs, or drug combinations, that calm patients and provide analgesia decrease struggling and discomfort during diagnostic and minor therapeutic procedures. Procedures can be carried out in less time and with greater precision when performed on cooperative patients. Therefore, it is an advantage to both the veterinary surgeon and the patient to provide sedation and analgesia for most diagnostic and therapeutic procedures.

Chemical restraint for diagnostic procedures and minimally invasive surgery can be accomplished with sedation or general anaesthesia. In some cases, sedation may be preferred to general anaesthesia. In other cases, a well controlled general anaesthetic may be more beneficial than heavy sedation. If minor surgery is planned, the use of local anaesthetic techniques in addition to sedation will make patients more comfortable and facilitate the procedure.

Combining two or more drugs from different classes often potentiates desired drug effects and minimizes unwanted side effects. Individual drug doses can be reduced and patients still exhibit appropriate sedation and analgesia. Balanced drug combinations are preferred to large doses of a single drug. Whenever potent sedative or analgesic drugs are used, patients must be carefully monitored and supported. Equipment for resuscitation should be available.

The administration of intravenous fluids to all patients that are heavily sedated is appropriate, even if they are apparently healthy. Intravenous fluid support is recommended in all cases when geriatric and paediatric patients are heavily sedated as well as in those patients that have decreased organ function or limited organ reserve. The incidence of cardiovascular complications and long-term effects on organ function will be reduced by this simple measure.

In general, any of the drug combinations discussed in the preanaesthetic section would be appropriate for physical restraint. Patient age, size, temperament and physical condition and the diagnostic or surgical procedure, its duration, anticipated complications, adverse effects and post-procedural analgesia should all be considered when choosing drugs for sedation.

Route of drug administration influences the time necessary before peak drug effects are observed. Drugs given subcutaneously may take 30 to 60 minutes, drugs given intramuscularly may take 15 to 30 minutes, and drugs given intravenously may take 1 to 5 minutes before peak effect. To avoid inadvertent overdose, additional drugs should not be given until peak effects are observed. If additional drugs are necessary to sedate a patient, initial drug effects may be waning while additional sedatives are taking effect. It may be wise to postpone a procedure if adequate sedation does not occur after the first or second dose of sedatives. A quiet environment is essential for any sedative combination to be effective.

In all cases where restraint is used, patients must be positioned comfortably and padded appropriately. This decreases the amounts of drugs necessary to keep patients from moving during procedures. Patients may initially resist positioning, but gentle quiet physical restraint will usually settle patients and they go on to tolerate the procedure without additional tranquillizers.

It is important to consider all drug effects when choosing protocols for sedation. Some drug effects may alter the results of diagnostic procedures. Opioids may cause panting, and motion will be increased during radiography. Xylazine may cause the accumulation of gastric gas in large breed dogs and influence upper gastrointestinal radiography. Acepromazine has no analgesic effects and is not suitable on its own for painful procedures such as wound debridement or skin biopsy.

Some seemingly innocuous diagnostic procedures can precipitate pain, such as radiography of the hip. A patient with severe coxofemoral arthritis may be in pain on recovery due to positioning and manipulation during radiography. It is appropriate to provide analgesia during and after procedures that may aggravate existing conditions or cause pain. Oral analgesics, such as non-steroidal anti-inflammatory drugs (NSAIDs), can be prescribed for patients after release from the veterinary hospital. Potential side effects of these drugs should be discussed with clients. It is generally assumed that any procedure that causes pain in humans will cause pain in animals. It is considered unethical to withhold analgesics from patients receiving veterinary care, and the addition of analgesic drugs to sedative protocols is appropriate in most patients.

Neuroleptanalgesic combinations (those that combine tranquillizers with analgesics) are usually good combinations for procedures that require sedation. Their disadvantage is that patients who seem asleep may startle at loud noises. A quiet environment is essential when using these combinations. They are generally used in young healthy patients, but may be used with caution in elderly or sick patients. Use of local anaesthetic techniques such as line, ring, conduction and regional blocks or extradural analgesia may greatly enhance patient comfort for minimally invasive surgical procedures.

The addition of an anticholinergic may be appropriate with any of the following combinations. The dose ranges given in the premedication section are applicable for sedative protocols. Doses should always be adjusted to meet individual patient needs.

Examples of neuroleptanalgesic combinations include:

- Oxymorphone and acepromazine
- Butorphanol and acepromazine
- Fentanyl and fluanisone
- Fentanyl and droperidol
- Morphine and acepromazine
- Pethidine and acepromazine
- Buprenorphine and acepromazine.

Combinations of benzodiazepines and opioids may be more appropriate in paediatric, geriatric or compromised patients. Benzodiazepines have very little effect upon the cardiovascular system and can be used in patients with decreased organ reserve. With the addition of a local anaesthetic technique, these combinations are good choices in geriatric patients undergoing skin biopsy. The addition of an anticholinergic may be appropriate with any of the following combinations. The dose ranges given in the premedication section are applicable for sedative protocols. Doses should always be adjusted to meet individual patient needs.

Examples of benzodiazepine–opioid combinations include:

- Midazolam and butorphanol
- Midazolam and buprenorphine
- Midazolam and oxymorphone
- Diazepam and butorphanol
- Diazepam and buprenorphine
- Diazepam and oxymorphone.

Diazepam should be administered intravenously and should not be mixed in syringes with any other drugs

The α_2-adrenergic agonists, especially medetomidine, may provide adequate sedation and analgesia when used alone. If sedation or analgesia are not adequate with xylazine or medetomidine, combinations with opioids or benzodiazepines may be used. Use caution when combining α_2-agonists with other potent tranquillizers, and their use with acepromazine is not recommended. The pre-emptive use of an anticholinergic may be appropriate with any of the following combinations. The dose ranges given in the premedication section are applicable for sedative protocols. Doses should always be adjusted to meet individual patient needs.

Examples of α_2-agonist combinations include:

- Xylazine and butorphanol
- Xylazine and buprenorphine
- Xylazine and butorphanol and midazolam
- Medetomidine and midazolam
- Medetomidine and butorphanol
- Medetomidine and butorphanol and diazepam (diazepam should be administered intravenously and should not be mixed in syringes with any other drugs).

Ketamine (see also Chapter 8)

In cats, ketamine is frequently used in combinations designed for chemical restraint. The use of ketamine for chemical restraint in dogs is not recommended. When used in sedative and premedication combinations, effective doses of ketamine in cats range from 3 to 11 mg/kg i.m. or 2 to 4 mg/kg i.v. Ketamine is a dissociative drug that has anaesthetic and analgesic properties. Administration of ketamine results in a central release of catecholamines that indirectly stimulates cardiovascular function. Ketamine increases cardiac output, heart rate and blood pressure in normal patients. However, catecholamine-depleted patients will experience negative inotropic effects due to the direct effects of ketamine on the heart.

Increased muscle tone and hypersalivation are also associated with ketamine. Pinnal, palpebral, laryngeal and pharyngeal reflexes are not abolished. The eyes remain open and should be protected with sterile lubricant. Ketamine can also cause increases in intracranial and intraocular pressures. It should be avoided in patients with a pre-existing seizure disorder or uncontrolled hyperthyroidism. Recover-

ies from ketamine sedation can be quite stormy and it is recommended that a tranquillizer be used in combination with ketamine.

Ketamine is reportedly *compatible* when mixed in syringes or intravenous tubing with:

- 5% Dextrose in water
- 0.9% Saline
- Xylazine.

Ketamine is reportedly *incompatible* when mixed in syringes or intravenous tubing with:

- Barbiturates
- Diazepam (it is, however, common practice to mix diazepam (or midazolam) and ketamine in the same syringe immediately before administration, with no apparent adverse effects. Solutions in which a precipitate has formed should not be given).

The pre-emptive or concurrent use of an anticholinergic may be appropriate with any of the following drug combinations. The dose ranges given in the premedication section are applicable for sedative protocols. Doses should always be adjusted to meet individual patient needs. Examples of ketamine combinations used in cats for sedation include:

- Midazolam and ketamine
- Butorphanol and ketamine
- Xylazine and ketamine
- Acepromazine and ketamine
- Medetomidine and ketamine
- Oxymorphone and ketamine
- Oxymorphone and acepromazine and ketamine
- Butorphanol and midazolam and ketamine.

SUMMARY

There are many drug combinations that can be used to sedate patients for diagnostic and minor procedures. Drug dosages and combinations should be tailored for each individual patient based on their physical status and the requirements of the procedure. The goal of sedation is to provide adequate analgesia and tranquillization so that the procedure may be accomplished without unnecessary stress or physiological compromise to the patient.

FURTHER READING

Booth NH (1982) Drugs acting on the central nervous system. In: *Veterinary Pharmacology and Therapeutics, 5th edn*, ed. NH Booth and LE MacDonald, pp. 149–352. Iowa State University Press, Ames

Gleed RD (1987) Tranquilizers and sedatives. In: *Principles and Practice of Veterinary Anesthesia*, ed. CE Short, pp. 16–27. Williams and Wilkins, Baltimore

Lin HC (1996) Dissociative anesthetics. In: *Lumb and Jones' Veterinary Anesthesia, 3rd edn*, ed. JC Thurmon *et al.*, pp. 241–298. Williams and Wilkins, Baltimore

Plumb DC (1995) *Veterinary Drug Handbook, 2nd edn*, ed. DC Plumb. Pharma Vet Publishing, White Bear Lake

Short CE (1987) Anticholinergics. In: *Principles and Practice of Veterinary Anesthesia*, ed. CE Short, pp. 8–15. Williams and Wilkins, Baltimore

Short CE (1987) Neuroleptanalgesia and alpha-adrenergic receptor analgesia. In: *Principles and Practice of Veterinary Anesthesia*, ed. CE Short, pp. 47–57. Williams and Wilkins, Baltimore

Stoelting RK (1991) *Pharmacology and Physiology in Anesthetic Practice, 2nd edn*, ed. RK Stoelting. JB Lippincott, Philadelphia

Thurmon JC, Tranquilli WJ and Benson GJ (1996) Preanesthetics and anesthetic adjuncts. In: *Lumb and Jones' Veterinary Anesthesia, 3rd edn*, ed. JC Thurmon *et al.*, pp. 183–209. Williams and Wilkins, Baltimore

CHAPTER EIGHT

Intravenous Anaesthetics

Jacky Reid and Andrea M. Nolan

INTRODUCTION

Indications

- For induction of anaesthesia when followed by inhalational agents
- As a sole anaesthetic agent for short-term minor procedures such as radiography, suturing, suture removal or ear examination
- As part of a total intravenous anaesthetic (TIVA) technique, where an appropriate intravenous agent is given by repeated boluses or by infusion, often in conjunction with analgesics
- As a supplement to inhalation anaesthesia
- To aid in the treatment of conditions such as tetanus and status epilepticus
- Occasionally to provide long-term sedation of animals in intensive care units.

Advantages

- Simple
- Cause a rapid onset of anaesthesia
- Relatively pleasant for the animal
- Do not require special equipment (except in the case of infusion techniques)
- Pose no danger from explosion or pollution
- Non-irritant to airways.

Disadvantages

- Superficial veins may be difficult to find
- Intravenous access may be difficult to maintain unless an intravenous catheter is used
- Drug may be irritant if given perivascularly
- Once injected the drug cannot be removed
- Drug may be cumulative
- If the animal is not intubated, the airway is unprotected and there may be a risk of aspiration of foreign material – tracheal intubation is mandatory for long procedures and for emergency resuscitation
- Possible apnoea on injection
- Possible hypotension on injection
- Possible excitement in recovery.

Techniques

- Single dose
- Topping up with increments
- Continuous infusion.

PRACTICAL ASPECTS OF INTRAVENOUS INJECTION

Proper preanaesthetic medication should preclude the necessity for forceful restraint for intravenous injection. In seriously debilitated or aged animals, where sedative premedication may be minimal or omitted altogether, gentle handling by a competent assistant should be all that is required.

Site

The easiest vein for injection is the cephalic (radial) vein. The recurrent tarsal (saphenous) vein may be used, but restraint is more difficult and the animal's response to the anaesthetic agent cannot be observed so easily. The external jugular vein is not recommended for injection unless it is catheterized, since it is much more difficult to ensure that all the drug is deposited slowly intravenously, and therefore there is a tendency to administer drugs too rapidly by this route. In the cat, should attempts to obtain intravenous access fail in both cephalic veins, there is an easily accessible superficial vein on the inner aspect of the thigh (medial saphenous vein). In dogs with large external ears, such as Basset Hounds, there are veins on the pinnae that are an option for catheterization should the veins on the legs prove inaccessible.

Equipment

For a single injection, a suitable gauge hypodermic needle will suffice, but if repeated injections or an infusion are contemplated, an over-the-needle catheter should be used. This will ensure that the vein is not damaged and that the drug is not injected perivascularly. There are a wide variety of Teflon catheters available and choice depends on personal preference. It is worth emphasizing, however, that for successful placement of these it is best to make a small nick in the skin so that the point of the catheter is not damaged as it passes through the skin. As the inner needle enters the vein, blood 'flashes back' into the hub of the needle, and the catheter should then be advanced into the vein while the needle is held firmly. The catheter should then be capped, flushed with heparinized saline and secured by adhesive tape.

To facilitate the infusion of intravenous anaesthetic agents, it is advisable to use either a volumetric infusion pump or a syringe driver – many of which are available. Volumetric infusion pumps are generally used for the administration of fluids in veterinary practice. While they can be used to infuse intravenous anaesthetic drugs, they are not ideal, and frequently drugs have to be diluted or given through a burette giving set. Syringe drivers are more flexible and are ideal for giving drugs by infusion. They take a selection of syringe sizes and afford excellent control over the administration rate (see Chapter 4).

BARBITURATES

Thiopentone sodium (thiopental)

Thiopentone is a highly lipid-soluble weak organic acid supplied as its sodium salt in powder form which, once made up with sterile water, is stable for 3–7 days depending on temperature. It is licensed for use in dogs and cats. The solution is very alkaline (pH 14) and is highly irritant if the concentration is greater than 2.5%. It is not miscible with acidic drugs as precipitation occurs. Once injected into blood (pH 7.4), the drug repartitions from its almost totally ionized form. At pH 7.4, 61% of a given dose of thiopentone exists in the unionized form. Thiopentone is approximately 80–85% bound to plasma proteins. As with all anaesthetic drugs, only the unbound unionized fraction of the drug is able to penetrate cell membranes and thus produce its effect. Therefore, the response to a given dose of the drug may vary depending on the pH of the blood. At normal blood pH, 39% of a given dose is ionized, but this percentage decreases as pH falls. Thus the non-ionized fraction increases and consequently acidosis will enhance penetration of the blood–brain barrier. The concentration of plasma proteins will also affect dose requirements. Hypoproteinaemia or uraemia (which results in displacement of the drug from binding sites) will increase the percentage of unbound, and therefore active, drug and, in severely affected animals, dose requirements will be reduced. Thiopentone crosses the placenta readily, and fetal tissues will rapidly equilibrate with the maternal blood.

Properties

- Thiopentone crosses the blood–brain barrier rapidly and, like other ultra-short-acting barbiturates, causes rapid loss of consciousness. The principal factor that limits the time to the onset of anaesthesia is the circulation time from the site of injection to the brain
- Thiopentone causes respiratory depression and, occasionally, apnoea
- Thiopentone causes cardiovascular depression. Hypotension and a reduction in cardiac output are observed after intravenous injection. The overall effect depends on the rate of drug administration and the total dose administered, the animal's condition (blood volume, acid-base balance etc.) and concurrent administration of drugs that affect the cardiovascular system e.g. acepromazine. Thiopentone has a direct myocardial depressant action, which is minimal at normal clinical doses but can be severe with high plasma concentrations of the drug. Hypovolaemia makes animals very susceptible to the myocardial depressant action of the barbiturates. Peripheral vasodilation is the primary reason for arterial hypotension. Cardiac arrhythmias may be noticed during induction of anaesthesia, but are generally innocuous in healthy animals
- Recovery from thiopentone anaesthesia is dependent upon redistribution of the drug to other tissues. After a single injection of thiopentone, plasma concentrations decline rapidly in a tri-exponential manner, as the drug is redistributed from the brain to other tissues of the body. Initially, the drug is taken up by relatively well perfused tissue such as brain, heart and kidney. Thus anaesthesia is induced (as brain concentrations increase) and the plasma concentration starts to decrease. Soon after, moderately perfused tissues, such as muscle, take up drug and this contributes to a further decrease in plasma thiopentone concentrations. At this time the plasma concentrations may be sufficiently low to reverse the concentration gradient between the brain and the plasma in favour of drug leaving the brain, when consciousness soon returns. Poorly perfused tissues, such as adipose tissue, take up drug slowly, as the blood flow to them is poor. However, the total capacity of fat for lipid-soluble drugs such as thiopentone is high and so this tissue can 'store' thiopentone. Metabolism of thiopentone occurs slowly in the liver. Animals recover from anaesthesia (after a single bolus dose) when most of the drug present in the body is partitioned into tissues. As this leaches out into plasma, dogs and cats may seem to be 'groggy', and full recovery may appear long, since the liver cannot metabolize the drug re-emerging from tissues fast enough to prevent some depression of the central

nervous system (CNS). Low clearance values of 1.5–3.2 ml/kg/min have been reported in the dog, and the drug is unsuitable for use to maintain anaesthesia. Repeated administration leads to cumulation of the drug because tissue sites become saturated. This causes potentially serious cardiovascular and respiratory effects and delayed recovery from anaesthesia

- Thiopentone is an irritant if injected perivascularly. It should be used in as dilute a solution as is compatible with a reasonable injection volume (1–2.5% in small animals)
- Thiopentone has poor analgesic properties. It was considered to be hyperalgesic, i.e. lowered the threshold to painful stimuli, although recent work has cast doubt upon this. Relatively deep anaesthesia is required with thiopentone to suppress responses to surgical stimulation
- Thiobarbiturates should be used with care in Greyhounds and other 'sight' hounds. Recovery from anaesthesia is longer in Greyhounds than in mixed-breed dogs. This correlates with high plasma thiobarbiturate concentrations reported in this species
- Thiopentone may be displaced from plasma protein binding sites by drugs that are more strongly protein bound, such as the non-steroidal anti-inflammatory agents, e.g. phenylbutazone and flunixin. In theory this may lead to an increased pharmacological effect
- Thiopentone reduces intracranial pressure in humans with elevated intracranial pressure, and may be indicated in patients with intracranial tumours. However, attention must be paid to avoiding hypoventilation, which may be induced by the barbiturates, as the resulting hypercapnia will have the effect of increasing intracranial pressure. Barbiturates produce no significant alteration in intracranial pressure in normal patients
- Thiopentone is an effective anticonvulsant (but the side effects of hypotension and respiratory depression mean that animals need to be carefully monitored).

Use

Thiopentone is used as an induction agent in all species. It is important to give the drug to effect and not to give a computed dose, since each individual's requirements will vary. However, as a guide, in unpremedicated fit animals, a dose of around 20–25 mg/kg may be required to produce unconsciousness sufficient to permit endotracheal intubation. This dose is halved by the use of premedicants. The dose should be given slowly (over 30–40 seconds) so that the injection may be stopped once the desired effect is obtained. The optimal method for administering thiopentone to induce anaesthesia is to give between one-half and two-thirds the calculated dose, and to wait to obtain the maximum effect before proceeding with increments. An even slower rate of injection should be used in sick animals (60 seconds or more). In cats it may be necessary to give the drug slightly more quickly as they tend to struggle more while being restrained. After a single intravenous dose, anaesthesia lasts 5–15 minutes. Its use for the maintenance of anaesthesia is not recommended due to the slow metabolism of the drug. This leads to cumulation of thiopentone in various body tissues, including fat, and consequently a prolonged recovery time. Apnoea on induction of anaesthesia with thiopentone is common. If this persists, the animal should be ventilated until spontaneous breathing resumes. Thiopentone should be used with extreme care in cardiovascularly compromised animals, when both the dose and the rate of administration should be reduced. Rapid intravenous injection of a full dose of thiopentone in these animals results in a precipitous fall in arterial blood pressure. If thiopentone is used to induce anaesthesia after xylazine or medetomidine premedication, the dose should be markedly decreased (around 75–90% reduction).

Methohexitone sodium (methohexital)

This oxybarbiturate is supplied as its sodium salt in a powder, which when made up in sterile water is relatively stable for about 6 weeks. It is highly alkaline, twice as potent as thiopentone and is generally administered as a 1–2.5% solution. Protein binding is similar to that measured for thiopentone (80–85%).

Properties

- Ultra-short-acting barbiturate that induces a rapid loss of consciousness
- Post-induction apnoea is more common than after thiopentone
- Cardiovascular depression similar to thiopentone. Some work has suggested that in cats the hypotensive effect is greater than with thiopentone, while the opposite is the case in humans. In both species the differences are small
- Recovery from anaesthesia is dependent on both redistribution and metabolism (three times as fast as thiopentone in the dog; clearance around 11 ml/kg/min). Redistribution of drug occurs in a manner similar to that of thiopentone. However, as drug diffuses out of tissues, hepatic metabolism clears the plasma of methohexitone considerably more rapidly than it does with thiopentone, and consequently there is less of a 'hangover' effect
- It is less irritant than thiopentone if injected perivascularly
- It has poor analgesic properties, similar to thiopentone

- Muscular twitching is often seen at induction and recovery
- Spiking activity seen on an electroencephalogram (EEG) is of questionable significance. Although methohexitone is not contraindicated in epileptic patients, thiopentone would be a better choice.

Use

Methohexitone, like thiopentone, should be given to effect. On average, approximately 5 mg/kg is required to produce unconsciousness in premedicated animals, but it is best to give approximately half this initially and then top up, incrementally, to effect. Methohexitone is mainly used as an induction agent, but due to its rapid metabolism it can be used to maintain anaesthesia with incremental dosing or by infusion, without prolonging recovery. Approximately 0.3 mg/kg/min will generally maintain anaesthesia.

Methohexitone does not cause prolonged recovery in Greyhounds and related breeds and is therefore preferred to thiopentone for these animals. It tends to be used selectively in small animals where a rapid recovery is required, e.g. brachycephalic dogs. Excitement and muscular twitching at recovery may be evident. This may be reduced by the use of adequate premedication. As with thiopentone, caution should be exercised when using methohexitone in animals in shock, and in animals premedicated with α_2-adrenoceptor agonists such as xylazine and medetomidine.

Pentobarbitone (pentobarbital)

Pentobarbitone is an oxybarbiturate, very similar in structure to thiopentone. It is less lipid soluble and is available as pentobarbitone sodium as a 6% solution (60 mg/ml), which is alkaline. Binding to plasma proteins is low (around 40%). It is licensed for use in dogs and cats as a sedative and as a general anaesthetic.

Properties

- Slow onset of action (60–90 seconds) due to lower lipid solubility compared with thiopentone and methohexitone
- Post-induction apnoea and respiratory depression are features of this drug when it is used as a sole anaesthetic agent
- Cardiovascular depression can be profound
- Recovery from anaesthesia is slow due to a combination of limited redistribution (as a consequence of low lipid solubility) and slow metabolism
- An irritant if injected perivascularly
- Poor analgesic properties.

Use

Pentobarbitone is not recommended for general anaesthesia in small animals. It has been used to control

convulsions. Care must be taken to ensure adequate ventilation. Induction of anaesthesia should be performed slowly to allow time for the drug to cross into the brain before topping up.

STEROID ANAESTHETICS

Alphaxalone/alphadolone

Alphaxalone/alphadolone is a mixture of two progesterone derivatives, alphaxalone (9 mg/ml) and alphadolone acetate (3 mg/ml). Alphaxalone is a considerably more potent anaesthetic than alphadolone. These drugs are not water soluble and are therefore solubilized by the use of 20% 'Cremophor EL' (polyoxyethylated castor oil). The solution is clear but viscous and of a neutral pH. Once opened, vials should be used at once since no bacteriostatic agent is included in the preparation. The solution should not be stored in the refrigerator, as the steroids tend to precipitate out of solution. The drugs are not highly plasma protein bound (<50%) and so the effects of a given dose of alphaxalone/alphadolone are not likely to be enhanced by the presence of hypoproteinaemia. The drug is not licensed for use in dogs, as they may exhibit a potentially fatal anaphylactoid reaction to the castor oil. The reported use of the drug, in combination with large doses of antihistamines, seems an unnecessary and dangerous choice when other safer drugs are available for dogs. In cats, birds and small laboratory animals alphaxalone/alphadolone is administered by intravenous or intramuscular injection.

Properties

- High therapeutic index and wide safety margin
- Short acting. Both steroid components are metabolized rapidly by the liver. The duration of action of a single dose of the drug is therefore short (5–20 minutes depending on the dose) and recovery is rapid. However, in cats with hepatic dysfunction, metabolism is likely to be delayed and the drug will have a prolonged duration of action. Renal dysfunction may delay recovery. Rapid loss of consciousness after intravenous injection (as for thiopentone and propofol) or deep intramuscular injection. Suitable for use in total intravenous anaesthesia
- Cardiovascular depression – hypotension similar to thiopentone
- Mild respiratory depression, although apnoea is rare
- Good muscle relaxation
- Little tissue toxicity if injected perivascularly
- Anaphylactoid reactions occur in some cats given alphaxalone/alphadolone. The severity of

these reactions varies from mild subcutaneous oedema of the paws and pinnae to more severe laryngeal and pulmonary oedema and profound hypotension. Although fatalities are rare, it is probably best to avoid using the drug when airway surgery is contemplated or if the animal has a history of atopy
- Like all anaesthetic agents, alphaxalone/ alphadolone will cross the placenta and cause fetal depression. In cats requiring Caesarian section, its use should therefore be confined to the induction of anaesthesia. Sufficient time should be allowed for redistribution of the drug from the kittens before they are delivered (see Chapter 18).

Use

Widely used in the cat, small laboratory animals and birds. Its high therapeutic index makes it a useful anaesthetic for induction and maintenance of anaesthesia in the cat.

Intramuscular route: Inject into a suitable muscle mass. The quadriceps group is usually preferred to other leg muscles because there are fewer intermuscular spaces into which the drug may be deposited inadvertently, and from which absorption will be so slow as to reduce the effectiveness of the drug.

The intramuscular dose can range from 4 mg/kg (suitable for premedication before topping up by the intravenous route some 10 minutes later) to 18 mg/kg, which will induce full anaesthesia within 10–15 minutes. However, the highest dose represents a considerable volume, which can be difficult to inject. A median dose of around 9 mg/kg is used more usually and this will produce sufficient restraint, with the option of increasing the depth of anaesthesia by giving further drug intravenously. More than one injection site may be required in large cats.

Intravenous route: As with all induction agents, alphaxalone/alphadolone is best administered intravenously, to effect. In healthy animals, approximately 6 mg/kg will induce anaesthesia sufficient to permit endotracheal intubation. For a short period of anaesthesia, sufficient for minor procedures (10 minutes), a further 3 mg/kg may be administered slowly until the desired depth of anaesthesia is achieved. In debilitated or old animals, this further dose is not usually required. If alphaxalone/ alphadolone is used as the sole anaesthetic agent, small (around 0.5 ml) increments may be injected as necessary to maintain anaesthesia, or an infusion may be set up to deliver the drug at a rate of around 0.24 mg/kg/min (i.e. 0.02 ml/kg/min). Because the drug is eliminated rapidly by hepatic metabolism, repeated doses do not prolong recovery, even after 24 hours anaesthesia/sedation, provided normal homeostasis has been maintained (i.e. fluid balance,

acid-base balance, respiratory and cardiovascular function and body temperature).

DISSOCIATIVE AGENTS

Ketamine

Ketamine hydrochloride is presented in aqueous solution. It is a weak organic base and the hydrochloride solution has a pH of 3.3–5.5, so that it is not miscible with alkaline solutions. The drug is formulated at a concentration of 100 mg/ml in 5 ml or 10 ml multidose vials. It is relatively stable for 3 years, but bottles should be protected from light and excessive heat. The preparation is a racemic mixture, with the stereoisomers producing different spectra of actions. Ketamine can be administered by intramuscular, intravenous, subcutaneous or intraperitoneal injection, and also it can be given orally.

Dissociative anaesthetics depress the cerebral cortex before causing medullary depression. Dissociative anaesthesia is a state whereby profound somatic analgesia is combined with a light plane of unconsciousness, but the animal seems to be dissociated from its environment. Pharyngeal, laryngeal, corneal and pedal reflexes, the abolition of which are conventionally used to assess depth of anaesthesia, persist relatively unimpaired, and the eyes remain open. In humans, dreams and emergence hallucinations are features of its use, and the administration of dissociative agents is largely restricted to young children. This picture can be modified by the use of α_2-adrenoceptor agonists (xylazine, medetomidine) or benzodiazepines (diazepam, midazolam) as premedicants. Ketamine is rapidly metabolized in the dog and cat by hepatic microsomes. The main metabolite, norketamine, has hypnotic properties (approximately one-fifth as potent as ketamine in this respect) and has a half-life longer than that of ketamine. This may explain the occasional drowsiness and prolonged recoveries in animals when large doses of ketamine have been given.

Properties

- Rapid induction following parenteral administration, although the rate of onset after intravenous injection is markedly slower than after thiopentone
- Little cumulation reported, although infusions of ketamine have not been widely used in dogs and cats. Clearance values are high (38–40 ml/kg/ min). Ketamine is metabolized rapidly by the liver, and both parent compound and metabolites are excreted in bile and via the kidneys. Hepatic dysfunction affects elimination of the drug and prolongs its action considerably. Renal dysfunction may delay the excretion of norketamine, which may contribute to drowsiness

- The respiratory effects of ketamine in the dog and cat are interesting. There is a degree of respiratory depression initially and often periodic breath-holding on inspiration, giving rise to a so-called 'apneustic' pattern of respiration. Generally, arterial blood oxygen tensions are well maintained (compared with barbiturates), and the preservation of cardiac output also allows tissue oxygenation to be well maintained
- Cardiovascular effects are dose related. Central stimulation of the sympathetic system leads to a tachycardia and increase in blood pressure and cardiac output. Large doses given intravenously may produce a transient fall in blood pressure as the drug produces a direct but transient depression of the myocardium. Normally the hypertensive effects predominate unless very large doses are used. Peripheral resistance does not increase. Studies in dogs and cats have indicated that ketamine does not induce cardiac arrhythymias and may be anti-arrhythmic. The increase in blood pressure produced by ketamine makes it unsuitable for intraocular surgery
- Good analgesia. Ketamine has been used successfully in humans as an analgesic for phantom limb pain and also for burns. In veterinary medicine, it may also prove useful at subanaesthetic doses for intractable pain and as an adjunctive analgesic in TIVA techniques (see Chapter 6)
- Causes increase in muscle tone. Spontaneous involuntary muscle movements, which may progress to tonic-clonic spasm of limb muscles, are frequently observed after administration of ketamine alone in small animals
- Salivation and lacrimation are increased
- Laryngeal and swallowing reflexes tend to persist
- If used as a sole agent in dogs (unlicensed for such use), convulsions are frequently observed. It is interesting to note that ketamine has been shown to have anti-epileptic properties in some species
- Ketamine increases cerebral blood flow and cerebral oxygen consumption, which may have serious adverse consequences in animals with raised intracranial pressure.

Use

It is doubtful if ketamine alone is of use for surgical procedures in veterinary practice, although it is licensed for such use in cats and subhuman primates. The increased muscle tone and incidence of convulsions at high doses, particularly in the dog, are undesirable properties and, clinically, ketamine is used in combination with a sedative or tranquillizer to offset these and other side effects. In the dog, combinations of midazolam/ketamine and diazepam/ketamine have been used for short-term anaesthesia and also for induction of anaesthesia before maintenance with an inhalational agent. The minimal cardiovascular and respiratory effects produced by this combination make it suitable for use in poor risk cases. Other sedatives that have been combined with ketamine for use in dogs include acepromazine and the α_2-adrenoceptor agonists, xylazine and medetomidine. More recently, the combination of medetomidine, butorphanol and ketamine has been advocated as suitable for use in dogs. Ketamine seems to reduce the undesirable cardiovascular effects of medetomidine in small animals. In the cat, ketamine is generally combined with xylazine or medetomidine or with a benzodiazepine tranquillizer such as midazolam. The combination produces satisfactory anaesthesia for many surgical procedures. It may be useful in uncontrollable cats, where its rapid absorption from any site (including the oral mucosa) allows for ease of administration (see Chapter 7 for further details).

Cats

Sedation/anaesthesia in combination with midazolam:

- By intramuscular injection: 0.2 mg/kg midazolam and 10 mg/kg ketamine
- By intravenous injection: 0.2 mg/kg midazolam and 5 mg/kg ketamine – given slowly to effect.

General anaesthesia in combination with medetomidine:

- By intramuscular injection: medetomidine 80 µg/kg and ketamine 2.5–7.5 mg/kg
- By intravenous injection: medetomidine 40 µg/kg with ketamine 1.25 mg/kg.

General anaesthesia in combination with medetomidine and butorphanol:

- By intramuscular injection: butorphanol 0.4 mg/kg, medetomidine 80 µg/kg and ketamine 5 mg/kg
- By intravenous injection: butorphanol 0.1 mg/kg, medetomidine 40 µg/kg and ketamine 1.25–2.5 mg/kg.

Dogs

Sedation/anaesthesia in combination with diazepam:

- By intravenous injection: 1 ml/10 kg of a 50:50 mixture of diazepam and ketamine (0.25 mg/kg diazepam, 5 mg/kg ketamine) given slowly to effect works well after sedative premedication (premedication smooths recovery).

General anaesthesia in combination with medetomidine:

- By intramuscular injection: medetomidine 40 μg/kg and ketamine 5.0–7.5 mg/kg.

General anaesthesia in combination with medetomidine and butorphanol:

- By intramuscular injection: butorphanol 0.1 mg/kg and medetomidine 25 μg/kg, followed 15 minutes later by ketamine 5 mg/kg.

Problems

- Recovery from ketamine alone can be stormy, especially in cats. Disturbances such as noise, lights and handling may precipitate seizures
- Hypothermia and delayed recovery may occur, especially in cats, which is probably related to large doses given intramuscularly. It is important to keep the ambient temperature high in the recovery area
- The depth of anaesthesia may be difficult to judge, and inexperienced observers may conclude, wrongly, that supplementary drugs (including volatile agents) are required. Any additional anaesthetic drug may produce marked respiratory depression and must be administered with great care
- Corneal drying may occur because the eyes remain open, and a bland ophthalmic ointment should be applied
- The administration of xylazine or medetomidine in combination with ketamine carries the risk of vomiting at induction, and this combination must not be used in those cases with gastrointestinal obstruction.

Tiletamine

Tiletamine is chemically very closely related to ketamine and its pharmacodynamic effects are similar, but it is longer lasting, more potent and has more pronounced side effects (muscle rigidity and tonic-clonic seizures) than ketamine. Consequently it is marketed for clinical use in combination with zolazepam, a benzodiazepine tranquillizer, which is an effective anti-convulsant and muscle relaxant. The combination is available in the USA but not in the UK. In the dog, the tranquillizing effects of the zolazepam seem to wane before the effects of the tiletamine, and so recoveries can be stormy, especially with high doses and in the absence of sedative premedication. In the cat, the reverse applies because of the long plasma half-life of zolazepam, and recoveries are twice as long as those seen in the dog. Tachycardia with zolazepam/tiletamine occurs more frequently in the dog than in the cat.

Respiratory depression and irregular breathing patterns are dose related.

Dose of combination

Wide dose ranges have been described, depending on the physical status of the animal, the degree of restraint required (low doses produce chemical restraint) and the duration of the surgical procedure. The following are intended as a guide.

Dogs

- 2–13 mg/kg i.m. or i.v.: onset time 30–60 seconds after intravenous injection and within 5–12 minutes after intramuscular injection.

Cats

- 2–15 mg/kg i.m. or i.v.: onset time as for the dog. Some cats show pain on intramuscular injection.

Increased salivation is a feature of its use, but this can be prevented by the prior administration of atropine or glycopyrrolate.

PROPOFOL

Propofol is a substituted phenol, presented as an emulsion (10 mg/ml) and administered intravenously. It is licensed for use in the dog and cat, both for bolus administration and for incremental injection.

The pharmacokinetics of propofol have been well described in humans and reasonably well described in healthy dogs, but not in cats. The pharmacokinetic properties of propofol are unique and contribute to its clinical advantages. Propofol is rapidly cleared from the body (clearance >40 ml/kg/min) by metabolism, approximately 10–20 times faster than thiopentone. Evidence is accumulating that extrahepatic metabolism of propofol occurs in humans, sheep, goats and dogs. After bolus intravenous injection of propofol, plasma concentrations decrease rapidly due to redistribution of drug to the brain and other highly perfused tissues, such as muscle (similar to thiopentone). Thereafter, the decrease in propofol plasma concentration is faster than for thiopentone due to rapid metabolism of the drug. The elimination half-life of propofol is long (values up to 330 minutes in dogs have been reported), but this is not clinically relevant and probably reflects the slow elimination of propofol from fat. Propofol, like thiopentone, has a large volume of distribution, i.e. it distributes widely through body tissues, as would be expected for a lipophilic drug. Propofol is metabolized to sulphate and glucuronide conjugates of a quinol derivative of propofol, which are inactive.

Properties

- Short acting (anaesthesia lasts approximately 5–8 minutes after bolus injection); rapid onset of anaesthesia, as for thiopentone
- Respiratory depression (post-induction apnoea is frequently observed)
- Cardiovascular depression – hypotension due to mild myocardial depression and peripheral vascular dilation
- Rapid and smooth recovery – due to redistribution and rapid metabolism of the drug. The same principles of redistribution of this lipophilic drug apply as for thiopentone. The lack of 'hangover' effect, which is a key feature of recovery from propofol anaesthesia, is due to the rapid metabolism of propofol as it returns from tissue sites into blood
- Suitable for use as a maintenance agent. Infusions of propofol for up to 4 hours have been reported in dogs, and shorter infusions have been reported in cats. The pharmacokinetics of propofol make it particularly attractive for use by infusion and, for infusions of less than 2 hours, propofol has been shown to be highly satisfactory. In humans, maintenance of anaesthesia for prolonged periods (8 hours) has been associated with fast return of conciousness
- Fair muscle relaxation, but occasionally muscle rigidity is observed
- Not irritant if injected perivascularly
- May have some analgesic properties
- Propofol decreases cerebral blood flow and cerebral oxygen consumption, and it seems that the autoregulatory capacity of the cerebral circulation remains intact during propofol anaesthesia. It reduces intracranial pressure in both normal patients and patients with raised intracranial pressure, although cerebral perfusion pressure may be decreased
- Propofol showed anti-convulsant properties similar to thiopentone in animal models of status epilepticus. However, the UK Committee on Safety of Medicines has advised anaesthetists to use propofol with care in humans with epilepsy, because of reports of increased EEG epileptiform activity in some patients.

Use

Propofol is used to induce anaesthesia in dogs and cats. It provides a rapid smooth induction of anaesthesia and a fast excitement-free recovery with no 'hangover' effect. In humans, propofol has rapidly become the drug of choice for induction of anaesthesia in outpatients, because of these properties. Anaesthesia may be maintained with top-up doses or by an intravenous infusion of propofol, without altering the quality or duration of recovery. Apnoea at induction is frequently observed, since propofol, like thiopentone and methohexitone, is a respiratory depressant. This may be related to the speed of injection of the drug; the slower the injection, the lower the incidence of apnoea. Where necessary, the animal should be ventilated slowly until spontaneous breathing recommences.

Old animals have a reduced dose requirement for propofol. Preliminary evidence suggests that propofol induces respiratory depression in puppies delivered by Caesarian section when the bitch has been anaesthetized with propofol. However, provided low doses are used, it is probably satisfactory (see Chapter 18). It should be used with care in animals in shock, i.e. the dose and speed of injection should be reduced to avoid a sudden decrease in peripheral vascular resistance and myocardial depression, leading to cardiovascular collapse. The authors use propofol in animals with severe hepatopathy at a reduced dose rate with few complications. After induction of anaesthesia with propofol, there is little reduction in renal blood flow. This is in contrast to thiopentone and all the volatile anaesthetic agents, and therefore propofol is probably the agent of choice in animals with compromised renal function. Experience has shown that it is a satisfactory induction agent in puppies as young as 4 weeks. Because of its renal sparing effects and lack of anaesthetic 'hangover', it is the drug of choice for induction of anaesthesia in geriatric animals.

Dog

Induction

- Propofol alone: 5–6 mg/kg i.v. (males seem to require a slightly higher dose than females)
- In premedicated dogs: 3–4 mg/kg i.v. (the dose must be reduced markedly where premedication used an α_2-adrenoceptor agonist (approximately 1–2 mg/kg)).

Maintenance

- Incremental doses or by infusion (see below).

Cats

Induction

- 6–7 mg/kg i.v. (the dose does not seem to be influenced by prior sedation with acepromazine). A single dose produces anaesthesia lasting only approximately 10–15 minutes. The dose must be reduced markedly where premedication used an α_2-adrenoceptor agonist.

Maintenance

- Infusion rates of 0.2–0.5 mg/kg/min have been used to maintain anaesthesia. However, there are few data on the use of propofol by infusion in cats. Some cats exhibit retching and sneezing and may paw their faces during recovery.

Problems

- Occasional transient profound bradycardia after intravenous administration
- Due to increased sensitivity in debilitated or old animals, the dose rate needs to be reduced considerably (2–3 mg/kg)
- Enhanced effect and prolonged duration of action is likely in animals with hypoproteinaemia
- Repeat anaesthesia with propofol in cats (daily anaesthesia for 30 minutes for up to 7 days) has been associated with haematological toxicity (increasing Heinz body production), increased recovery times from anaesthesia and anorexia.

ETOMIDATE

The imidazole derivative etomidate is recommended for induction of anaesthesia for Caesarian section, for traumatized patients and for those with myocardial disease, liver disease or unstable haemodynamics. It decreases intracranial pressure in animals with severe intracranial lesions, decreases brain oxygen consumption and may have protective properties in the face of global ischaemia, making it a good agent to use for neurosurgical procedures. When etomidate is used alone in dogs at doses that produce general anaesthesia (1.5–3 mg/kg i.v.), heart rate, mean arterial blood pressure and myocardial performance remain stable. Side effects include sneezing, retching, myoclonus, pain on injection and phlebitis, but these can be minimized by the use of adequate sedative premedication. It is rapidly metabolized to inactive metabolites in the liver, and its pharmacokinetic characteristics should make it suitable for administration by repeat bolus or continuous infusion. Nevertheless, etomidate has been implicated in the development of Addisonian crises in intensive care patients during long-term infusion for sedation, and it also inhibits adrenal steroidogenesis in dogs. While this is unlikely to be a problem with a single induction dose of 3 mg/kg, long-term infusion may have serious endocrine effects. In practice, continuous infusion of etomidate is precluded by haemolysis that is probably caused by the 35% (v/v) propylene glycol in which it is supplied.

TOTAL INTRAVENOUS ANAESTHESIA

Total intravenous anaesthesia offers many advantages to the anaesthetist and veterinary surgeon. It is relatively easy to administer, although intravenous access must be secure, and consequently the animal must have an intravenous cannula placed before induction of anaesthesia. Recovery is primarily determined by the pharmacokinetic profiles of the drugs used and can be faster than after inhalation anaesthesia, where recovery is largely governed by physicochemical properties such as the blood/gas solubility coefficient. The use of TIVA eliminates any possible hazards to people associated with exposure to trace concentrations of volatile and gaseous anaesthetic agents.

Of all the anaesthetic drugs currently licensed, propofol has a pharmacokinetic profile that makes it the most suitable drug for maintenance of anaesthesia by continuous infusion. It has a short duration of action, which is related to its redistribution within the body and its rapid metabolism to inactive substances. Pharmacokinetic data from dogs have shown that it is cleared rapidly from the body indicating that, on recovery from anaesthesia, a considerably smaller proportion of propofol than, for example, thiopentone, is present in the body. It is because of this high clearance rate that propofol can be used successfully to maintain anaesthesia.

Propofol infusions of up to 2 hours have been used by several groups to maintain anaesthesia in dogs undergoing a variety of surgical procedures. Dose rates of between 0.3 and 0.5 mg/kg/min seem to be necessary in premedicated spontaneously breathing dogs to ensure surgical anaesthesia. In Greyhounds, slower recovery from anaesthesia by up to 2 hours has been reported after propofol infusion. Delayed recovery can arise if anaesthesia is prolonged and the propofol infusion is not reduced in a stepwise manner over time. Propofol infusions in cats have not been studied in detail. A recent report showing that propofol induced toxic side effects in cats when infused for 30 minutes repeatedly over a 7-day period, may have significance clinically where prolonged infusions are necessary.

Propofol may have some analgesic properties, but for surgery, supplemental analgesia is recommended. This can be provided by intermittent administration or continuous infusion of an opioid drug such as alfentanil. However, there are limited data available on the use of propofol/alfentanil infusions clinically in small animals, and although this combination is used frequently in humans, it is not yet recommended for dogs or cats. It may prove to be a successful technique in mechanically ventilated animals, but it is unlikely to be used where spontaneous breathing is desired. Alternatively, pethidine (meperidine) or morphine may be given as a premedicant and topped up as required during the perioperative period, while the use of 67% nitrous oxide will also reduce the propofol requirement and provide analgesia. Maintenance of anaesthesia with propofol has depressant effects on the cardiovascular and respiratory systems. However, in healthy animals maintained in a light plane of surgical anaesthesia, these effects are mild. The blood propofol concentration required to maintain anaesthesia has been reasonably well defined and seems to be similar across a range of species (approximately 3-7 µg/ml, with nitrous oxide, depending on the severity of the surgical procedure; 5-10 µg/ml when propofol is used alone).

More recent advances in anaesthesia have included the development of target controlled infusions (TCI) of propofol. The anaesthetist uses a computer programmed syringe driver that infuses propofol to achieve the desired blood propofol concentration. This system is now used in humans. It is simple to use and gives excellent control over the depth of anaesthesia. Recent work in dogs in the authors' hospital has shown the usefulness of this technique, and this represents a new method of anaesthesia for development in animals in the near future.

NEUROLEPTANAESTHETIC MIXTURES

Neuroleptanalgesic mixtures may be administered in large doses so that the animal becomes virtually unconscious, at which point they may then be loosely termed neuroleptanaesthetic mixtures. Such mixtures are combinations of a potent opioid and a sedative/tranquillizer drug, and are therefore used only in dogs. In animals that are old, debilitated or have moderate to severe systemic disease, the use of proprietary combinations should be avoided. Proprietary combinations should not be confused with home made neuroleptanalgesic mixtures (e.g. acepromazine and pethidine for sedation/premedication, or fentanyl and diazepam for induction of anaesthesia). Further details on the use of neuroleptanalgesic mixtures may be found in Chapter 7 and in the specific chapters on anaesthetic management.

Proprietary neuroleptanalgesic combinations

Advantages

- Ease of administration may be considered an advantage
- Potential for administration of an antagonist.

Disadvantages

- The narcotic component of some combinations produces such marked respiratory depression and cardiovascular impairment that it is essential to provide a secure airway and an oxygen enriched atmosphere if hypoxia is to be avoided. Moreover, intermittent positive-pressure ventilation may be required to avoid severe hypercapnia. Bradycardia is frequently a feature in dogs, and arterial hypotension occurs
- The potent narcotic provides good analgesia but, unfortunately, administration of a narcotic antagonist at the end of surgery not only reverses anaesthesia but also abolishes all pain relief and renders the further administration of any narcotic analgesic virtually useless for a considerable period of time
- Poor muscle relaxation
- In the UK, these are controlled drugs under the Misuse of Drugs Act, 1971. In the USA, they are regulated under the Controlled Substances Act, 1970
- Potential for accidental or deliberate self-administration, which may be fatal (applies to etorphine hydrochloride-methotrimeprazine (see below))
- Sensitivity to noise and lights
- May cause defecation and vomition.

Etorphine and methotrimeprazine

This combination includes 0.074 mg/ml etorphine hydrochloride and 18 mg/ml methotrimeprazine. It is marketed with its antagonist, which contains 0.295 mg/ml diprenorphine hydrochloride.

Dose

- 0.05 ml/kg i.v.
- 0.1 ml/kg i.m.

Onset

- Immediate after intravenous administration
- Five minutes after intramuscular administration.

Duration

- 60-90 minutes
- Full recovery takes up to 2 hours.

Use of etorphine hydrochloride and methotrimeprazine in small animals

Atropine may be given to counteract bradycardia, although this may precipitate cardiac arrhythmias, particularly if supplemental oxygen is not being administered.

There is a considerable degree of risk associated with its use in elderly dogs and in debilitated or sick animals.

Not recommended for use.

Fluanisone/fentanyl citrate

This combination includes the butyrophenone tranquillizer fluanisone, 10 mg/ml, and the potent opioid, fentanyl citrate, 0.315 mg/ml. It is licensed for use in rats, rabbits, guinea pigs and mice. It is not licensed for use in dogs.

Further details of its use may be found in Chapter 7 and in specific chapters on anaesthetic management.

CONCLUSIONS

Despite seeming to offer the advantages of simplicity, the use of intravenous anaesthetic agents alone without proper regard for normal good anaesthetic management cannot be condoned. It is always vital to ensure that the airway is open and secure from inhalation of foreign material. Hypoventilation and hypoxia must be avoided, and equipment for artificial ventilation with oxygen must be available. Lack of these basic facilities can no longer be defended.

In addition, proper care must be taken to ensure that hypothermia does not occur, fluid balance is maintained and that no animal should be discharged from the care of a veterinary surgeon until fully recovered from the effects of anaesthesia.

FURTHER READING

Andress JL, Day TK and Day DG (1995) The effects of consecutive day propofol anesthesia on feline red blood cells. *Veterinary Surgery* **24**, 277–282

Brearley JC, Kellagher REB and Hall LW (1988) Propofol anaesthesia in cats. *Journal of Small Animal Practice* **29**, 315–322

Cullen LK and Jones RS (1977) Clinical observations on xylazine/ketamine anaesthesia in the cat. *Veterinary Record* **101**, 115–116

Hall LW and Chambers JP (1987) A clinical trial of propofol infusion anaesthesia in dogs. *Journal of Small Animal Practice* **28**, 623–637

Hall LW and Clarke KW (1983) *Veterinary Anaesthesia, 8th edn.* Baillière Tindall, London

Hall LW, Lagerweij E and Nolan AM (1993) Effects of medetomidine premedication on propofol infusion anaesthesia in dogs. *Journal of Veterinary Anaesthesia* **20**, 78–83

Haskins SC, Patz JD and Farver TB (1986) Xylazine and xylazine-ketamine in dogs. *American Journal of Veterinary Research* **47**, 636–641

Jones RS (1979) Injectable anaesthetic agents in the cat: a review. *Journal of Small Animal Practice* **20**, 345–352

Lin HC, Thurmon JC, Benson GJ and Tranquilli WJ (1993) Telazol – a review of its pharmacology and use in veterinary medicine. *Journal of Veterinary Pharmacology and Therapeutics* **16**, 383–418

Nolan AM and Reid J (1993) Pharmacokinetics of propofol given by intravenous infusion in dogs undergoing surgery. *British Journal of Anaesthesia* **70**, 546–551

Robertson SA, Johnston S and Beemsterboer J (1992) Cardiopulmonary, anesthetic and postanesthetic effects of intravenous infusions of propofol in greyhounds and non-greyhounds. *American Journal of Veterinary Research* **53**, 1027–1032

Thurmon JC, Tranquilli WJ and Benson GJ (1996) *Lumb and Jones' Veterinary Anesthesia, 3rd edn.* Williams and Wilkins, Baltimore

Watkins SB, Hall LW and Clarke KW (1987) Propofol as an intravenous anaesthetic agent in dogs. *Veterinary Record* **120**, 326–329

CHAPTER NINE

Inhalant Anaesthetics

John W. Ludders

INTRODUCTION

Since their discovery and subsequent use in veterinary medicine, general anaesthetics have made it possible for veterinarians to manage animal patients surgically in a manner that is humane and relatively safe. However, it is the inhalant anaesthetics that have made it possible for veterinary surgeons to extend the boundaries of the surgical sciences. It is these drugs that have enabled veterinarians to anaesthetize animals more safely and for longer periods of time, thus enabling surgical procedures that would have been impossible 20 years ago. This chapter discusses the inhalant anaesthetics in most common use in veterinary medicine today.

PHYSICOCHEMICAL PROPERTIES

The physical and chemical properties of inhalant anaesthetics determine how and why these drugs are used. Figure 9.1 summarizes these properties. These anaesthetics are either halogenated hydrocarbons (halothane), halogenated ethers (desflurane, enflurane, isoflurane, methoxyflurane and sevoflurane) or inorganic gases (nitrous oxide). Nitrous oxide (N_2O) will be discussed as a special case at the end of this section.

Preservatives

Only enflurane, isoflurane and sevoflurane are stable in the presence of light and do not require preservatives for storage. Both halothane and methoxyflurane can be degraded by sunlight to toxic end products, and for this reason they are supplied in dark coloured bottles. In addition, a preservative (0.01% thymol) is added to halothane to increase its stability. As halothane vaporizes within a vaporizer the thymol accumulates as a residue, which can affect the mechanical operation and output characteristics of the vaporizer. For example, a halothane vaporizer that has not been cleaned for some time may have a turnstile that rotates with difficulty mainly due to the sticky nature of the thymol residue. To ensure proper function, it is recommended that all vaporizers should be periodically cleaned and calibrated in accordance with the manufacturer's guidelines.

Reaction with metal and carbon dioxide absorbent

Halothane and methoxyflurane react with certain metals such as aluminium and brass. Thus, anaesthetic equipment should be built with alternative materials.

Carbon monoxide

To some degree, all inhalant anaesthetics react with soda lime to produce carbon monoxide (CO), but the magnitude of CO production is greatest with desflurane and enflurane, intermediate with isoflurane and least with halothane and sevoflurane (Fang *et al.*, 1995). The toxicity of CO is well known, and its accumulation in breathing circuits should be avoided. This interaction is not quantitatively sufficient to preclude the use of inhalant anaesthetics; however, to reduce the accumulation of CO in circle and to-and-fro systems, inhalant anaesthetics should not be used with dry carbon dioxide (CO_2) absorbent and thus the absorbent should be periodically and regularly replaced with fresh moist absorbent. Furthermore, since prolonged contact of inhalant anaesthetics with absorbent enhances the production of CO, a system that has not been used for several days, for example over a weekend, should be flushed with oxygen before using the breathing circuit.

Compound A

Compound A (CF_2=C(CF_3)-O-CH_2F) is a degradation product that results from the interaction of sevoflurane with CO_2 absorbent. There is some controversy about the toxicity of Compound A as it has been shown to produce renal failure in rats, but not in humans or other animals, including dogs (Bito and Ikeda, 1994; Bito *et al.*, 1997; Muir and Gadawski, 1998). Baralyme produces a four-fold greater degradation of sevoflurane vapour to Compound A than does soda lime (Liu *et al.*, 1991). Others have concluded that the variability in concentrations of Compound A found in clinical practice may be due to a number of factors, including fresh gas flow rate and degree of rebreathing, sevoflurane concentration and the temperature and dryness of the absorbent (Fang *et al.*, 1996). The effect of dry CO_2 absorbent on the production of Compound A seems to be complex – fresh but dry absorbent destroys Compound A as it is made while dry absorbent that has been exposed to sevoflurane

Property	Enflurane	Halothane	Isoflurane	Methoxyflurane	Desflurane	Sevoflurane	Nitrous oxide
Formula	$CHFCl-CF-O-CHF_2$	$CBrClH-CF_3$	$CF_3-CHCl-O-CF_2H$	$CHCl_2-CF_2-O-CH_3$	$CF_3-CHF-O-CF_2H$	$CFH_2-O-(CF_3)_2$	N_2O
Type of volatile anaesthetic	Ether	Halogenated hydrocarbon	Ether	Ether	Ether	Ether	Inorganic gas
Molecular weight	184.5	197.4	184.5	165.0	168.0	187.0	44.0
Specific gravity @ 25°C	1.52	1.86	1.50	1.41	–	–	–
Preservatives	Not needed	Required	Not needed	Required	Not needed	Not needed	Not needed
Reacts with:							
Soda lime	No	Yes	No	Yes	No	Yes	No
Ultraviolet light	No	Yes	No	Yes	–	–	–
Metal	No	Yes	No	Yes	No	No	–
Boiling point (°C) @ 760 mmHg	56.5	50.2	48.5	104.7	23.5	–	-89
Vapour pressure (mmHg)							
20°C	171.8	244.1	239.5	22.8	681	170	–
22°C	188.6	265.5	261.8	25.5	743	–	–
24°C	206.6	288.3	285.8	28.4	–	–	–
Vapour concentration							
% saturation @ 20°C	22.6	32.1	31.5	3.0	89.6	22.4	–
% saturation @ 22°C	24.8	34.9	34.4	3.3	97.8	–	–
Millilitres of vapour/ml of liquid @ 20°C	197.5	227	194.7	206.9	209.7	182.7	–
Solubility coefficients:							
Blood/gas	2.0	2.5	1.5	15.0	0.42	0.68	0.47
Oil/gas	96.0	224.0	91.0	970.0	18.7	47.0	1.4
Fat/gas	83.0	51.0	45.0	902.0	27.0	48.0	1.08

Figure 9.1: Physicochemical properties and some solubility characteristics (solvent/gas) of volatile anaesthetics.

Adapted from Quasha et al. (1980) and Steffey (1996) with permission.

for a period of time can produce unusually high concentrations of Compound A (Fang *et al.*, 1996).

Vapour pressure and vaporizers

Each inhalant anaesthetic has a unique range of vapour pressures that depend on its temperature (Figure 9.1); as temperature increases so does vapour pressure. At a comfortable room temperature of 20°C, the range of vapour pressures varies widely, from 23 mmHg for methoxyflurane to 681 mmHg for desflurane. From this information can be derived the maximum possible concentration for a given anaesthetic. For example, at 20°C and 760 mmHg (barometric pressure at sea level), the maximum concentration of methoxyflurane is 3% (23/760 x 100) while, under the same conditions of temperature and pressure, desflurane can achieve a concentration of 89%. Since only fractions of the maximum possible concentration of any inhalant anaesthetic are needed to maintain anaesthesia safely in a patient, a method is needed to control the delivery of clinically useful concentrations to a patient. Vaporizers are designed to regulate and control factors that influence the vaporization of liquid anaesthetics, and a number of design characteristics are used to define vaporizers. Other sections in this manual describe vaporizers that are uniquely designed and calibrated for specific anaesthetics. However, there are other vaporizers that can volatilize any anaesthetic, but that require the anaesthetist to calculate gas flows to determine the concentration of delivered anaesthetic.

Measured flow vaporizers

The use of a measured flow vaporizer requires that the anaesthetist know the temperature of the liquid anaesthetic and calculate the carrier and diluting gas flows needed to deliver a desired concentration of anaesthetic to a patient. In the past, when these were the most common type of vaporizers, the manufacturers provided calculators like slide rules to assist anaesthetists, but these calculators are no longer made.

Some older Foregger anaesthesia machines have a Vernitrol vaporizer incorporated into the machine, which uses a thermal percentage system for determining anaesthetic delivery to the patient. The diluent gas flowmeter has two scales: one showing the gas flow in millilitres per minute and the other showing temperature in degrees centigrade. The flowmeter controlling gas flow to the vaporizer also has two scales: one showing gas flow to the vaporizer in millilitres per minute and the other showing the percentage of anaesthetic vapour to be delivered to the patient. Vaporizer output is determined by setting the diluent flowmeter to the temperature of the vaporizer and the vaporizer flowmeter to the desired anaesthetic vapour concentration.

For other measured flow vaporizers, such as the Copper Kettle or side-arm Vernitrol, output can be determined by using the formula:

$$F = \frac{C \times D \times (1-Z)}{Z - C}$$

where F is flow through the vaporizer, C is desired anaesthetic concentration, D is total fresh gas flow and Z is the ratio of anaesthetic vapour pressure to barometric pressure.

For example, using a Copper Kettle, an anaesthetist wants to deliver 1% halothane to a patient and wants the total fresh gas flow (D) to be 3 l/min of oxygen. Barometric pressure is 760 mmHg and the temperature of the liquid anaesthetic is 20°C (a halothane vapour pressure of 244 mmHg). Using the above formula, where $C = 0.01$, $D = 3000$ ml/min and $Z = 244/760 = 0.32$

$$F = \frac{0.01 \times 3000 \times (1 - 0.32)}{(0.32 - 0.01)}$$

$F = 65.8$ ml/min through the vaporizer.

Finally, mental calculations can be used (easy to do with halothane and isoflurane). From the example above the ratio of halothane vapour pressure (at 20°C) to barometric pressure is 0.32, or roughly 33%. This means that about one-third of the vaporizer output is halothane and two-thirds are the gas delivered to the vaporizer (in this case oxygen). More specifically, the output from the vaporizer consists of 33 ml of halothane vapour per minute and 66 ml of oxygen per minute. To dilute the 33 ml of halothane vapour from 33% to 1% requires a diluent flow of about 3000 ml/min.

Another example: if 100 ml of oxygen is delivered to a Copper Kettle containing halothane at 20°C, how much diluent gas flow is required to achieve a 1% halothane vapour concentration? The input to the vaporizer of 100 ml represents two-thirds of the eventual output. Thus total output will be 150 ml/min of which 50 ml is halothane vapour. To dilute the halothane vapour to 1%, about 5000 ml of diluent gas flow will be needed. This approach works just as well for isoflurane because it has nearly the same vapour pressure as halothane.

These mental exercises serve to show why anaesthetic vaporizers have moved away from the measured flow design. Although the math is easy, a miscalculation (not unlikely under stressful circumstances) can be fatal for the patient. Furthermore, the design of these older machines and their lack of safety devices makes it possible to turn on the gas flow to the vaporizer without the diluent gas flow and thus deliver very high and potentially lethal concentrations of anaesthetic.

Nitrous oxide

Critical temperature is that temperature above which the molecules of a substance are too active to be compressed into the liquid state; above critical temperature the substance is a gas. Because the boiling point for N_2O at 760 mmHg is -89°C and its critical temperature is 36°C, it is a vapour at room temperature (20°C). At room temperature, N_2O is provided as a liquid in full cylinders under 750 p.s.i. (about 50 atmospheres; 5000 kPa). For gases such as oxygen, the volume remaining in a cylinder can easily be determined by looking at the pressure gauge on the cylinder. This is not the case for N_2O because the pressure gauge will read full as long as there is liquid N_2O remaining in the cylinder. It is only after all of the liquid has volatilized that the gauge starts to decrease and indicates the amount of vapour left in the cylinder. To determine how much liquid N_2O remains in a cylinder, the full and empty weights of the cylinder must be known; by subtracting the known empty weight from the current weight it is possible to determine how much liquid N_2O remains in the cylinder. Further details may be found in Chapter 4.

Nitrous oxide has some physical characteristics that distinguish it from other inhalant anaesthetics. It has a very low coefficient of solubility in blood, oil and fat, so that its uptake and equilibration throughout the body is very rapid. Because it is used in large volumes and its uptake is rapid during the induction phase of anaesthesia, it enhances the uptake of a second anaesthetic gas (second gas and concentration effects), especially the more soluble inhalants. Clinically, this means that the speed of induction can be enhanced by using N_2O during induction of anaesthesia with an inhalant, a feature that is particularly helpful during mask inductions. The down side of using N_2O is the phenomenon of dilutional (diffusion) hypoxia. This typically occurs at the time when the N_2O is turned off and the patient is disconnected from the breathing circuit and starts to breathe room air consisting of 20% oxygen. Nitrous oxide, however, is used in large volumes during anaesthesia (usually 50% or greater), and when it is turned off its uptake is reversed and it moves from the blood to the alveoli. Thus, during the first 5 to 10 minutes after discontinuing the N_2O, the volume moving into the lung is large and dilutes the oxygen in the alveoli. This may not be clinically significant in animals with adequate pulmonary function or those inhaling high concentrations of oxygen, but in patients with reduced pulmonary reserves and breathing air or with additional demands for oxygen (e.g. shivering), the dilutional hypoxia can be life threatening. The best solution is to keep patients attached to the breathing circuit and to allow them to breathe 100% oxygen for the first 5 to 10 minutes after discontinuing N_2O.

MAC AND ITS APPLICATION TO CLINICAL PRACTICE

The term MAC refers to the minimum alveolar concentration of an anaesthetic at one atmosphere that produces immobility in 50% of subjects exposed to a supramaximal noxious stimulus (Steffey, 1996); hence, it is a measure of anaesthetic potency. It is also a standard measurement that is applicable to all inhalant anaesthetics and makes it possible to compare equipotent doses of inhaled anaesthetics in terms of their effects, and to quantify factors that influence anaesthetic requirements (Figure 9.2). When applying the concept of MAC to clinical practice it must be kept in mind that MAC is usually determined in healthy unmedicated animals and that a number of patient-related factors may increase or decrease MAC (Figure 9.3). For example, the MAC of a given inhalant is reduced by the concomitant use of analgesics (opioids), sedative hypnotics (α_2 agonists) or tranquillizers. Morphine administered to dogs reduces MAC by 17–33%, depending on the dose used; acepromazine (0.02–0.2 mg/kg i.m.) reduces halothane MAC by about 40%

Species	Enflurane	Methoxyflurane	Halothane	Isoflurane	Desflurane	Sevoflurane	Nitrous oxide
Cat	1.2	0.23	1.14	1.63	9.8	2.58	255
Dog	2.06-2.2	0.23	0.87	1.28	7.2	2.1-2.36	188-297
Horse	2.12	2.8	0.88	1.31	7.6	2.31	205
Swine	—	—	0.91	2.04	10.0	2.66	162-277
Sandhill Crane	—	—	—	1.34	—	—	—
Duck	—	—	1.03	1.30	—	—	—
Rabbit	—	—	0.82	—	8.9	3.7	—
Monkey (Stump-tailed macaque)	—	—	0.89	—	—	—	200
Rat	—	0.27	1.11-1.17	1.38	5.7-7.1	2.45	136-235

Figure 9.2: *Minimum alveolar concentrations (MAC) (volume %) for inhalant anaesthetics in selected animals.*

Adapted from Quasha et al. (1980) and Steffey (1996) with permission.

Factors affecting MAC
• Circadian rhythms
• Metabolic acidosis – causes a slight decrease in MAC (methodology affects the results)
• Hypoxia – MAC is decreased when PaO_2 is below 38 mmHg
• Anaemia – when oxygen (O_2) content is <4.3 ml O_2/100 ml blood (haematocrit = 13%), MAC is decreased
• Hypotension – decreases MAC
• Neurotransmitter release – increases MAC
• Age – older animals require less anaesthetic
• Temperature – increasing temperature increases the cerebral metabolic rate of the brain and increases MAC
• Thyroid function – whole body O_2 consumption minimally affects MAC; in dogs, changing from gross hypothyroidism to gross hyperthyroidism increases MAC by only 20%

• Electrolytes and osmolality – in general, changes in serum electrolytes or osmolality alter anaesthetic requirement when they are accompanied by changes in brain sodium concentrations
 	
     Lithium – decreases MAC
 	
     Calcium – very high cerebrospinal fluid (CSF) calcium ion concentrations produce a state resembling general anaesthesia
 	
     Bromine – decreases MAC
 	
     Sodium
 	
         Hypernatraemia – increases MAC
 	
         Serum and CSF hypo-osmolality dilute CSF sodium and decrease MAC

• Narcotics – decrease MAC
• Sedatives and tranquillizers – decrease MAC
• Local anaesthetics – decrease MAC
• Pregnancy – decreases MAC
• Other inhalant anaesthetics (nitrous oxide) – decrease MAC

Factors NOT affecting MAC
• Type of stimulation
• Duration of anaesthesia
• Species – from species to species MAC varies by 10–20%. Interspecies variation may be explained by variations in techniques
• Sex
• Hypocarbia and hypercarbia within the range of 14–95 mmHg
• Metabolic alkalosis
• Hypoxia and hyperoxia – within the range of 38–500 mmHg, oxygen does not affect MAC. Below 38 mmHg, hypoxia induces progressive narcosis and reduces MAC
• Hypertension

• Electrolytes and osmolality
 	
     Potassium – no effect
 	
     Hyperosmolality – no consistent change in MAC

Figure 9.3: Patient-related factors that do and do not affect minimum alveolar concentration (MAC).

Reproduced from Quasha et al. (1980) with permission.

Species	Halothane AI	Isoflurane AI
Dog	2.9	2.51
Cat	–	2.40
Horse	2.6	2.33
Duck	1.51	1.65

Figure 9.4: *Anaesthetic index (AI) for halothane and isoflurane in four animal species.*

(Heard *et al.*, 1986); and medetomidine (30 µg/kg i.v.) reduces isoflurane MAC by 53% (Ewing *et al.*, 1993) Disease states also affect MAC. In a rodent model of sepsis, isoflurane MAC was reduced by 57% (Gill *et al.*, 1995).

Anaesthetic index

The anaesthetic index (AI) is derived by dividing the end-tidal concentration of an anaesthetic that produces apnoea by the MAC for the anaesthetic (Figure 9.4). Thus AI is a measure of the tendency for an inhalant anaesthetic to cause respiratory depression and apnoea. The lower the AI for an anaesthetic, the greater is its depressant effect on ventilation.

MAC and N_2O

The MAC for N_2O in the dog and cat ranges between 188% and 297% (see Figure 9.2), whereas its MAC in humans is 105%. Thus the MAC for N_2O cannot be achieved at normal barometric pressures. Furthermore, N_2O is not as potent an anaesthetic in animals as it is in humans and cannot be used by itself to produce general anaesthesia. However, when N_2O is used at concentrations of 50% to 66%, the MAC of a concomitantly used primary anaesthetic, such as halothane or isoflurane, can be reduced by 20% to 35%. Since these inhalant anaesthetics depress cardiopulmonary function in a dose-dependent manner, N_2O-mediated reduction in MAC can be used to spare cardiopulmonary function.

When using anaesthetic gas mixtures that include N_2O, the anaesthetist must make certain that the inspired concentration of oxygen is at least 30%. This is easy to do when using relatively high gas flows as all that is required is to make sure that the oxygen flow is 30% or more of the total fresh gas flow. However, if a low flow closed circuit technique is used, then either N_2O should not be used as part of the gas mixture or an oxygen analyser must be used to ensure that the fraction of inspired oxygen is ≥ 30% (see Chapter 4).

PHYSIOLOGICAL EFFECTS OF INHALANT ANAESTHETICS

Cardiopulmonary effects

All inhalant anaesthetics, except N_2O, depress cardiopulmonary function in a dose-dependent manner, as shown by decreases in cardiac output, arterial blood pressure and glomerular filtration rate and increases in the partial pressure of CO_2 in arterial blood ($PaCO_2$). The degree to which inhalants depress cardiopulmonary function, however, varies from anaesthetic to anaesthetic, and it is these differences that usually guide selection of one inhalant over another.

Myocardial contractility

All anaesthetic inhalants depress myocardial contractility to some degree or another, and it seems that the mechanism of action is interference with calcium flux and content within the sarcoplasmic reticulum of myocardial cells. Myocardial contractility is affected most by halothane, then enflurane and least by isoflurane (Simpson, 1993). Desflurane and sevoflurane seem to affect contractility in a manner similar to isoflurane.

Systemic vascular resistance

Isoflurane, desflurane and sevoflurane are more potent vasodilators than either halothane or enflurane. The typical cardiac response to vasodilation is an increase in heart rate, and this probably explains the higher heart rate observed with isoflurane compared with halothane.

Cardiac arrhythmias

The threshold for adrenaline (epinephrine)-induced cardiac arrhythmias is lower with halothane than with enflurane, methoxyflurane or isoflurane. In fact dogs or cats that develop ventricular premature contractions during halothane anaesthesia often can be converted to normal sinus rhythm when they are switched to enflurane or isoflurane anaesthesia. Again, in terms of their arrhythmic effects, both desflurane and sevoflurane seem to be similar to isoflurane.

Pulmonary function

Isoflurane is a more potent respiratory depressant than halothane (see above).

Hepatic effects

Halothane has been implicated as a causative agent of hepatitis, but the relationship is multifactorial and requires other contributing factors such as hypoxia, drug-induced induction of hepatic enzymes or immune-mediated factors. Methoxyflurane and enflurane, although they have received less bad press concerning hepatitis than halothane, have been associated with anaesthesia-induced hepatitis. Isoflurane seems to be much less likely to do so, and this may be due to the lack of toxic metabolites associated with its non-pulmonary metabolism and excretion as well as to its low blood/gas solubility.

Renal effects

All of the inhalant anaesthetics can indirectly affect renal function by depressing cardiovascular function and, thus, glomerular blood flow and filtration. In addition, metabolism of the fluorinated ethers (methoxyflurane, isoflurane, sevoflurane and desflurane) produces fluoride ions as metabolites that can cause renal tubular damage. However, the rate of metabolism and the concentrations of fluoride ions achieved varies with the agent. Following methoxyflurane anaesthesia in humans, plasma fluoride concentrations achieved sufficiently high levels to produce renal tubular damage and high output renal failure. However, this phenomenon has not been observed in dogs (Pedersoli, 1977a,b; Fleming and Pedersoli, 1980), possibly because the canine kidney is more resistant to the effects of fluoride ions than is the human kidney. Studies of the other fluorinated ethers have shown that the rate of metabolism is considerably less than that of methoxyflurane. For example, sevoflurane metabolism is approximately one-third that of methoxyflurane, and 1.5–2 times that of enflurane, while that of desflurane is minimal (Kharasch, 1996) as is the case for isoflurane. Although the canine kidney may be more resistant to the effects of fluoride ions, it is reasonable not to use methoxyflurane for a patient with renal disease. If there is no other option, then recommendations from the human literature suggest that methoxyflurane anaesthesia should be limited to no more than 2 MAC hours, i.e. the end-tidal concentration should not exceed MAC (0.23% in the dog) for more than 2 hours.

Central nervous system effects

The major concerns for properly managing anaesthesia in patients with intracranial disease is to prevent clinically significant increases in intracranial pressure while preserving cerebral perfusion pressure and cerebral blood flow, so that the metabolic needs of the brain are met (see Chapter 20). Halothane, isoflurane, sevoflurane, desflurane and methoxyflurane all decrease the metabolic rate of the brain ($CMRO_2$). However, isoflurane and sevoflurane seem to decrease $CMRO_2$ more than they decrease cerebral blood flow, thus preserving a positive or near normal energy state in the brain. This is not the case for halothane. Enflurane at increasing levels of MAC produces seizures.

COST CONSIDERATIONS

The choice of which anaesthetic to use in practice is often influenced by cost considerations. The purchase price of an anaesthetic is certainly important, but the total cost of using a given anaesthetic is also determined by the drugs that are used to premedicate patients (premedicated patients need lower concentrations of anaesthetics), and the gas flows that are used. Figure 9.5 compares the cost of halothane with isoflurane at three fresh gas flows and two vaporizer dial settings. As can be seen, by using a low flow

Method for calculating millilitres of vapour and millilitres of liquid anaesthetic						
millilitres of vapour = (vaporizer dial setting (%) ÷ 100) x flow to vaporizer (ml/min) x time (min);						
millilitres of liquid anaesthetic = millilitres of vapour ÷ millilitres of vapour/ml of liquid @ 20°C (see Figure 9.1)						
Anaesthetic	**Vaporizer setting (%)**	**Fresh gas flow through vaporizer (l/min)**	**Time (min)**	**Millilitres of vapour**	**Millilitres of liquid**	**Cost £ ($) (1998)**
Halothane	2	3	120	7200	31.7	4.43 (1.98)
United Kingdom:	2	1	120	2400	10.6	1.48 (0.63)
£34 per 250 ml or	2	0.14*	120	336	1.5	0.21 (0.09)
£0.14 per ml	1	3	120	3600	15.9	2.23 (0.95)
United States:	1	1	120	1200	5.3	0.74 (0.31)
$15 per 250 ml or $0.06 per ml						
Isoflurane	2	3	120	7200	37.0	17.76 (16.65)
United Kingdom:	2	1	120	2400	12.3	5.98 (5.54)
£119 per 250 ml	2	0.14*	120	336	1.7	0.82 (0.77)
or £0.48 per ml	1	3	120	3600	18.5	8.88 (8.33)
United States:	1	1	120	1200	6.2	2.98 (2.79)
$45 per 100 ml or $0.45 per ml						

Figure 9.5: Cost comparison of halothane and isoflurane at three gas flows and two vaporizer settings.

* This flow could be used in a low flow technique (7 ml/kg/min) for a dog weighing 20 kg.

CHAPTER TEN

Neuromuscular Blockade

Ronald S. Jones

INTRODUCTION

It has been known for many centuries that, when hunting for food, South American indians used compounds on the tips of their arrows that could paralyse animals. These people showed great perception in developing this hunting technique and, in particular, taking advantage of the fact that curare is not absorbed from the gastrointestinal tract. This meant that animals killed by this technique could be eaten without any problems from the mode of slaughter.

The first recorded administration of curare to animals was by Sir Benjamin Brody, in 1811. He was also the first person to show that artificial ventilation could maintain life in an animal paralysed by curare.

The first clinical attempt to use curare in canine anaesthesia was by Pickett, in 1951. He administered the pure alkaloid, but there were three reasons why his results were unimpressive. First, the preparation was crude, second, he did not appreciate that the compound released histamine in the dog and, third, the dogs were allowed to breathe spontaneously. The first report on the use of the depolarizing muscle relaxant, suxamethonium, was by Hall, in 1952.

Following the initial description of the technique by Gray and Halton, Gray and another colleague, Rees, divided general anaesthesia into three components and developed the triad concept. This was based on the effects that were required in the patient, i.e. narcosis, muscle relaxation and analgesia. Later, Gray suggested that the word analgesia was a misnomer and that the correct term should be 'freedom from harmful reflex responses to the trauma of operation'. This was based on the view that as analgesia means freedom from pain and, as the unconscious individual cannot 'feel' pain, it is incorrect. It implied that actions such as movement and an increase in heart rate in response to a painful stimulus could not occur in the unconscious individual. Reflex depression was, therefore, the preferred and more accurate term.

Most individual general anaesthetics, when used at conventional doses, inadequately fulfil at least one component of the triad of anaesthesia. All general anaesthetic agents depress central nervous function to produce narcosis. Unfortunately, at clinically useful doses they also tend to depress the protective reflexes that compensate for factors such as blood loss. They also depress the cardiovascular and respiratory systems and may affect liver and kidney function. To minimize these untoward side-effects it is usual to minimize the dose of general anaesthetic used. Under these circumstances it may be necessary to use specific drugs to fulfil the other components of the triad of anaesthesia. Neuromuscular blocking agents may be used to provide muscle relaxation; their use is discussed in detail below.

To ensure that reflex depression is adequate during surgery under anaesthesia using a muscle relaxant technique, it is usual to give an analgesic drug as part of the premedication. In addition, agents that are used to supplement N_2O, either other inhalational agents or opioid analgesic drugs, will produce reflex depression.

PHYSIOLOGY OF NEUROMUSCULAR TRANSMISSION

In order to appreciate the action of drugs that act at the neuromuscular junction (NMJ, Figure 10.1), it is essential to be familiar with the physiology of neuromuscular transmission. A large myelinated nerve from the ventral horn of the spinal cord carries impulses to the muscle, branching extensively as it approaches the muscle. The nerve carries stimuli to several muscle fibres that must be activated simultaneously to produce a muscle contraction. As the nerve approaches the muscle cell, its branches lose their myelin sheaths. The nerve terminals lie in grooves on the surface of the muscle fibre and are covered by a Schwann cell. The area where the nerve ending lies in close proximity to the muscle fibre is the NMJ. The muscle fibre membrane, which forms the groove in which the nerve terminals lie, is deeply corrugated, and these corrugations are called secondary clefts. Deeper to the secondary clefts is a region rich in mitochondria, which covers

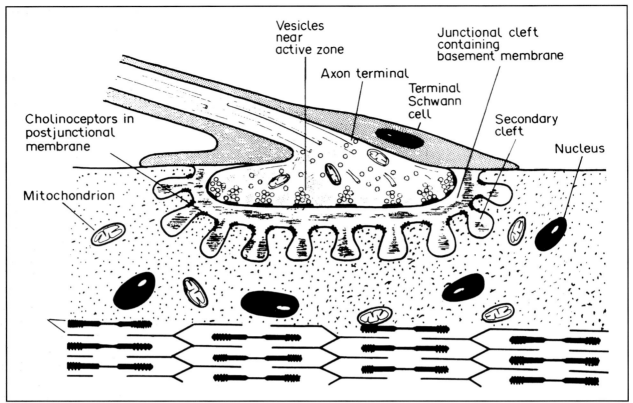

Figure 10.1: *Neuromuscular junction. The axon terminal contains mitochondria, microtubules and acetylcholine-containing vesicles.*

Reproduced from Jones and Payne (1988) with permission of the Royal Society of Medicine.

the contractile mechanisms of the muscle. The small gap between the nerve terminals and the muscle membrane, which is up to 60 nm wide, is known as the junctional cleft.

An action potential travelling along the motor nerve produces depolarization of the nerve terminal and triggers the release of acetylcholine, which crosses the junctional cleft to stimulate nicotinic cholinoceptors on the postsynaptic muscle membrane. Acetylcholine is synthesized in the nerve terminal from choline and acetate in the presence of the enzyme acetyltransferase. The acetylcholine molecules are contained in uniformly sized vesicles, which are mobilized down the nerve fibre to the presynaptic membrane where they are concentrated in areas called active zones. The active zones lie directly opposite high concentrations of cholinoceptors, located on the shoulders of the secondary clefts of the postsynaptic muscle membrane. Thus, when the acetylcholine is released, it travels a minimal distance across the junctional cleft to reach the receptor. Interaction between acetylcholine and the receptor triggers an end-plate potential, which is converted to a muscle action potential and then into a muscle fibre contraction.

After activating the receptor, acetylcholine is rapidly hydrolysed by acetylcholinesterase to choline and acetate. Some of the choline is taken up by the nerve terminal for the resynthesis of acetylcholine.

MUSCLE RELAXANT DRUGS AND THEIR PHARMACOLOGY

Muscle relaxant drugs are of two distinct types: depolarizing or non-depolarizing (competitive). They are considerably different in their effects.

The non-depolarizing drugs are mainly mono- or biquaternary salts and are very hydrophilic. They do not produce muscle fasciculations and have a relatively slow onset. Their effects are reversible with anticholinesterases. The relaxed muscle is still responsive to other stimuli, e.g. electrical stimulation. During partial paralysis, monitoring of the blockade shows fade and post-tetanic facilitation followed by exhaustion and depression of muscle twitch. The effects are potentiated by volatile anaesthetic agents and magnesium ions. Repeated bursts of tetanus cause their effect to wear off. Acidosis increases the duration and degree of non-depolarizing block.

The depolarizing drugs produce initial muscle fasciculations and their action is relatively rapid in onset. Depolarized muscle fibres are unresponsive to other stimuli. Their action is not reversed by anticholinesterases. In partial paralysis, neuromuscular monitoring shows depression of the muscle twitch, no fade and no post-tetanic facilitation. The effects of suxamethonium are potentiated by isoflurane, respiratory alkalosis, hypothermia and magnesium ions. Effects are antagonized by halothane, acidosis and non-depolarizing relaxants. Repeated or continuous use will produce either a phase II (non-depolarizing) or dual block.

Depolarizing muscle relaxants

The only muscle relaxant in this group currently available is suxamethonium (succinylcholine, U.S.P.) chloride. It is the dicholine ester of succinic acid and is hydrolysed by cholinesterase and pseudocholinesterase to choline and succinic acid. It is not possible to predict the sensitivity of animals to suxamethonium by measuring the concentration of cholinesterase in the blood. As cholinesterase is synthesized in the liver, however, it is likely that severe liver damage, cachexia or malnutrition may prolong the duration of action of the drug. The activity of pseudocholinesterase is depressed by organophosphorus compounds (which may be used as ectoparasiticides) and suxamethonium should not be used in animals that have been recently treated with these agents. Administration of suxamethonium causes transient muscle fasciculations, which are due to initial depolarization of the muscle end-plate. It is suggested that the drug produces actual muscle injury, which is associated with release of potassium into the blood. A rise in serum potassium concentration may be associated with cardiac irregularities. Prolonged administration may, however, produce a large decrease in serum potassium concentration.

Administration of suxamethonium may produce an increase in arterial blood pressure. Variable changes in pulse rate have been reported. Both bradycardia and tachycardia have been observed and often the rate will not change.

It has been shown that a single dose of 0.3 mg/kg, when given intravenously to dogs, will have a duration of action of 25–30 minutes to complete recovery. It has also been suggested that incremental doses of the drug or even infusions may be used. However, monitoring of neuromuscular block (see below) is essential in these circumstances, as tachyphylaxis and so-called phase II (or dual) block may occur. With the onset of phase II block, a more prolonged return of neuromuscular activity can be expected, but, when it is fully developed, it can be reversed by anticholinesterase drugs. There does not seem to be any connection between the development of tachyphylaxis and phase II block in the dog. It has also been shown that, when a dose of 0.3 mg/kg of suxamethonium is given to the dog, phase II block begins to develop after a single dose but is not fully developed until after a third or fourth dose.

Non-depolarizing muscle relaxants

There are a number of drugs in this group but, despite recent developments in this area, there are only a few drugs which are worthy of full discussion. Non-depolarizing muscle relaxants are either quaternary ammonium or steroid compounds. They are discussed in order of their historical discovery.

Tubocurarine chloride

This is the original non-depolarizing muscle relaxant and is derived from the *Chondrodendron tomentosum* tree. It is still used to a variable extent in humans. As indicated earlier, it does have profound cardiovascular effects in the dog and hence its use is contraindicated.

Gallamine triethiodide

Gallamine was the first synthetic muscle relaxant to be produced for clinical use. It has an atropine-like effect on the postganglionic nerve endings of the heart, which produces a tachycardia. It may also block the muscarinic effects of acetylcholine and have a direct effect on cardiac β-receptors. It frequently produces a rise in arterial blood pressure and, combined with the tachycardia, this may lead to greater haemorrhage than normal during surgery. The drug should not be used in animals in which renal function is compromised because virtually all of an admini-stered dose of gallamine is excreted via the kidneys. However, it has been shown that it is redistribution, from postjunctional receptor sites to non-specific tissue acceptors, rather than renal excretion, which limits the duration of action of gallamine. A 1 mg/kg dose produces neuromuscular block for ~29 minutes.

Pancuronium bromide

Pancuronium is a biquaternary amino-steroid, which is devoid of hormonal activity. While up to 30% of an administered dose of pancuronium may be metabolized, the rest is excreted as the unchanged parent compound. Only 10% is excreted in the bile and the remainder by the kidney. Hence, the administration of the compound is contraindicated in animals with impaired renal function, and extreme care is needed in animals with liver disease. Pancuronium has a minimal effect on the cardiovascular system but it can stimulate the myocardium and produce a rise in heart rate and in blood pressure. It shows relatively little cumulative effect and is readily reversed by anticholinesterases. A dose of 0.06 mg/kg has a duration of action of ~31 minutes.

Vecuronium bromide

Vecuronium is a steroid agent. It was developed from pancuronium and differs from it only in the nature of the 2 β-atom, which is tertiary as distinct from quaternary. This modification produces a drug molecule that is significantly different in both physical and chemical properties. It has an increased selectivity of pharmacological profile, shorter time course of action and relative lack of cumulation when compared with pancuronium. It is not sufficiently stable to be supplied and stored in solution. It is presented in a lyophilized form that dissolves readily in water and is stable at room temperature for up to 24 hours. Unlike pancuronium, the drug is not dependent on renal excretion as its principal route of elimination from the body and it can, therefore, be used in animals with compromised renal function. The principal route of elimination would seem to be the liver and, therefore, the drug should be used with considerable caution in animals with impaired hepatic function. Metabolism of the drug is relatively insignificant, as it is primarily eliminated in an unchanged form in the bile.

Vecuronium is virtually free from ganglion blocking activity, and extremely large doses are required to produce inhibition of cardiac muscarinic receptors. Administration of the drug is associated with minimal cardiovascular effects. Even at high doses, it has very little effect on heart rate and arterial blood pressure. It does not seem to release histamine. It has been shown that, in the absence of halothane, an initial dose of 0.1 mg/kg has a duration of action of ~18 minutes. However, under clinical conditions, when halothane was employed as part of the anaesthetic technique, that dose of the drug had a duration of action of ~25 minutes. It was also shown that the drug was non-cumulative and the mean time interval between subsequent increments of 0.04 mg/kg was 18 minutes. It can also be given by intra-venous infusion at a rate of 0.01 mg/kg/h.

Atracurium besylate

Atracurium is a novel compound, as it is mainly broken down in the plasma by a self-destruction process known as the Hofmann elimination. This reaction occurs under physiological conditions at body pH and temperature and proceeds independently from hepatic and renal function. Hence, atracurium is the drug of choice in animals with impaired function of either the liver and/or kidneys. As the compound does release histamine under certain circumstances, it should be used with care in animals with a history of anaphylaxis. Under conditions of clinical anaesthesia in the presence of halothane, a dose of 0.5 mg/kg has a duration of action of 40 minutes. Incremental doses of 0.2 mg/kg are non-cumulative and have a mean duration of action of 17.5 minutes. In view of its unique metabolism and lack of cumulation, atracurium is an ideal drug for giving by infusion. A dose of 0.5 mg/kg/h has been used after an initial bolus dose of 0.5 mg/kg.

Cisatracurium besylate

Atracurium is a mixture of 10 isomers, six of which were isolated and tested for their pharmacological activity. Cisatracurium is the R-*cis*, R-*cis* isomer. It is considered to be about five times as potent as the parent compound in most experimental species. It does not produce histamine-like cardiovascular effects or any increase in plasma histamine concentrations. It is metabolized mainly by the Hofmann elimination and is less dependent on plasma esterases than the parent mixture. To date, no information seems to exist on its use under clinical conditions in domestic animals.

Mivacurium

This is a benzylisoquinoline compound with one third to half the potency of atracurium in primates. In humans, it has a short duration of action because of its rapid hydrolysis by pseudocholinesterase. Acetylcholinesterase metabolism and spontaneous hydrolysis are minimal. It has a relatively slow onset and offset of action in the dog. A dose of 0.03 mg/kg has been used in the dog. It can be reversed by anticholinesterase drugs but there is very little published information on its use.

Rocuronium

This is a monoquaternary steroidal compound of low potency, which has a rapid onset of action. The duration of action in equipotent doses is similar to that of atracurium and vecuronium. It has minimal cumulative effects and is potentiated by isoflurane. It has similar cardiovascular effects to vecuronium and is readily reversible with anticholinesterase drugs.

Doxacurium

This is a very potent, long-acting agent. It is of limited potential use in veterinary anaesthesia. Its use has been described in experimental dogs and this has illustrated the difficulties that are inherent in a relaxant with these properties.

Interaction between depolarizing and non-depolarizing relaxants

This is a somewhat complex subject. The effects may vary from species to species and also with the stage of block produced by one particular drug when the other is given.

In the dog, it has been shown that prior administration of all the common non-depolarizing muscle relaxants significantly reduces the duration of action of suxamethonium. Prior administration of suxamethonium significantly reduces the duration of action of alcuronium, gallamine and pancuronium. With atracurium, no significant effect is observed but, with vecuronium, there is much slower recovery.

MONITORING OF NEUROMUSCULAR BLOCKADE

The monitoring of neuromuscular function, during and after anaesthesia, provides the anaesthetist with valuable information. The data contribute to improved patient care and a more predictable approach to the use of relaxants, not only during routine clinical use but also where the response may be modified by drug treatment, or disease. Monitoring also permits detection of partial blockade, when redosing and, in the case of non-depolarizing agents, reversal are best accomplished.

In humans, attempts were made to assess muscle relaxation in the clinical situation by observation of clinical signs. A number of these techniques have been applied to the dog but, in general, have not been satisfactory, as they require the active cooperation of the patient. A commonly used method of assessing relaxation during anaesthesia is by noting the changes in pressure in the anaesthetic reservoir bag when intermittent positive-pressure ventilation (IPPV) is being performed. Onset of relaxation is characterized by an increase in compliance, while return of muscle tone may be detected by a decrease in compliance. The method is of limited value because respiratory obstruction may result in similar pressure changes. In the clinical situation, small portable nerve stimulators are the only useful and effective equipment for assessing neuromuscular blockade.

Stimulation of the peroneal nerve in the hindlimb, or the ulnar nerve in the forelimb, with recording of the movement or twitchings of the foot, have been described. A technique of stimulating the facial nerve and recording the movement of the nose has also been documented.

A number of different patterns of nerve stimulation have been described, and the evoked muscle response depends on the particular pattern chosen. Single twitch stimulation is only considered to be useful as a screening test to differentiate between central and peripheral apnoea. The height of the evoked twitch produced by a given single stimulus varies over time and with the frequency at which the stimulus is applied. Hence, the single twitch method is not a good indicator of the extent of neuromuscular blockade.

Tetanic stimulation, not exceeding a frequency of 50 Hz, is of value in assessing deep neuromuscular blockade. In this technique, tetanus is applied for 5 seconds and the response to post-tetanic stimulation observed. A single tetanic burst of 50 Hz for 5 seconds may also be used. If the tetanus is sustained, then reversal of blockade may be considered adequate. If fade occurs, then a non-depolarizing block is present.

The train-of-four technique is a suitable technique for monitoring neuromuscular block, under clinical conditions, in the dog. Four supramaximal stimuli are applied at a frequency of 2 Hz, and each such train is repeated at an interval of 10 seconds. Absence of any visible response to the four stimuli characterizes complete blockade. Four twitches with equally reduced amplitude suggest partial conventional depolarizing blockade. When the four twitches appear in order of descending amplitude, this suggests partial non-polarizing blockade. Under the latter conditions the ratio of the amplitude of the fourth to the first response provides a convenient method for assessment of neuromuscular transmission. By simply counting the twitches that can be observed, the extent of the block can be roughly assessed and the dose of relaxant adjusted. When two or three twitches are visible, redosing may be used to prolong neuromuscular blockade or administration of an anticholinesterase used to reverse non-depolarizing neuromuscular blockade. Reversal is occasionally incomplete or unsuccessful if it is attempted prior to reappearance of at least one twitch.

The visual assessment of muscle responses to train-of-four stimulation in human patients is inaccurate; therefore, in the absence of recording equipment, double-burst stimulation is considered to be superior. An initial burst of three impulses to the nerve at a frequency of 50 Hz (one impulse every 20 ms) followed by a second after an interval of 750 ms allows visualization or manual detection of small amounts of residual neuromuscular block under clinical conditions. In the absence of muscle relaxation, two short muscle contractions of equal strength are produced; in the partially paralysed muscle, the second response is weaker than the first, i.e. the responses fade. Absence of fade in response to double-burst stimulation means that clinically significant residual neuromuscular block is absent.

Distinguishing features of neuromuscular block

In the presence of partial neuromuscular block, the mechanical muscle responses to different patterns of nerve stimulation display features characteristic of the type of block present. Responses to single-twitch stimulation show depression of twitch height in all types of block. However, the degree of train-of-four fade, tetanic fade and post-tetanic twitch potentiation differ in the presence of depolarizing and non-depolarizing block. The evoked muscle responses, after initial doses of suxamethonium, show characteristics of a depolarizing block but, when high doses are given or its action is prolonged, the characteristics of the block change to resemble those of a non-depolarizing block. This is known as phase II block. Spontaneous recovery from the phase II block takes longer than that from the initial depolarizing block.

The train-of-four ratio has been used to characterize the suxamethonium neuromuscular block in humans and dogs. Initially, the depolarizing block is indicated by minimal train-of-four fade; however, the development of phase II block is indicated by marked fade. In the dog, phase II block begins to develop after a single dose of 0.3 mg/kg of suxamethonium. Tachyphylaxis, defined as 'a diminishing paralysing action in response to an equivalent dose of relaxant,' is evident early in the depolarizing phase.

FACTORS AFFECTING THE ACTION OF RELAXANTS

There are a wide variety of factors that may influence the action of muscle relaxants. These will, of course, affect the sensitivity to the drugs and may explain some of the variation seen in the response to these drugs in clinical practice.

Age
While it is generally accepted that young animals are sensitive to the old competitive muscle relaxants, they are usually more resistant to atracurium and vecuronium. It is also suggested that they require larger doses of suxamethonium than older animals. Elderly animals with some reduction in cardiovascular, renal and hepatic function are usually more sensitive to the old non-depolarizing relaxants, whereas old age seems to have little effect on the action of atracurium, vecuronium and suxamethonium.

Temperature
Changes in body temperature affect the response to muscle relaxants in a complex manner. For example, hypothermia changes regional blood flow and reduces plasma clearance, renal and biliary excretion and the metabolic rate. The onset of neuromuscular block is delayed during hypothermia, so that extreme care is needed to prevent overdosage. The duration of action is also likely to be increased. Conversely, it has been shown that hyperthermia increases the requirement for atracurium in the dog, probably because of an effect on the Hofmann elimination reaction.

Muscle disease
Although muscle disease is relatively rare in animals, it is well known that myasthenia gravis occurs in dogs. Dogs with myasthenia gravis are sensitive to non-depolarizing muscle relaxants, but it has been shown that both atracurium and vecuronium can be used at one-tenth to one-fifth of the normal dose. Neuromuscular monitoring is essential. Myotonia has been described in the dog, but there are no recorded cases of the use of relaxants in these animals. It is suggested that these animals are likely to be normal in their responses to non-depolarizing muscle relaxants and sensitive to depolarizing drugs, which tend to provoke a generalized muscle spasm. Animals that have suffered severe trauma are likely to show resistance to the non-depolarizing drugs.

Anaesthetic agents
The majority of injectable anaesthetic agents and N_2O have very little effect on the actions of muscle relaxants. However, ketamine has been shown to potentiate some of the non-depolarizing drugs. It is well established that fluorinated inhalational anaesthetic agents potentiate the non-depolarizing muscle relaxants. The effect pro-duced by isoflurane and enflurane is somewhat greater than that produced by halothane. These agents increase the intensity and duration of the block via both a central and peripheral action. The peripheral effect is caused by a depressant action on the motor end-plate and depression of acetylcholine release from the motor nerve terminal. Alteration in muscle blood flow could also be important, but the inhalational agents do not seem to affect the pharmacokinetics of the relaxants.

Antibiotics
Several classes of antibiotics have neuromuscular-blocking properties and several mechanisms have been described. The antibiotics may either have a synergism with muscle relaxants or may produce paralysis in their own right.

Aminoglycoside antibiotics, such as streptomycin, gentamicin and tobramycin, decrease acetylcholine release (i.e. have a magnesium-like action) and lower post-junctional sensitivity to acetylcholine. The block is reversed by the administration of calcium, but only partially by neostigmine. Calcium may be used prophylactically. Polypeptide antibiotics, such as the polymyxins, may decrease acetylcholine release and have a direct effect on muscle. They are very potent in producing neuromuscular block in their own right. The block is not reliably reversed by calcium or 4-aminopyridine, and anticholinesterase administration seems to enhance the block. The exact mechanism of the effects of tetracycline antibiotics on muscle relaxants is not known. They have a prejunctional blocking action in addition to an effect on muscle contractility. While they chelate calcium, the action is not thought to be due to a decrease in calcium ions at the end-plate. Calcium is only partially effective in reversing the block produced by tetracyclines, and anticholinesterases have no effect. Lincomycin and clindamycin have a pre- and postjunctional effect. Calcium and anticholinesterases are only partially effective reversal agents, and 4-aminopyridine is the drug of choice. Metronidazole would not seem to have an effect at the NMJ but has a secondary effect on the distribution and/or metabolism of relaxants.

Care should always be exercised when using the above antibiotics with relaxants, and it should be emphasized that rapid absorption of these drugs could occur from the pleural or peritoneal cavities when they are used intraoperatively. Careful monitoring is essential under such circumstances.

Other drug treatment
A wide variety of other drugs have been shown to affect the action of muscle relaxants. A number of anticholinesterase drugs are known to prolong the duration of action of suxamethonium. These include a number of organophosphate preparations that are used widely as anthelmintics and pesticides in animals and are also incorporated into flea collars. Ecothiophate

drops, which are used in the treatment of glaucoma, may also prolong the duration of action of suxamethonium. Anti-arrhythmic drugs and local anaesthetics may potentiate both non-depolarizing and suxamethonium block, due to pre- and postjunctional effects. Diuretics that produce a hypokalaemia may also potentiate the non-depolarizing relaxants. The calcium channel blockers, such as verapamil, are being increasingly used in the treatment of heart disease in veterinary practice and are reported to potentiate non-depolarizing relaxants and possibly suxamethonium.

Acid–base balance

The effect of changes in acid–base balance on the action of relaxants is complex. The effects may be due to a number of factors, including changes in protein binding and in ionization of the drug. The most consistent changes are produced by changes in carbon dioxide (CO_2) tensions, either as a respiratory acidosis or alkalosis. Respiratory acidosis prolongs, and alkalosis reduces, the effects of atracurium, tubocurarine and vecuronium. However, respiratory acidosis decreases, and alkalosis increases, the effects of gallamine and suxamethonium. Pancuronium block is prolonged by hypercapnia. In view of the complexity of these changes, laboratory studies and predictions may differ from the clinical situation.

Electrolyte disturbance

Hypokalaemia and hypernatraemia may potentiate the actions of the non-depolarizing drugs, while hyperkalaemia and hyponatraemia may have the opposite effect but potentiate suxamethonium block. Hyper-magnesaemia and hypocalcaemia may potentiate non-depolarizing relaxants by decreasing acetylcholine release. Calcium is frequently effective in antagonizing block associated with muscle relaxants and magnesium.

It is advisable to correct any major electrolyte imbalances before using muscle relaxants, but if this is not possible, to use them extremely sparingly or not at all.

Hepatic and renal disease

The presence of hepatic and renal disease used to be an absolute contraindication to the use of muscle relaxants. However, there is considerable evidence to show that this does not apply to the use of atracurium, with its novel metabolism, which is independent of hepatic and renal mechanisms.

INDICATIONS FOR USE OF MUSCLE RELAXANTS

There are a number of indications for the use of relaxants in canine anaesthesia and, as further experience is gained, their use will be widened. Their main indications are listed below:

- To relax skeletal muscle for easier surgical access, during such procedures as laparotomies, thoracotomies and laminectomies. They are also indicated for orthopaedic procedures, particularly to facilitate reduction of dislocated joints. While it has been suggested that the reduction of fractured bones may not be influenced by the use of muscle relaxants, clinical experience would suggest that, particularly in the large breeds of dog, they are extremely valuable in a number of orthopaedic procedures
- In the initiation of IPPV. This is not only essential for intrathoracic surgery but is also essential to produce anaesthesia with minimal hypercapnia and no hypoxia. This is particularly important in animals with compromised cardiovascular or respiratory systems undergoing relatively major surgery. This enables minimal amounts of anaesthetic agents to be given with maximum effect
- During delicate procedures, such as intraocular surgery, so that sudden reflex movements can be prevented
- They may also be employed to provide improved conditions (including relaxed jaw muscles) for bronchoscopy and oesophagoscopy
- As developments occur in the intensive care of animals, long-term ventilation in animals with head or thoracic injuries will increase. This is greatly facilitated by the use of muscle relaxants such as atracurium, given by infusion.

CONTRAINDICATIONS

Muscle relaxants should never be used in the absence of adequate facilities for the provision of IPPV. In practice, this means the availability of endotracheal tubes (ETTs) and anaesthetic equipment and circuitry, with a rebreathing bag that can be used to provide manual ventilation. While mechanical ventilators are extremely useful, they are certainly not essential. One of the most important factors in the correct use of muscle relaxants is to appreciate that it is essential to give anaesthetic agents to ensure unconsciousness (see below). When there are doubts about the ability to assess and ensure unconsciousness during the whole procedure, then muscle relaxants should not be used.

In addition to the above absolute contraindications, there are a number of other factors that should be borne in mind and careful consideration given to them before deciding to use muscle relaxants. IPPV increases mean intrathoracic pressure, reducing venous return to the heart. In normal animals, a compensatory reflex increase in venous tone occurs. In animals where venous tone does not compensate, problems can occur, and this is particularly important in shocked and hypovolaemic patients. An increase in mean intrathoracic pressure above atmospheric pressure can cause cardiovascular failure in animals with hypovolaemia.

CLINICAL USE OF MUSCLE RELAXANTS

There are a number of general principles that are extremely important when muscle relaxants are being used as part of an anaesthetic technique in dogs. Endotracheal intubation, preferably with a cuffed tube, is essential. This is to ensure a clear airway throughout the whole of the procedure. As the oesophageal muscle relaxes and the protective reflexes of the larynx and pharynx are abolished, the stomach contents are likely to be regurgitated and may be inhaled if an ETT is not in place. If any means other than an ETT are used to facilitate the administration of anaesthetic gases to an animal, such as a mask, then the stomach and even the intestines may be inflated by the passage of gas down the oesophagus by positive pressure applied at the mouth and/or nose.

It is important to appreciate that the stated doses of muscle relaxants are only guides to their use, and the duration of action and the intensity of block are variable. In view of the many factors that may influence the action of these drugs, it is essential to treat each patient on an individual basis and to monitor neuromuscular block. Incremental doses of relaxants should be about one-tenth to one-fifth of the original dose of relaxant.

It is essential to ensure an 'open vein' for the whole of the procedure. An intravenous catheter should be placed in a cephalic vein before the induction of anaesthesia. If the animal resents attempts to place the catheter, anaesthesia should be induced by the intravenous route using a needle, and the catheter placed as soon as possible after induction.

Induction of anaesthesia is normally performed by the intravenous route. As soon as anaesthesia is induced and the jaws relaxed, the trachea is intubated with a cuffed ETT and the animal connected to an anaesthetic circuit or ventilator. It is preferable, at this stage, to inflate the lungs with oxygen for three or more breaths. After administration of the muscle relaxant, IPPV is begun either manually or with a ventilator. A carrier gas of 33% oxygen and 66% N_2O should be used, although this may be changed to 50:50 during intrathoracic surgery when lung collapse may occur either accidentally or electively. Low concentrations of halothane or isoflurane are added to the carrier gases; the usual delivered concentration from a calibrated vaporizer is in the region of 0.5–1.5%, which should be adjusted to meet the requirements of the animal. If anaesthesia tends to become light, or analgesia is inadequate, then small incremental doses of either fentanyl or alfentanil may be given.

Intermittent positive-pressure ventilation

Ventilation may be manual or mechanical. For the small dog (up to about 10 kg), a Jackson Rees modification of the Ayre's T-piece is the circuit of choice. The modified Bain circuit can be used in dogs more than 10 kg in weight. While the commonly used rebreathing circuits, such as the Waters to-and-fro and the circle absorber, have been used for IPPV with muscle relaxants, they can pose problems with control of the concentration of CO_2 in the circuit unless end-tidal CO_2 can be monitored (Chapter 5). If, however, the circle system is used with the absorber out of circuit and with a fairly high fresh gas flow, it is extremely useful for controlled ventilation in the dog. In this system, the absorber is bypassed or the soda lime removed and ventilation performed.

A number of mechanical ventilators have been used in dogs weighing more than 10 kg, but one of the most satisfactory is the Manley, which is a minute volume divider and is operated by the gas flow delivered to it.

Tidal volumes that have been recommended vary from 20 to 30 ml/kg and minute volumes from 400 to 600 ml/kg. The actual pulmonary ventilation produced by intermittent positive pressure can be monitored by measuring the end-tidal CO_2 tension of the patient. In general, it is recommended that a state of mild hypocapnia should be maintained, i.e. an end-tidal CO_2 concentration of 35–38 mmHg (4.6–5 kPa).

If it is not possible to monitor end-tidal CO_2, a non-rebreathing circuit may be used with relatively high fresh gas flows and CO_2 added to the fresh gas mixture at a concentration of 4%. It is, therefore, possible to utilize the technique of hyperventilation without the accompanying deleterious effects of hypocapnia.

Monitoring of anaesthesia
While a number of the signs that are commonly used to monitor anaesthesia are abolished when muscle relaxants are used, it is still essential to monitor the depth of anaesthesia to prevent the scenario of an 'awake but paralysed' animal. It is essential that the anaesthetist is fully conversant with the effects of anaesthetic agents during those procedures when relaxants are not employed. Indications that the depth of anaesthesia during neuromuscular blockade is insufficient include:

- Increases in pulse rate unrelated to haemorrhage, or signs of vasovagal syncope (bradycardia with pallor of the mucous membranes)
- Dilation of the pupils. Normally the pupils are constricted at levels of surgical anaesthesia. They can dilate again with either increasing or decreasing depth of anaesthesia
- Lacrimation and increased salivation
- Despite the presence of neuromuscular block, twitching of the tongue and of the facial muscles.

REVERSAL OF NEUROMUSCULAR BLOCK

Reversal of non-depolarizing neuromuscular block is achieved by pharmacological means. The aim is to establish a high concentration of acetylcholine at the binding site of the post-synaptic cholinoceptors. This is achieved by using drugs that inhibit the enzyme cholinesterase, thus preventing the breakdown of endogenous acetylcholine and allowing its accumulation at the synaptic cleft to restore neuromuscular transmission and normal muscle function.

Three drugs have been used for anticholinesterase activity: pyridostigmine, edrophonium and neostigmine. However, it is only the last two drugs that have been used extensively in veterinary anaesthetic practice.

There are a number of factors that influence reversal of neuromuscular block, and they should be investigated when reversal is considered to be incomplete. If the drugs are given during deep neuromuscular block, as indicated by the absence of a response to peripheral nerve stimulation, then reversal will be slower. The speed of the reversal will also depend on which drug is chosen (edrophonium has the most rapid onset) and is directly proportional to the dose of reversal agent. It is likely to be slower in the elderly patient. Respiratory acidosis tends to prolong the duration of action of most non-depolarizing relaxants and impair reversal by neostigmine. Non-depolarizing block is potentiated by either high serum concentrations of magnesium or by low concentrations of calcium and potassium, and hence blood electrolyte levels should be checked if there are reversal problems, particularly if the animal is on diuretic treatment.

The response to an anticholinesterase can vary considerably with the degree of block present. In an investigation of the reversal of atracurium with neostigmine, the dose required varied by a factor of 5 when it was given at 10% block as opposed to 50% block.

It has been reported that the recommended dose of neostigmine and edrophonium can vary widely. This may be partly due to a lack of standardization of the procedures when determining the dose. The dose of neostigmine varies from 0.01 to 0.1 mg/kg and edrophonium from 1 to 2 mg/kg. In the clinical situation using the train-of-four response, it is recommended that at least two twitches should be present before attempting to reverse the block.

Before administering the anticholinesterase, an anticholinergic drug such as atropine or glycopyrrolate should be given intravenously to block the muscarinic effects of acetylcholine. Doses of 0.04 mg/kg of atropine or 0.01 mg/kg of glycopyrrolate should be used. In some centres, these drugs are given at least 1 minute before the anticholinesterase, in other institutions they are given together in the same syringe and administered by slow intravenous injection. Doses of either 0.1 mg/kg of neostigmine or 1 mg/kg of edrophonium are recommended. IPPV should be continued until recovery is adequate. Monitoring of the neuromuscular block should be continued until the train-of-four responses are all considered to be of equal force. The reversal drugs are given at about 5 minutes before the projected termination of the procedure. Care is necessary with an extensive wound closure and with inexperienced surgeons. If an inhalational agent is being given, it is discontinued once the reversal agents have been given.

FURTHER READING

Cullen LK (1996) Muscle relaxants and neuromuscular block. In: *Lumb and Jones Veterinary Anaesthesia, 3ʳᵈ edn*, ed. JC Thurmon *et al.*, pp. 337–364. Williams and Wilkins, Baltimore

Hall LW and Clarke LW (1991) *Veterinary Anaesthesia, 9ᵗʰ edn*. Baillière Tindall, London

Jones RM and Payne JP (1988) *Recent Developments in Muscle Relaxation: Atracurium in Perspective*. Royal Society of Medicine, London

Jones RS (1992a) Muscle relaxants in canine anaesthesia 1: History and the drugs. *Journal of Small Animal Practice* **33**, 371–375

Jones RS (1992b) Muscle relaxants in canine anaesthesia 2: Clinical application. *Journal of Small Animal Practice* **33**, 423–429

CHAPTER ELEVEN

Fluid Therapy and Blood Transfusion

Paula F. Moon

INTRODUCTION

Fluid therapy is indicated for the treatment or prevention of decreased oxygen delivery, hypotension, hypovolaemia, and electrolyte, metabolic and acid–base disorders. As a patient's health status decreases, the importance of selecting the most compatible fluid increases. This chapter reviews the decision making process for designing an appropriate fluid plan for the anaesthetized small animal patient.

FLUID DYNAMICS

In an emergency, fluids are often administered intravenously for the sole purpose of improving blood volume and restoring cardiac output to levels that, at the least, can sustain life. Definitive fluid selection, however, depends on matching the patient's needs with a fluid composition and volume of distribution equivalent to the deficit. Therefore, it is essential to know the composition of each solution (Figure 11.1) and how it equilibrates within the different fluid compartments of the patient (Figures 11.2 and 11.3). Equilibration of intravenous fluid depends on a balance of hydrostatic, osmotic and oncotic pressures as well as the permeability characteristics of the capillaries themselves (Starling's law). Normal vascular endothelium is permeable to small ions or electrolytes but impermeable to large proteins. Hydrostatic pressure is rarely an important factor in determining the fluid type chosen. Fluid osmotic and oncotic pressures are more important criteria when choosing an intravenous fluid.

Osmotic pressure

Osmosis is the net movement of water across a semipermeable membrane caused by the concentration differences of impermeable solutes. Osmotic pressure – the pressure exerted by the particles within the solution – prevents the movement of water across the membrane. Tonicity refers to the osmotic pressure of a fluid when compared with plasma. An isotonic solution has the same proportion of particles and water as that found in plasma. Therefore, isotonic fluid administration produces no change in the osmotic pressure of plasma and

no fluid shift between compartments. Sodium, the primary ion present in extracellular fluid (ECF), is also the main component of most electrolyte or crystalloid solutions (see Figure 11.1). Sodium freely crosses capillary boundaries, taking water with it as it distributes throughout the entire ECF volume (ECFV). Similarly, all isotonic electrolyte solutions will distribute themselves throughout the ECFV.

A solution that is hypotonic has fewer osmotically active particles than plasma. Because the addition of a hypotonic solution decreases the plasma osmotic pressure, a pressure difference is established between intravascular and extravascular spaces. For equilibrium to be re-established, water moves out of the intravascular space (low osmotic pressure) and into the interstitial space and tissue cells (high osmotic pressure). Conversely, when a hypertonic solution is administered, water moves from the interstitial space and tissues (low osmotic pressure) and into the intravascular space (high osmotic pressure). The more hypertonic the solution, the larger the driving pressure, and the more rapidly the water will move in and expand the plasma volume. This is the principal mechanism for the rapid plasma volume expansion after hypertonic saline administration and explains why a smaller volume of hypertonic saline causes a larger expansion of the plasma volume than an equivalent volume of isotonic saline. Eventually, the shifting water results in no osmotic pressure difference between compartments, and the volume of administered electrolyte fluid redistributes evenly throughout the ECF compartment. Hence, hypertonic saline is transient in its effect.

Some crystalloid solutions consist entirely, or partially, of glucose and water. Glucose molecules are unique because they only have a transient osmostic effect. Because 5% dextrose in water is isotonic and 10% dextrose in water is hypertonic, they produce initial shifts in water between the ECF and plasma as predicted based on osmotic pressures. However, cellular transport and metabolism rapidly reduce the amount of osmotically active glucose. Consequently, 5% dextrose in water is ultimately hypotonic and should only be administered to provide free water throughout all fluid compartments. Hypotonic solutions, including

Solution	Colloid oncotic pressure (mmHg)	Osmolarity (mOsm/l)	pH	Sodium (mmol/l)	Chloride (mmol/l)	Potassium (mmol/l)	Calcium (mmol/l)	Magnesium (mmol/l)	Buffer (mmol/l)
Isotonic crystalloids									
0.9% Saline (NaCl)	0	308	5.0–5.7	154	154	0	0	0	0
5% Dextrose in water	0	252–278	4.0–6.5	0	0	0	0	0	0
Isolyte-S*	0	295	7.4	141	98	5	0	3	29 Acetate/23 gluconate
Lactated Ringer's solution†	0	273	6.5	130	109	4	3	0	28 Lactate
Plasma-Lyte‡ 148	0	294–310	7.4	140	98	5	0	3	27 Acetate/23 gluconate
Ringer's solution	0	310	5.8–6.1	147	156	4	4.5	0	0
Hypertonic crystalloids									
3% NaCl	0	1026	5.0	513	513	0	0	0	0
7.5% NaCl	0	2567	5.0–5.7	1283	1283	0	0	0	0
5% Dextrose in water/ lactated Ringer's solution	0	495–527	4–6	130	109	4	2.7	0	28 Lactate
Iso-oncotic colloids									
3% Plasmagel	No data	310	No data	120	147	0	Some	0	Some
6% Albumin	30	310	5.5	154	154	0	0	0	0
6% Hetastarch§	31	310	5.5	154	154	0	0	0	0
6% Pentastach¶	25	310	5.5	154	154	0	0	0	0
Haemaccel**	25–29	No data	7.3	145	145	5.1	6.25	No data	No data
Oxypolygelatin††	45–47	200	7.4	145	100	0	1	0	30 Carbonate
Hyperoncotic colloids (in normal saline)									
6% Dextran 70†	75	309	5.0	154	154	0	0	0	0
10% Dextran 40‡‡	>100	310	3.5–7.0	154	154	0	0	0	0
10% Hydroxyethyl starch (HES)§§	>100	308	Acidic	154	154	0	0	0	0
20% HES	>100	310	Acidic	154	154	0	0	0	0
Hypertonic-hyperoncotic									
7.5% NaCl-20% HES	>100	2567	Acidic	1283	1283	0	0	0	0
7.5% NaCl-6% dextran 70	75	2567	~4–5	1283	1283	0	0	0	0

Figure 11.1: Electrolyte composition and physical properties of commonly available fluids.

*McGraw, Irvine, CA, USA. †Baxter Healthcare, Deerfield, IL, USA. ‡Travenol Labs, Deerfield, IL, USA. §Du Pont Pharmaceuticals, Wilmington, DE, USA and Du Pont, Stevenage, UK. ¶Du Pont Critical Care, Waukegan, IL, USA. **Hoechst Roussel Veterinary, Milton Keynes, UK. ††Marshallton Veterinary Group, West Chester, PA, USA. ‡‡Also available in dextrose: Cambridge Laboratories, Newcastle upon Tyne, UK. §§Fresenius Ltd, Runcorn, Cheshire, UK.*

Fluid type	Examples	Volume needed to increase plasma volume by 1 litre	Distribution	Examples of clinical indications
Colloid	Starch Gelatin Dextrans	1 litre	Plasma volume	Hypovolaemia, hypotension, normovolaemic haemodilution, hypoalbuminaemia
Hypertonic crystalloid	7.5% Saline (NaCl)	300 ml	Immediate plasma volume expansion causing ICFV reduction	Hypovolaemic shock, cerebral oedema
Hypotonic crystalloid	5% Dextrose	14 litres	Total body water	Free water deficit, hypernatraemia
Isotonic crystalloid	0.9% NaCl Lactated Ringer's solution	4 litres	ECFV (plasma volume and ISFV expansion)	Dehydration, hypovolaemia, hypotension, normovolaemic haemodilution

Figure 11.2: *Categories, distribution and clinical indications for commonly available fluids for intravenous fluid therapy.*

ECFV=extracellular fluid volume; ICFV=intracellular fluid volume; ISFV= interstitial fluid volume.

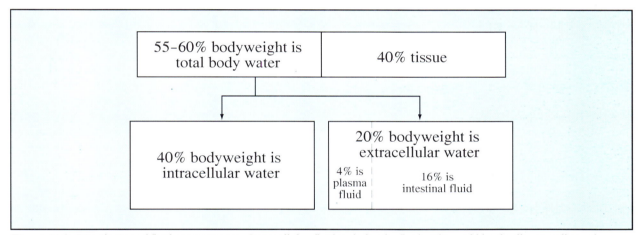

Figure 11.3: *Distribution of fluid compartments. Intracellular fluid includes the fluid within red blood cells, as well as other cells. Interstitial fluid volume includes fluid in the cerebrospinal fluid, pleural and peritoneal spaces and ocular fluids.*

dextrose solutions, do not adequately replace fluid losses under conditions of anaesthesia and surgery, because they will cause cellular and interstitial oedema faster than if an isotonic fluid is used to maintain an equivalent degree of plasma volume expansion. The movement of free water into cells may either treat cellular dehydration or produce cellular oedema, depending on the situation in a given patient. Thus, it is imperative to consider the effects of a fluid's tonicity on the patient's fluid compartments.

Oncotic pressure

The second important property in selecting a fluid is its oncotic pressure. Oncotic pressure – the pressure exerted by the large molecules that do not cross the capillary membranes – influences the distribution of

water between the vascular and interstitial spaces. The normal colloid oncotic pressure of plasma is 20–25 mmHg and, in most situations, it is assumed that plasma oncotic pressure is adequate if the serum albumin concentration is ≥2.5 g/dl and the total protein (TP) concentration is ≥5 g/dl. The contribution that proteins (albumin, globulins) make to the total plasma osmotic pressure is small (around 4%), but is sufficient to cause an osmotic pressure difference with the interstitial fluid that retains water preferentially in the intravascular space.

A normal capillary is impermeable to molecules with molecular weights >35,000 daltons. Solutions containing these large molecules are considered colloids. Iso-oncotic colloids have the same oncotic pressure as plasma, and hyperoncotic colloids have a higher oncotic pressure. Hyperoncotic fluid administration will increase plasma oncotic pressure and will draw water into the vascular compartment, as will hypertonic saline. However, unlike such crystalloid solutions that are composed of permeable particles, colloid molecules cannot cross normal capillary membranes. Therefore, the plasma volume expansion is maintained for a longer period of time than after administration of an equivalent crystalloid solution.

FLUID TYPES

Isotonic crystalloids

Isotonic crystalloids (e.g. lactated Ringer's solution) are inexpensive methods of expanding both the vascular and the interstitial fluid compartments. They are commonly used to maintain plasma volume in uncomplicated anaesthetized patients, to replace deficits in dehydrated patients, to restore third space losses and to promote urinary flow. Within 30 to 45 minutes after administration, around 75–80% of the administered volume has left the plasma volume and has redistributed primarily into the interstitial space. This property of crystalloids usually prevents sustained improvement in plasma volume and haemodynamic parameters unless they are administered as a continuous infusion. Large volumes of isotonic fluids, coupled with their large volume of redistribution, may promote peripheral and pulmonary oedema.

Hypertonic crystalloids

Advantages

The overwhelming advantage of hypertonic solutions is their potent plasma volume expansion (see above), and therefore they are useful in the initial treatment of hypovolaemic shock by rapid administration of only a small volume of fluid. Replacement of a quarter to one-third of the lost volume of blood with hypertonic solution rapidly restores cardiovascular variables compared with three to four times the lost volume that is necessary with isotonic crystalloids. Hypertonic solutions are a stop-gap therapy and must be followed by the administration of appropriate follow-up fluids (crystalloids, colloids or blood products). In addition to the treatment of shock, slow infusions of hypertonic saline have been advocated for intraoperative use during cardiac surgery, to prevent tissue oedema from conventional fluid therapy. Hypertonic saline (3–5%) also decreases intracranial pressure and total brain water in experimental traumatic brain injury models, and it may be useful in treating cerebral oedema.

Hypertonic solutions rapidly expand the plasma volume, increase cardiac output and improve blood pressure. Hypertonic saline may directly increase myocardial contractility and decrease systemic vascular resistance. Hypertonic solutions also improve microcirculatory blood flow because of a reduction in endothelial cell size and a lower blood viscosity. For a more sustained effect, hypertonic crystalloids can be administered with a colloid.

Disadvantages

Most of the adverse effects of hypertonic saline are transient but can be clinically relevant. The most important side effects are hypernatraemia, hyperchloraemia, hypokalaemia, hyperosmolarity and a metabolic acidosis. For example, at the standard shock dose (4 ml/kg i.v. over 10 minutes), a hyperchloraemic metabolic acidosis can cause a transient decrease of 0.05 units in pH that lasts around 10 minutes. New hypertonic solutions have attempted to prevent some of these side effects, and both hypernatraemic-isochloraemic-acetate solutions and isonatraemic hyperchloraemic solutions are being developed. Because of its hyperosmolarity, hypertonic saline administered through a small peripheral vein to a patient with poor perfusion may result in intravascular haemolysis and haemoglobinuria. Hypertonic saline also produces haemodilution of all blood components. Finally, ventricular dysrhythmias can occasionally be observed during fluid administration, and their incidence may increase with the severity of the patient's condition.

The use of hypertonic saline in dehydrated patients or patients with ongoing uncontrolled blood loss continues to be a controversial topic. Certainly, with pre-existing cellular dehydration, hypertonic saline causes a further decrease in cell size, and it is especially important to administer an isotonic crystalloid promptly to replace this aggravated cellular fluid deficit. However, some evidence suggests that mild cellular dehydration does not compromise the efficacy of a single dose of hypertonic saline for treatment of hypovolaemia. Cardiovascular improvement is not sustained, however, with a second dose of hypertonic saline in these patients. In more severely dehydrated patients, mortality may actually increase with the use of hypertonic saline.

The other concern with hypertonic saline is that uncontrolled bleeding will worsen (due to the rapid increase in blood pressure) and the likelihood of mortality may increase. This issue is still being debated, with data supporting both views. As with any fluid therapy, aggressive volume restoration to normotension can promote continued blood loss if the source of the haemorrhage is not controlled. Therefore, it seems rational to provide only enough fluid to prevent tissue ischaemia and maintain life support as an initial measure. It must be realized that striving for a normal blood pressure in such situations may not be an appropriate end point until the bleeding has been controlled.

Synthetic colloid solutions

Indications for colloid administration are hypoalbuminaemia, blood loss, hypovolaemia, third space fluid accumulation, sepsis and persistent hypotension. Colloids do not cross normal capillary walls and have a more sustained effect on plasma volume than crystalloid solutions. Compared with plasma, synthetic colloids have a longer storage time and there is no risk of transmission of infectious diseases and no long-term sensitization effect. Colloids are less expensive than plasma, but more costly than crystalloids.

Ordinarily, the volume of colloid administered should be equal to, or slightly greater than, the lost volume of blood. Compared with isotonic crystalloids, this translates into less total fluid administered, less fluid distributed into extravascular spaces and less risk of peripheral oedema. However, both colloids and crystalloids have been associated with pulmonary oedema in patients with permeable capillaries. Diseased capillaries may leak both colloids and fluid into the interstitial space when gaps in the endothelium become large enough, resulting in oedema. Colloids that are larger than the gaps, however, may impede transport of water and small proteins through permeable capillaries. Pentastarch, in particular, may be useful in plugging leaky capillaries in patients with sepsis, pulmonary dysfunction, burns and other diseases with increased capillary permeability.

Typically, synthetic colloids are categorized as a type of dextran, gelatin or starch (Figure 11.4). The plasma half-life is proportional to the size of the molecules. Molecules ≤50,000 daltons are rapidly filtered unchanged by the kidneys, while larger molecules are degraded, metabolized and excreted through both renal and gastrointestinal pathways. Diseases that alter renal function or vascular permeability will alter the duration of plasma volume expansion. In addition, if high doses of the smaller colloids are administered to a patient with renal dysfunction, renal tubular obstruction may occur, potentially causing acute renal failure.

Disadvantages

Three potential disadvantages of all synthetic colloids are circulatory overload, anaphylactic reactions and coagulation disorders. Because of slow fluid redistribution, circulatory overload and haemodilution may occur if the patient is not properly monitored. Since errors in fluid loading with colloids have a prolonged effect, the volume of colloid used should be carefully titrated and central venous pressure, systemic blood pressure, pulmonary capillary wedge pressure, and urine output should be monitored in patients with pulmonary oedema, congestive heart failure or renal failure.

Historically, anaphylactic and anaphylactoid reactions have been reported in humans for all three classes of colloids; the incidence is estimated to be about 0.033% overall. This incidence is small compared with the extent of reactions after administration of blood, penicillin, barbiturates or contrast media. The incidence in veterinary medicine is unknown, although adverse reactions to dextrans have been reported in both dogs (rarely) and rats (commonly). Reactions are usually immediate, after administration of even a small volume. Therefore, initial slow administration with careful monitoring is justified. Signs of an adverse reaction include hypotension, ischaemia, flushing, urticaria, respiratory compromise, pulmonary oedema and gastrointestinal disturbances. In a few extremely rare instances, administration of a colloid has been fatal.

Although all colloids affect coagulation, gelatins are the least detrimental, followed by starches and then dextrans. For dextrans, the effects have been attributed to platelet coating, precipitation of coagulation factors, increased fibrinolytic activity and decreased functional von Willebrand factor. The effect on coagulation with dextrans seems to be dose related. The manufacturer's recommended dose for 6% dextran 70 is up to 20 ml/kg the first day and half this dose for the following two days. Higher doses may increase blood viscosity, vascular resistance and afterload. A rate of 2 ml/kg/h is not associated with bleeding problems in humans, while large doses given rapidly may cause haemorrhagic diathesis. There are no controlled data on the maximum safe dose for dextrans in veterinary medicine. Empirical doses of 5–10 ml/kg/h have been suggested for the treatment of hypoproteinaemia, while doses of 5–15 ml/kg as a rapid bolus up to 40–50 ml/kg/h have been suggested for acute hypovolaemia. One veterinary study (Concannon et al., 1992) reported that at doses of 20 ml/kg over 30 or 60 minutes, there were minimal haemostatic abnormalities in clinically normal dogs, but there were enough alterations to suggest dextrans may precipitate bleeding in dogs with marginal haemostatic function. The coagulation changes that can occur with hetastarch, although measurable, are not as pronounced. Hetastarch slightly prolongs partial thromboplastin and prothrombin bleeding times. Clotting factor VIII function is decreased 25–50%, and there is altered fibrin formation with hetastarch (Conroy et al., 1996). Since both dextrans and starches have documented haematological effects that are due to more than simple haemodilution, one should consider avoiding them and using a gelatin or plasma in patients with coagulopathies or von Willebrand's disease or when massive blood loss is expected.

PRIORITIES IN FLUID THERAPY

The primary goal in any fluid therapy plan is to maintain oxygen delivery to, and oxygen consumption by, vital organs, thereby sustaining aerobic metabolism. Oxygen

Colloid % solution Trade name	Albumin 5%	Polygeline 3.5% Haemaccel	Plasmagel 3%	Oxypolygelatin Vetaplasma	Dextran-40 10% Rheomacrodex	Dextran-70 6% Macrodex	Hetastarch 6% Hespan	Pentastarch 10% Pentaspan
Category	Protein	Gelatin			Dextran		Starch	
Substance		Polypeptide			Polysaccharide		Amylopectin (branched polysaccharide)	
Source	Blood	Cattle bone			Bacteria		Maize or sorghum	
Molecular weight (mean (range) in Daltons)	69,000	35,000 (5000–50,000)	35,000 (10,000–100,000)	30,000 (5600–100,000)	40,000 (15,000–75,000)	70,000 (20,000–175,000)	450,000 (10,000–1,000,000)	264,000 (150,000–350,000)*
Oncotic pressure (mmHg)	20	25–29		45–47	40	40	30–35	30–40
% Interstitial	20	50	50	50	0	0	0	0
% Intravascular	80	50	50	50	100	100	100	100
Plasma half-life (hours)	>16	2–4	2–4	2–4	2–6	6–12	>24	3–8
Total elimination		Very rapid	Very rapid	Very rapid	Very rapid	Rapid	Protracted	Prolonged
% Adverse reactions (in humans, after 1980)	Fewest (0.001)		Some (0.78)		Few (0.2),† common in rats		Extremely rare (0)	
Coagulopathies		Rare			Reported		Reported	
Manufacturer		Hoechst Roussel Veterinary, Milton Keynes, UK	Marshallton Veterinary Group, West Chester, PA, USA	Abbott Laboratories, North Chicago, IL, USA	Cambridge Laboratories, Newcastle-upon-Tyne, UK	Baxter HealthCare, Deerfield, IL, USA	Fresenius Ltd, Runcorn, Cheshire, UK	

Figure 11.4: Comparison of commonly available colloid solutions.

*Average molecular weight of pentastarch is higher than hetastarch although weight average molecular weight is lower, i.e. pentastarch has a narrower range of medium weight molecules.
†If pretreated with dextran 1.

Variable	Normal range
Arterial haemoglobin saturation (SaO_2) (%)	>95
Base deficit (mmol/l)	+2 to -2
Blood lactate (mmol/l)	<2
Cardiac index (ml/kg/min)	100-150
Central venous pressure (cm H_2O)	Awake: -3 to +4 Anaesthetized: 2-7
Gastric intramucosal pH	7.35-7.41
Heart rate (beats/min)	Dog: 70-180 Cat: 145-200
Haematocrit (%)	Dog: 37-55 Cat: 25-45
Mean arterial blood pressure (mmHg)	80-110
Mixed venous haemoglobin saturation ($S\bar{v}O_2$) (%)	>65
Oxygen delivery (DO_2) (ml/kg/min)	20-30
Oxygen extraction (%)	20-30
Oxygen uptake ($\dot{V}O_2$) (ml/kg/min)	4-10
Pulmonary artery wedge pressure (mmHg)	3-9
Urine output (ml/kg/h)	1-2

Figure 11.5: *Normal values of cardiopulmonary variables used for monitoring fluid therapy.*

delivery is primarily based on cardiac output, arterial oxygen saturation of haemoglobin and haemoglobin content. The determinants of oxygen consumption ($\dot{V}O_2$) are found in the equation:

$$\dot{V}O_2 = CO \times Hb \times 14.4 \times (SaO_2 - S\bar{v}O_2)$$

where CO is cardiac output, Hb is haemoglobin concentration and SaO_2 and $S\bar{v}O_2$ are arterial and mixed venous oxygen saturation, respectively.

A $\dot{V}O_2$ that falls below the normal range (Figure 11.5) is evidence of impaired tissue oxygenation.

In situations such as acute haemorrhage, both cardiac output and total red cell mass decline. Initially, the consequences of low cardiac output far outweigh the consequences of low red cell mass. Therefore, treating hypovolaemia is more important than treating anaemia, and restoring volume is more important than maintaining haemoglobin concentration. A dog's blood volume is 80-90 ml/kg and a cat's blood volume is 60-70 ml/kg. A rough estimate for determining the fluid volume needed to restore the patient's blood

volume can be calculated based on the final distribution of the chosen fluid type: when administering whole blood, give a volume equal to the volume deficit; when administering a colloid, give a volume equal to 1-1.5 times the volume deficit, and, when administering an isotonic crystalloid, give a volume equal to 3-4 times the volume deficit (Figure 11.6).

After volume restoration, the second priority is restoration of haemoglobin concentration. However, a haematocrit, by itself, gives no information about oxygen delivery or oxygen uptake by the tissues. If it did, then a dehydrated patient with an increased haematocrit would have an increased oxygen delivery, and fluids would not be needed. This rationale is obviously incorrect, implying that the common practice of transfusing red blood cells based on a specific haematocrit alone has little scientific basis. A more rational approach to determining if red cell transfusions are necessary is to evaluate oxygen delivery variables and look for evidence of inadequate $\dot{V}O_2$ (see Figure 11.5). For example, in situations of normovolaemic anaemia (following crystalloid fluid therapy or if the patient has chronic anaemia), a red cell transfusion may not be necessary because blood volume is adequate and a compensatory increase in cardiac output may have occurred. However, red cell administration may be indicated if oxygen delivery is below normal, if lactate is being produced (suggesting anaerobic metabolism) or if oxygen extraction is much greater than normal (suggesting tissue oxygen needs are greater than delivery). A normalization of these variables and, especially, an increase in oxygen consumption after a unit of blood or packed red cells, should be considered a positive response, and transfusions should be continued until oxygen consumption is no longer dependent on haemoglobin content.

Other priorities in fluid therapy include the correction or prevention of acid-base, electrolyte and metabolic disorders. These are tailored to the individual patient and can be addressed either by selecting a fluid of appropriate pH and electrolyte composition (see Figure 11.1) or by adding a supplement to the fluid (Figure 11.7). Chronic abnormalities should be corrected slowly; acute changes more quickly.

The pH of the common solutions varies greatly, i.e. some are acidifying and others alkalinizing, depending on whether or not buffers are added (see Figure 11.1). Chloride or lactate, the anions associated with the sodium and potassium cations in most fluids, can be used interchangeably for most patients. When there is concern about acidosis, the clinician should select a fluid of the appropriate pH with a metabolizable buffer (acetate, gluconate or lactate).

Calcium-free solutions, such as saline (0.9% NaCl), Isolyte and Plasmalyte can be administered simultaneously with blood products. Solutions that contain calcium, such as lactated Ringer's, cannot be combined with blood products as microprecipitates may occur.

Calculation of fluid volume needed:

1. Calculate the patient's normal blood volume (BV)
2. Estimate the per cent blood loss, based on clinical signs and history
3. Calculate the volume deficit, VD = BV x % blood loss
4. Determine the resuscitation volume, based on
     whole blood volume = VD
     colloid volume =1.5 x VD
     isotonic crystalloid volume = 4 x VD

Normal blood volume (ml/kg): Dog: 80–90; Cat: 60–70

Normal plasma volume (ml/kg): Dog: 36–57; Cat: 35–53

Shock fluid rates
Isotonic crystalloid fluids: Dog: 80–90 ml/kg/h; Cat: 60–70 ml/kg/h
7.5% Hypertonic saline ± colloid: 4 ml/kg over 10 minutes

Blood replacement
Millilitres of blood to administer =

$$\frac{\text{(desired Hb - existing Hb)} \times \text{(ml/kg BV} \times \text{recipient kg weight)}}{\text{donor Hb}}$$

Plasma replacement
Millilitres of plasma to administer =

$$\frac{\text{(desired TP - existing TP)} \times \text{(ml/kg PV} \times \text{recipient kg weight)}}{\text{donor TP}}$$

Cryoprecipitate*
Millilitres of cryoprecipitate to administer =

$$\frac{\text{recipient kg weight} \times \text{BV (l/kg)} \times \text{(1-Hct(l/l))} \times \text{(desired - current factor level (U/ml))}}{\text{Factor level in plasma product (U/ml)}}$$

Platelet-rich plasma*
Expected 1-hour platelet count (x 10^9/l) =

$$\text{Platelet count before transfusion (x } 10^9/\text{l)} + \frac{\text{Unit platelet count (x}10^9/\text{l)} \times \text{unit volume} \times 0.51†}{\text{recipient kg weight} \times \text{BV (l/kg)}}$$

Figure 11.6: Guidelines for calculating replacement of fluid and blood components.

BV=Blood volume; Hb=haemoglobin; Hct=haematocrit; TP=total protein.
*Adapted from Mathews KA (1996) with the permission of LifeLearn. †Corrects for splenic sequestration of transfused platelets.

PREANAESTHETIC FLUID CONSIDERATIONS

In a healthy adult, the body is composed of 55–60% water, divided unequally into cellular (40%) and extracellular (20%) volumes (see Figure 11.3). The ECFV can be subdivided into the interstitial fluid volume and the plasma volume. With disease, any combination of fluid compartments may be increased or decreased, and every attempt should be made to predict the individual patient's needs. An estimate of the fluids needed should be calculated to replace the fluid deficit, provide maintenance fluids and replace ongoing losses. In addition, the anaesthetist should plan to replace fluid lost through additional evaporative losses, surgical blood loss and third space fluid loss.

Preoperatively, a minimum database of haematocrit and concentrations of TP, glucose and urea (or creatinine) should be assessed, and the patient should be evaluated for signs of dehydration or haemodynamic compromise. Clinical assessment includes evaluating skin elasticity, pulse rate and quality, mucous membrane colour, capillary refill time, respiratory rate and character, temperature of extremities and behaviour and mentation. The ability to assess ECFV is important but often must be estimated based on these non-specific clinical signs and abnormalities such as haemoconcentration, oliguria, azotaemia and acid-base or electrolyte alterations. A history suggestive of ECF deficits may include protracted gastrointestinal losses (vomiting, diarrhoea, bowel obstruction), sepsis, trauma or chronic diuretic administration. In some cases, additional information such as percentage of

Supplement	Emergency dose	Osmolarity (mOsm/l)	pH	Composition (mmol/l)
Calcium chloride (10%)	0.05–0.1 ml/kg slowly	2040	5.5–7.5	34 calcium 68 chloride
Calcium gluconate (10%)	0.5–3 ml/kg slowly or 60–90 mg/kg/day	680	6–8.2	465 calcium gluconate (no data)
Dextrose (50%)	500 mg/kg diluted, for immediate bolus	2530	4.2	no data
Magnesium sulphate (1 g/2 ml)	0.15–0.30 mmol/kg over 5 minutes	4060	5.5–7.0	4.06 magnesium sulphate (no data)
Mannitol (25%)	0.25–3 g/kg diluted and slowly over 30 minutes	1373	4.5–7.0	no data
Potassium chloride (2 mmol/ml)	0.5–1 mmol/kg/h	4000	4–8	2000 potassium 2000 chloride
Sodium bicarbonate (8.4%), (1 mmol/ml)	0.3 x body weight (kg) x base deficit (mmol/l) or 1 mmol/l immediately	2000	7.8	1000 sodium 1000 bicarbonate
Tromethamine* (0.3 M)	Millilitres needed = body weight (kg) x base deficit (mmol/l) x (1.1)	380	8.6	300 tromethamine

Figure 11.7: Fluid intravenous supplements.

Abbott Laboratories, North Chicago, IL, USA.

mixed venous blood oxygen saturation, blood gas tensions, buffer or base deficit calculations, blood lactate concentrations, urine output and urine specific gravity will assist in determining adequacy of tissue perfusion and severity of metabolic abnormalities.

Whenever time permits, stabilization of the patient's oxygen delivery, pH and electrolytes should occur in the preoperative period to optimize the patient's ability to tolerate the subsequent cardiopulmonary depressant effects of general anaesthesia. In an emergency, however, adequate oxygen delivery still must be restored but mild metabolic, electrolyte and acid-base disorders can be corrected during the intraoperative and postoperative periods. Treatment should always be initiated preoperatively for extreme hyperkalaemia (≥ 8 mmol/l), acidaemia (pH ≤ 7.20) or hypoglycaemia (≤ 60 mg/dl, 3.3 mmol/l). Fluids should be warmed before administration, because cold fluids will promote hypothermia and increase a patient's metabolic oxygen demands as they attempt to maintain body temperature.

For most routine surgical patients, a balanced isotonic crystalloid solution is an appropriate fluid administered at a rate of 5–10 ml/kg/h. Dehydration will decrease the cellular, interstitial and plasma fluid volumes, and such patients need volume expansion of all fluid compartments. Practically, however, the patient's own physiological mechanisms are relied on to control cellular fluid deficits. Therefore, for most dehydrated patients a balanced isotonic crystalloid is, again, an acceptable fluid choice. If it can be predicted that massive acute blood loss might occur, or that the patient may become severely hypotensive, a crystalloid is an acceptable initial fluid choice, provided that colloids and blood products are immediately available to maintain blood volume as soon as indicated during the procedure. In more chronic progressive types of hypovolaemia, the patient needs restoration of both blood volume and interstitial fluid volume and will benefit from a combination of both an isotonic crystalloid (to replace the interstitial fluid deficit, maintain urine output) and a colloid (to maintain plasma volume). Septic conditions or severe ischaemic episodes, from any cause, can decrease blood volume but increase cellular and interstitial volumes because of changes in capillary and cell membrane permeability and secondary fluid shifts. Such patients need fluids to support oxygen delivery, but those fluids should be chosen that will minimize further tissue or organ oedema. With a pre-existing metabolic acidosis or when there is concern for a future acidosis, the pH of the initial fluid should be near that of plasma (see Figure 11.1), and acetate and gluconate, which are easier to metabolize than lactate, may be a better choice in severely ill patients. In mild to moderate metabolic acidosis, efforts should be made to improve the circulating blood volume and oxygen delivery by either increasing the volume of fluid being administered or by restoration of erythrocytes to improve oxygen content. Stored blood and packed red cells are extremely acidotic, and fresh whole blood is preferred to prevent a worsening of the acidosis in critical patients. With a life-threatening acidaemia (pH <7.2), administration of an alkalinizing solution may be of temporary benefit while the underlying cause is being treated. Controversy exists over the usefulness of sodium bicarbonate, but other buffers, such as tromethamine, are commercially available and cause fewer side effects (see Figure 11.7). A buffer should not be administered through the same catheter as either a solution containing calcium (e.g. lactated Ringer's) or any type of blood product.

INTRAOPERATIVE FLUID CONSIDERATIONS

The two concerns for intraoperative maintenance fluids are whether or not to administer glucose, and how much water, sodium and potassium are necessary to replace losses. Glucose has, in the past, been given perioperatively to decrease protein catabolism and prevent hypoglycaemia. This may be a special concern for diabetic patients, patients with liver disease or paediatric patients. However, the stress response that results from anaesthesia and surgery produces an anti-insulin effect, making it difficult to predict the glucose requirements for an individual patient. Except where hypoglycaemia is likely, routinely administering glucose has two disadvantages. First, hyperglycaemia may occur, causing an osmotic diuresis and dehydration. Second, studies have indicated that hyperglycaemia may worsen neurological ischaemia and outcome after traumatic brain injury. This latter finding may have clinical relevance for critically ill patients as well. To prevent hypoglycaemia, a 2.5% dextrose infusion can be prepared by the addition of 5 ml of 50% dextrose to 100 ml of an isotonic crystalloid solution. This allows additional dextrose to be administered without the concern of also administering free water. Blood glucose concentration should then be re-evaluated and additional glucose added to the solution if necessary (glucose <80–100 mg/dl (4.5–5.7 mmol/l).

Sodium and potassium are two *electrolytes* that must be replaced in the perioperative period. To replace intraoperative fluid losses, the sodium and potassium content of the commonly administered fluids are similar in composition to the ECF (see Figure 11.1). Any whole body imbalance in these two electrolytes caused by such short-term fluid administration is generally well compensated by the kidneys. There are no short-term requirements for other electrolytes except in instances where severe derangement has occurred.

Water requirements include the need to replace gastrointestinal, renal and insensible losses (e.g. respiratory, cutaneous). Additional fluids are required to replace blood and third space fluid losses and to prevent hypotension from the vasodilation and myocardial depression of general anaesthesia.

Even the awake animal is intolerant to acute blood loss, and rapid intervention is essential. In hypovolaemic shock, the mortality rate is directly related to the magnitude and duration of the ischaemic insult (see Chapter 21). Since life-saving compensatory reflexes are obtunded or removed in patients under general anaesthesia, these patients are even more sensitive to acute blood loss and hypovolaemia. Furthermore, seemingly small volumes of blood loss may not be tolerated in sick, debilitated or traumatized patients.

The goal of fluid therapy after blood loss is to restore blood volume, as a first priority, but also to replenish interstitial fluid deficits that may have occurred due to compensatory flux into the vascular space. In emergency situations, restoration of blood volume and cardiac output will occur with any fluid that re-expands the plasma volume (crystalloids, colloids or blood products). However, colloids and crystalloids both flow faster through the administration system than blood products because a fluid's flow rate increases as its viscosity decreases. Hence, any acellular solution will flow faster than whole blood, and whole blood will flow faster than undiluted packed red cells. Practically, therefore, cardiac output is most rapidly restored with colloids and least rapidly restored with packed red cells. Due to differences in distribution, the volume of crystalloids must be at least three times greater than the volume of colloid infused to have an equivalent effect on cardiac output. In mild to moderate haemorrhage, crystalloids are beneficial because this type of fluid also replaces the interstitial fluid deficit. In severe haemorrhage, administering both a colloid and a crystalloid will restore both the blood volume and interstitial fluid volume more rapidly. In addition, acellular solutions will decrease the patient's haemoglobin concentration; and mild haemodilution, by decreasing blood viscosity, may improve microcirculatory blood flow without detrimental effects on oxygen delivery. Conventional shock doses of an isotonic crystalloid fluid are 90 ml/kg/h for dogs and 60 ml/kg/h for cats (i.e. one blood volume in an hour), with the fluid rate slowed as soon as favourable responses are observed. If the patient remains unstable, then additional fluids such as colloids and blood may be necessary to maintain intravascular volume during the critical period, with fluid rates dictated by the patient's clinical condition. For emergency blood volume expansion, hypertonic saline plus a colloid can be life saving. The standard emergency dose is 4 ml/kg i.v. of 7.5% hypertonic saline in 6% dextran-70 over 10 minutes, followed by conventional fluid therapy. If hypertonic saline is given more rapidly, hypotension due to direct vascular relaxation and vasodilation may occur. This hypotension, in the face of a life-threatening hypovolaemia, can be detrimental and even fatal. If hypertonic saline is administered more slowly than the shock rate, fluid shifting will still occur, but the onset may be slower and maximum effect may be obtunded. Lower hypertonic saline doses may be necessary in patients with cardiac disease to prevent circulatory overload and cardiac failure. The shock colloid dose is 5–20 ml/kg over 30 minutes. It should be noted that all these crystalloid and colloid shock doses are approximate starting doses. The safe maximum rate or volume that can be administered is undetermined for any fluid. In one study, 8–14% dehydrated but otherwise healthy dogs received lactated Ringer's solution intravenously at a dose of either 90 ml/kg/h (group A), 225 ml/kg/h (group B) or 360 ml/kg/h (group C) for 1 hour (Cornelius *et al.*, 1978). Clinical signs were absent or mild in groups A and B while group C showed marked serous nasal discharge, coughing and dyspnoea within 20 minutes of fluid administration. It may be concluded that isotonic crystalloid fluids probably can be administered faster than 90 ml/kg/h but slower than 360 ml/kg/h in otherwise healthy dogs (i.e. no pulmonary oedema, sepsis or heart disease). The rule of thumb is to infuse fluids as slowly as possible but as quickly as necessary to produce haemodynamic stability. While shock doses should be decreased as soon as the patient's clinical condition permits, it is equally important to be aggressive during initial resuscitation because duration of ischaemia affects outcome. Cellular oedema and injury to major organs can continue after apparently successful resuscitation due to the no-reflow phenomenon and reperfusion injury from sustained ischaemia.

Third spacing is the abnormal accumulation of fluid in normal extracellular locations. It is caused by expansion of the interstitial fluid space, ascites, hydrothorax or fluid accumulation around traumatized tissues (including excessive surgical manipulation). Loss of fluid into these spaces needs to be considered when calculating fluid replacement. This fluid loss may lead to hypovolaemia (if the fluid came from the vasculature), dehydration (if the fluid came from the extracellular space), hypoproteinaemia (if the fluid has high protein content) and ultimately, poor tissue perfusion. The fluid can accumulate in regions that may further compromise circulation to an organ or within an organ. In humans, guidelines for third space fluid losses are calculated based on extent of expected tissue trauma; these losses are corrected in addition to the fluids calculated to replace blood loss.

Keeping in mind that the greater the tissue damage, the more the third spacing of fluids occurs, estimated fluid rates for an anaesthetized patient are approximately 4 ml/kg/h for procedures with minimal trauma, 6 ml/kg/h for moderate trauma, and 8 ml/kg/h for extreme tissue trauma (Giesecke and Egberth, 1985). For all patients, clinical monitoring will determine if the rate is adequate or should be adjusted.

Special conditions

Cardiac function
Patients with decreased cardiac function do not tolerate excessive fluid administration. Large sodium loads should be avoided. Colloids are an acceptable alternative but must be titrated carefully because over-expansion of the plasma volume with colloids will not be corrected very quickly.

Oliguria
Patients with acute oliguria also need to be monitored carefully, as the oliguria may be renal or prerenal in origin. An acceptable plan would be to infuse an isotonic crystalloid while monitoring urine output, central venous pressure, blood pressure and heart rate. The patient's response to a small fluid challenge may help differentiate the origin of the oliguria. Signs of urine output >0.5 ml/kg/h indicate prerenal oliguria. If a fluid challenge causes neither signs of improvement nor toxicity, and there is concern that further fluids may result in an unacceptable risk, fluid rates should be decreased. In these patients, concurrent therapy may include dopamine or diuretic administration. If colloids are chosen, careful titration and monitoring is essential because many colloids are cleared by the kidneys and may have a prolonged effect or worsen the renal disease.

Cranial problems
Patients with traumatic brain injury and/or increased intracranial pressure are very fragile and respond quickly to insufficient or excessive fluid administration. Unfortunately, no single fluid is superior in this situation, and extreme care must be taken in evaluating the patient's response. The volume and type of fluid depend on whether or not the patient is haemodynamically stable and if the blood–brain barrier is thought to be intact. The goal is to provide a systolic blood pressure >90 mmHg without detrimentally affecting cerebral perfusion pressure. Paradoxically, cerebral perfusion pressure can decrease with fluid therapy due to the redistribution of water into the cerebral interstitial and cellular spaces, increasing cerebral oedema and causing secondary brain injury. The normal blood–brain barrier is relatively impermeable to both protein and sodium, causing water normally to move in or out of brain cells and interstitium in response primarily to capillary osmotic pressure and secondarily to oncotic pressure. Therefore, sodium changes are more important than protein changes in these patients. Thus, even a slightly hypotonic solution, such as lactated Ringer's, may promote cerebral oedema. Isotonic saline with supplemental potassium may be a more appropriate fluid. However, prolonged saline use is not advisable because the patient may become hypernatraemic or hyperchloraemic, and such a solution is devoid of other important electrolytes. Hypertonic (3–5%) saline solution lowers intracranial pressure and

may decrease cerebral oedema, as well as provide rapid intravascular volume expansion. Solutions containing colloids have been associated with lower intracranial pressure than with isotonic crystalloid solutions. Pentastarch, in particular, is composed of very large molecules and may be used to plug leaks in the blood-brain barrier. Solutions that should be avoided in patients with any type of neurological disease are those containing glucose. It is thought that patients with neurological conditions with increased plasma glucose concentrations have a worse neurological outcome because the glucose promotes cellular metabolism and leads to anerobic conditions and lactic acidosis. In addition, solutions containing only dextrose cause cerebral oedema due to the free water that remains after the dextrose is utilized (see above). If dextrose must be administered to treat hypoglycaemia, it is imperative to add the dextrose to an isotonic solution, and not to use dextrose in water.

POSTOPERATIVE FLUID CONSIDERATIONS

Most patients receive a high fluid rate preoperatively and intraoperatively to maintain intravascular blood volume. In the postoperative phase, this fluid may redistribute to extravascular spaces thus causing a decrease in intravascular volume, while at the same time the patient, awakening from anaesthesia, has an increase in blood pressure and glomerular filtration that promotes a diuresis. These patients may need additional fluids for several hours after the anaesthetic period to compensate for this inappropriate diuresis. The diuresis may mask signs of hypovolaemia, as it will seem that the patient has adequate urine production. Furthermore, patients that were not hydrated before anaesthesia may continue to be dehydrated at the end of the anaesthetic procedure and continue to require additional fluid volume. On the other hand, interstitial over-expansion may develop after administration of isotonic crystalloids. Once haemodynamic stability has returned, this sequestered fluid needs to be mobilized, returned to the plasma volume and eventually removed from the body. Mobilization of accumulated fluids tends to occur maximally around the third postoperative day, with continued fluid shifting for up to 10 days, depending on the circumstances and severity of the surgical trauma. Close monitoring of haemodynamic variables as well as urine output, electrolyte and acid-base status are important during this period for critically ill patients.

FLUID THERAPY MONITORING

The goal of monitoring is to evaluate for adequate oxygen delivery (see Figure 11.5), and to assess the effect of any changes made in the fluid management. In high-risk surgical patients, survivors frequently had supranormal oxygen delivery indices compared with those who later died (Bland *et al.*, 1985). Thus, intensive monitoring is necessary in critically ill patients, even if there are no outward clinical signs of hypoperfusion. The challenge, however, is that there is no practical way to measure oxygen delivery, blood volume, ECFV, etc. directly and continuously. Both subjective and objective information must be relied upon. Subjective signs include lethargy, mucous membrane colour, capillary refill time, temperature of extremities and other signs of perfusion. Useful objective data include heart rate, direct or indirect arterial pressure, pulse pressure, central venous pressure, temperature, pulse oximetry, blood pH and gas tensions, electrolyte concentration, haematocrit, TP concentration, urea concentration, urine output and response to fluid challenges, as well as calculation of oxygen indices (see Figure 11.5).

Many of the common cardiovascular monitoring techniques have limitations, of which the clinician should be aware. For example, changes in systemic blood pressure and heart rate are important but non-specific markers of hypovolaemia due to blood loss. Hypotension may just as easily be due to excessive anaesthetic depth, the type of anaesthetic used, cardiac dysfunction or decreases in systemic vascular resistance. Non-invasive methods for measuring blood pressure can yield equally low measurements in both hypovolaemic and hypothermic patients (presumably due to vasoconstrictive responses), and it is difficult to differentiate between these two, especially when they often co-exist in a patient. Cardiac filling pressures, such as central venous pressure and pulmonary artery wedge pressure, show a poor correlation to the presence and extent of blood loss until the blood loss is severe (>30%). Since the values themselves are normally small and quite variable (i.e. central venous pressures of 5–10 cmH$_2$0), their usefulness for detecting significant changes may be limited by the sensitivity of the monitoring equipment and the care with which the transducers are zeroed (see Chapter 5). Knowing the limitations of the various monitoring methods will permit these variables to be useful surveillance tools, as long as all detected abnormalities are critically evaluated and investigated further.

Periodic assessment of the patient's packed cell volume or haematocrit will detect acute anaemia and its direct effect on oxygen delivery. The haematocrit is often measured in patients with acute blood loss and during fluid therapy, but it should be remembered that the haematocrit by itself is not a reliable or appropriate method of evaluating blood loss. Since whole blood is lost during haemorrhage, the haematocrit of the patient will not change acutely, although the total volume of blood and red cell mass will decrease. After several hours, with transcapillary refill and the kidneys actively conserving sodium and water, the haematocrit of

Disorder	Fresh whole blood	Stored whole blood	Packed red cells	Platelet-rich plasma	Fresh frozen plasma	Cryoprecipitate	Stored or frozen plasma
Acute haemorrhage	x*	x	x (plus colloid)		x (plus red cells)		x (plus red cells)
Anaemia	x	x	x*				
Coagulopathy	x			x	x*	x	
Hypoproteinaemia					x		x*
Platelet function abnormality				x*	x		
Deficient specific clotting factors					x*	x*	
Thrombocytopenia	x			x*			
von Willebrand's disease	x			x	x	x*	

Figure 11.8: *Indications for blood component therapy.*

Best choice of blood component for that disorder.

a patient will decrease, but this decrease may not be maximal for up to 24 hours. If, simultaneously, the patient is treated with asanguineous intravenous fluids to promote normovolaemia, the haematocrit will decrease even further as a result of haemodilution of the remaining red cells. Neither of these causes of decreasing haematocrit are indications of ongoing blood loss. However, a decrease in haematocrit plus a dependency on continued fluid therapy to maintain haemodynamic stability suggests ongoing blood loss.

Even after apparently adequate intravenous fluid volume replacement, unrecognized tissue hypoperfusion may be present due to cellular and interstitial oedema that developed during the hypovolaemic crisis. This unseen hypoperfusion is the most likely cause of many postoperative complications that develop in critical patients, such as acute renal failure, hepatic failure or systemic inflammatory response syndrome. Monitoring oxygen indices (e.g. oxygen extraction, venous partial pressure of oxygen) is one method of evaluating the adequacy of tissue perfusion. In most situations where tissue oxygen delivery falls, tissue oxygen extraction will increase as a method of obtaining more oxygen. The normal SaO_2 is >95% and the $S\bar{v}O_2$ > 65%, for a normal extraction of 20–30%. The oxygen extraction will increase, and $S\bar{v}O_2$ will decrease, as tissues take out more and more oxygen from the inadequate amount of blood being delivered. At the point where extraction can no longer increase, oxygen consumption by the tissues becomes dependent on oxygen delivery (critical oxygen delivery threshold). Experience suggests that the transition from compensated hypovolaemia to uncompensated hypovolaemic shock takes place when the $S\bar{v}O_2$ falls below 50% and the oxygen extraction approaches 50–60%. Thus, an oxygen extraction >30% is a marker of profound tissue hypoperfusion, and an oxygen extraction >50% indicates hypovolaemic shock. Other possible differentials for increased oxygen extraction are anaemia and hypermetabolism. A rough estimate of oxygen extraction can be done using a pulse oximeter (in lieu of an arterial blood gas or arterial haemoximeter) and a mixed venous blood gas in which oxygen saturation values are provided. Monitoring blood lactate concentrations or the base deficit from a blood gas sample will provide additional information on the development of lactic acidosis from hypoperfusion. A lactate concentration >4 mmol/l or a base deficit > -10 mmol/l suggests profound oxygen debt.

BLOOD TRANSFUSION MEDICINE

The classical indications for blood transfusion are treatment or prevention of hypoproteinaemia, hypovolaemia, coagulation disorders and decreased oxygen delivery from acute blood loss or anaemia. With the increasing number of commercial animal blood banks in the United States, specific blood component therapy is possible for the general practitioner (Figure 11.8).

Blood volume

Blood volume is critical for homeostasis. Clearly, blood volume will decrease during haemorrhage, but it can also decrease with disease associated with hypoproteinaemia (due to decreased intravascular oncotic pressure). Initially, blood volume can be restored with either crystalloid or colloid therapy, as described above. However, there are two points to consider in deciding whether or not blood therapy is indicated: the haemoglobin content of the patient and the rate of blood loss.

Absolute minimums in haemoglobin content are controversial for both awake and anaesthetized patients and should be evaluated in conjunction with the other determinants of oxygen delivery. Cardiac output and blood flow may increase to compensate for a decrease in haematocrit, but at some point cardiac output and blood flow are maximal and a lower haematocrit becomes critical. Conventional wisdom suggests that a patient can tolerate a lower haematocrit when awake or if the anaemia is of chronic duration. For these patients, a haematocrit of 18-20% is often well tolerated. However, when anaesthesia is required, blood products are necessary sooner because of increased fluid needs during surgery, depressed compensatory reflexes, myocardial depression and vasodilation from the anaesthetics. Haematocrits <25-27% may limit oxygen delivery and delay wound healing. Therefore, depending on the length of anaesthesia and the invasiveness of the surgical procedure, the pre-anaesthetic haematocrit is recommended to be at least 30-34% in dogs and 25-29% in cats.

The most common indications for administration of a blood product during anaesthesia are acute blood loss or normovolaemic anaemia from acellular fluid administration. Signs of blood loss such as tachycardia and hypotension are inconsistent, imprecise and unreliable in anaesthetized patients; therapy should not be withheld until these signs are observed. Even in awake healthy patients, a 30-40% acute blood loss may cause the reflex tachycardia and vasoconstriction to be lost, with the sudden and profound onset of hypotension and hypovolaemic shock. In awake previously healthy patients, a >40% acute blood loss is usually fatal unless immediate volume and haemoglobin restoration occurs. Under anaesthesia, the amount of permissible blood loss is much less. An anaesthetized patient with an acute blood loss of ≥10% may require a blood transfusion, especially if the patient also becomes haemodynamically unstable, a prolonged anaesthesia time is predicted or additional blood loss is likely.

The actual blood volume of a patient should be calculated to determine the significance of fluids lost in the perioperative period as well as to predict the volume of fluid necessary to replace deficits. Calculating the exact blood volume in larger animals is often overlooked, but it is important to have an estimate.

Blood volume is generally calculated as 8-10% bodyweight in dogs (45% cells and 55% plasma), and around 6% bodyweight in cats (36% cells and 64% plasma). Therefore, a given volume of blood lost will be a greater percentage of a cat's blood volume than that of a dog of the same bodyweight. Also, loss of a given volume of blood will have a more profound effect on a smaller animal than on a larger animal. For small patients, counting Q-tips and gauzes that have become blood soaked during haemostasis may become essential to assess blood or fluid loss accurately.

Blood types and incompatibility reactions

A cross-matching test evaluates for serological incompatibility between donor and recipient blood, but it does not determine blood type. Cross-matching tests check for the presence of haemolysing or haemagglutinating antibodies in the plasma (or serum) that are directed against red blood cell antigens. Cross matching is performed in both dogs and cats to decrease the risk of transfusion reactions, and to decrease the risk of sensitizing the recipient. Transfusion reactions may occur in previously sensitized animals, animals with naturally occurring isoantibodies or those with neonatal isoerythrolysis. Sensitizing an animal should be avoided if more than one blood transfusion is predicted or if the animal is an intact breeding female. Blood typing reveals blood group antigens on the red blood cell surface. It is possible to obtain a blood typing card to classify dogs as DEA 1.1 positive or negative and another to classify cats as type A or type B.

Dog blood types

About 12 different dog blood types exist (Figure 11.9). The most antigenic is DEA 1.1, followed by DEA 1.2 and, possibly, DEA 7. In contrast to cats, dogs do not seem to have any clinically important naturally occurring antibodies to other dog blood types. The low incidence of DEA 1.1, 1.2 and 7, and the lack of naturally occurring antibodies, have two important clinical implications. First, if neither donor nor recipient has ever received a transfusion before, a cross match will not detect any alloantibodies even if the blood samples are of two different types. Second, a random, first-time transfusion is unlikely to cause an immediate incompatibility reaction because 4-14 days are required for the recipient to produce antibodies to the donor cells.

Blood type (DEA)	1.1	1.2	3	4	5	6	7	8
USA	33-45	7-24	5-10	87-98	12-25	67-99	8-45	40
Netherlands	38	4	5	56	8	74	31	17
Japan	44	22	24	No data	No data	60	No data	No data

Figure 11.9: *Population incidences (percentages) of canine blood types.*

Adapted from Giger et al. (1995) Journal of the American Veterinary Medical Association **206(9)**, 1358-1362, with permission.

Domestic shorthair cats*		Type A (%)	Type B (%)	Purebred cats	Type A (%)	Type B (%)
USA	Northeast	99.7	0.3	Abyssinian	84	16
	North Central	99.6	0.4	American Shorthair	100	0
	Southeast	98.5	1.5	Birman*	82	18
	Southwest	97.5	2.5	British Shorthair*	64	36
	West Coast	95.3	4.7	Burmese	100	0
Other countries	Australia (Brisbane)	73.7	26.3	Devon Rex	67	33
	Argentina	97.3	2.7	Exotic Shorthair	73	27
Europe	Austria	97.0	3.0	Japanese Bobtail	84	16
	England	97.1	2.9	Maine Coon	97	3
	Finland	100	0	Norwegian Forest	96	7
	France	85.1	14.9	Oriental Shorthair	100	0
	Germany	94.0	6.0	Persian	86	14
	Italy	88.8	11.2	Scottish Fold*	81	19
	Netherlands	96.1	3.9	Siamese	100	0
	Scotland	97.1	2.9	Somali*	82	18
	Switzerland	99.6	0.4	Sphinx*	83	17
				Tonkinese	100	0

Figure 11.10: Blood type A and B frequency in cats.

Reproduced from Giger U and Oakley D (1998) Current feline transfusion therapy: unique issues in cats. In: Proceedings of the VI International Veterinary Emergency and Critical Care Symposium, pp. 207–210, with permission.
*Breeds with isolated type AB cats.

For blood transfusions in dogs, it is recommended that blood donors be confirmed DEA 1.1, 1.2 and 7 negative (with DEA 1.1 the most important). These dogs can be considered universal donors because the other blood types cause minimal antigenic stimulation in unsensitized dogs. It is preferable to blood type the recipient as well, to prevent a delayed haemolytic reaction and to prevent sensitization (see below) but, in emergency situations, this can be foregone. Nevertheless, a blood type and cross match should always be performed if either the donor or recipient has previously received a blood transfusion.

Incompatibility reactions in dogs

An immediate or delayed reaction can occur with incompatible blood types. If a cross match is not available and the dogs are of different blood types, the recipient dog may destroy the donor red cells as antibodies develop. This delayed haemolytic transfusion reaction can be observed as a rapid decline in the haematocrit over 1–2 weeks after the transfusion and is easily overlooked or misdiagnosed on follow up blood work. The dog also is now sensitized to that blood type, and all future transfusions with blood of that type may cause an acute haemolytic reaction.

An acute haemolytic reaction occurs when mismatched blood is administered to a previously sensitized recipient. The most severe reaction will occur when a previously DEA 1.1 sensitized dog receives another DEA 1.1 blood transfusion. The signs of an acute transfusion reaction are variable and can develop within minutes to hours after the transfusion has begun. The severity of the signs is roughly proportional to the amount of incompatible blood received and the degree of incompatibility. Common signs include fever, vomiting, urticaria, haemoglobinaemia and haemoglobinuria. Although rare, the reaction can be fatal, with initial signs of severe hypotension, bradycardia and erratic respirations. If the animal survives this phase, a second phase may occur in which the patient becomes tachypnoeic, hypertensive and tachycardic and may develop other cardiac dysrhythmias. Stabilization, if it is to occur, generally follows within 30 minutes.

Cat blood types

Cats have an AB blood group system: the most common blood type is type A (Figure 11.10). A and B are alleles, with A being dominant. The third cat blood type, type AB, is inherited separately as a third allele that is recessive to A and co-dominant with B. In

		Packed cell volume of donated blood (including anticoagulant)										
Packed cell volume of recipient		30%	32%	34%	36%	38%	40%	42%	44%	46%	48%	50%
	4%	16.3	15.3	14.4	13.6	12.9	12.3	11.7	11.1	10.6	10.2	9.8
	6%	14.0	13.1	12.4	11.7	11.1	10.5	10.0	9.5	9.1	8.8	8.4
	8%	11.7	10.9	10.3	9.7	9.2	8.8	8.3	8.0	7.6	7.3	7.0
	10%	9.3	8.8	8.2	7.8	7.4	7.0	6.7	6.7	6.1	5.8	5.6
	12%	7.0	6.6	6.2	5.8	5.5	5.3	5.0	4.8	4.6	4.4	4.2
	14%	4.7	4.3	4.1	3.9	3.7	3.5	3.3	3.2	3.0	2.9	2.8

Example:	Packed cell volume of recipient	6%
	Packed cell volume of donated blood	46%
	Weight of recipient	7 lb
	Volume of blood needed per pound	9.1 ml (see above)
	Multiplied by weight of recipient	x 7 lb
	Total volume of blood needed	= 63.7 ml

Figure 11.11: Volume of blood (millilitres) needed for transfusion per pound (lb) bodyweight of recipient cat based on a post-transfusion packed cell volume of 18% (2.2 lb = 1kg).

Reproduced from Norsworthy GD (1977) Blood transfusion in the cat. Feline Practice 7, 29, with permission.

certain breeds, type B can be very common compared with the general population (see Figure 11.10), and historical information from owners or breeders may be important. Thirty five per cent of type A cats and 70% of type B cats have natural isoagglutinins against the opposite red blood cell antigens. Type AB cats do not have any alloantibodies against either type A or type B red blood cells. There is no universal donor.

For blood transfusions in cats, it is recommended that both donor and recipient cats be blood typed. Blood typing prevents acute or delayed transfusion reactions and prevents sensitizing a cat that may not have naturally occurring alloantibodies. If blood typing is not available, a major and minor cross match should be performed. Small test doses of blood to recipient should never be administered. Type A donors are preferred because of their common blood type, but access to a type B cat is advisable. Cats with type AB blood are best transfused with type AB blood or, at the very least, type A blood. The reason for not using a type B donor blood is because more type B cats have isoagglutinins than type A cats, and because any anti-A alloantibodies in the type B donor blood will recognize the A antigens in the recipient type AB blood, causing a more severe haemolytic reaction than using type A donor blood.

Incompatibility reactions in cats

Because naturally occurring alloantibodies are much more common in cats than in dogs, a random first-time blood transfusion will have a higher likelihood of a reaction (around 36%) (Kirk and Bistner, 1985). The mean survival half-life of feline red cells is around 30 days in cats that receive a matched blood type. Type A cats with anti-B serum that receive mismatched blood will have decreased red cell survival (half-life of around 2 days) and a mild, sometimes clinically inapparent, transfusion reaction. However, type B cats with anti-A serum that receive type A blood will have tremendously decreased red cell survival (half-life of around 1 hour) and will exhibit marked systemic reactions consistent with an acute intravascular haemolytic transfusion reaction. As little as 5 ml of blood can be fatal in such situations.

Calculating the transfusion volume needed

Formulas have been devised to estimate the volume of whole blood or blood component to administer to a patient (see Figure 11.6). Alternatively, some less precise rules-of-thumb are available. For whole blood, a dog can receive 10–40 ml/kg and a cat 5–20 ml/kg, and the patient's haematocrit should be remeasured. However, a volume of whole blood (in millilitres) equal to the (required haematocrit rise) x (the bodyweight in pounds) can be administered. These rough estimates are serviceable but do not take into account the haematocrit of the donor or the fact that cats and dogs have a different ratio of red cell mass to plasma volume. A precalculated chart is also available for cats (Figure 11.11). For plasma, it can be estimated that around 22 ml/kg of plasma will be necessary to increase albumin concentration by 5 g/l. The estimated initial dose of fresh frozen plasma for coagulopathies is 10–20 ml/kg bodyweight. This dose may be repeated several times to obtain the desired effect. If cryoprecipitate is needed, the standard dose is around 1 ml/kg, or 1 U/10 kg.

TRANSFUSION ADMINISTRATION AND COMPLICATIONS

Route of administration

Jugular, cephalic and saphenous veins and intraosseous femoral or humeral sites are all acceptable routes for blood administration. Intraperitoneal transfusions may be all that is available in neonates, but the rate of peritoneal absorption is slow.

Preparation

Refrigerated blood and blood products should be warmed gently to body temperature before transfusing (not to exceed 37°C or 98.6°F). Packed red cells can be diluted with 0.9% saline. Frozen bags of plasma must be handled carefully to prevent cracking during the thawing process. Thawing of frozen plasma, conducted with a circulating warm water bath with the temperature between 30 and 37°C (86–98.6°F), generally takes around 30 minutes. Frozen plasma can be microwaved and be ready to administer after about 3–5 minutes. To microwave frozen plasma, the plasma bag is placed in a container of water, without its sides touching the container, and the container is placed in the centre of a microwave oven (700 W setting). The plasma unit is microwaved in 5–10 second periods and is agitated for 3–5 seconds by hand between exposures (to prevent localized overheating). Microwave thawing of canine fresh frozen plasma does not alter the one-stage prothrombin time, factor VIII coagulant activity and von Willebrand factor antigen (Hurst *et al.*, 1987). Once frozen plasma has been thawed in the microwave it should be transferred into a water-bath for warming to body temperature. Thawed plasma should be used within 6–8 hours and should never be refrozen. Liquid plasma and other components should not be warmed all the way to body temperature in a microwave.

Stored blood and packed red cells become quickly acidotic and have higher ammonia concentrations than fresh whole blood. Citrate-phosphate-dextrose, the anticoagulant solution in most blood collection bags, has a pH of 5.5. Thus, even the pH of a freshly drawn bag of blood will decrease to approximately 7.0 or 7.1. With additional storage, lactic and pyruvic acids produced by red cell metabolism and glycolysis will accumulate, and the pH may decrease to 6.9 after 3 weeks of storage. A contributing factor to this acidosis of stored blood is hypercapnia. However, excess carbon dioxide is normally rapidly removed by patients with adequate ventilation. Considering these modifications of stored blood, fresh whole blood may be more appropriate for patients with pre-existing acidosis or hepatic encephalopathy, or in critically ill patients.

Autotransfusion

The best method of autotransfusion is to estimate the volume of blood transfusion needed preoperatively, and to harvest this volume of blood from the patient and store it several days to a week before the surgery. Alternatively, blood can be withdrawn from the patient immediately before the procedure and replaced with appropriate crystalloids or colloids, a technique termed normovolaemic haemodilution. This blood can then be given when needed intraoperatively without concern of an incompatible transfusion reaction. Intraoperative salvage techniques for autotransfusion have some definite drawbacks but can be done. Intraoperative salvage is preferably done with some type of automated cell saver or blood salvage system. The blood is aspirated from the surgical field, mixed with anticoagulant and transferred to a reservoir unit. In the reservoir it is filtered, centrifuged, washed and resuspended. Complications include haemolysis, coagulopathies, decreased calcium and air embolism. Salvaged blood should not be reinfused if the blood may contain tumour cells, urine, bile, faecal matter or other contaminants.

Desmopressin acetate

Desmopressin acetate (DDAVP) is used to release factor VIII and von Willebrand factor transiently from a patient's endothelial stores. It is administered to humans with selected types of von Willebrand's disease before surgery. The recommended dose is 0.1–0.3 mg/kg i.v., using human intranasal drops diluted with sterile saline and administered over 10 minutes. The peak effect is obtained 30–50 minutes after administration, and the duration of response is transient (about 6 hours). In dogs, a dose of 1–5 mg/kg has been used empirically as an alternative to transfusion therapy for some patients with von Willebrand's disease, or to increase factor VIII concentrations in the blood donor dog 30 minutes before collection (Turrentine *et al.*, 1988). Limitations to DDAVP include its transient effect, failure of some dogs to respond (presumably because some dogs have inactive or minimal von Willebrand factor, even in storage) and refractory patients after repeated treatments. Thus, DDAVP can only be considered adjunct therapy in some specific patients and cannot be considered a reliable substitute to transfusion therapy.

Administration and rate

A blood filter must always be used to remove microthrombi from blood products. A human adult filter is generally acceptable, but when small volumes of blood are being administered, a 170 μm micropore filter can also be used safely, with less blood being trapped in the filter apparatus.

Always administer blood products in a separate line or, at the least, with compatible fluids that do not contain calcium or bicarbonate (e.g. 0.9% NaCl). Do not administer drugs through the blood line, and do not add any drugs to the blood bags. Gently oscillate the bag to mix the contents periodically during administration.

An extremely slow rate of administration is initially indicated to observe for signs of an acute transfusion reaction. Even with appropriate serological screening, non-immunological transfusion reactions can occur due to improper storage or transfusion technique, contamination with infectious organisms, etc. As already mentioned, a transfusion reaction can have a wide variety of signs but, should any occur, the transfusion has to be aborted immediately. If no transfusion reaction develops, the subsequent rate should be as slow as possible to obtain the desired result over 4–8 hours. A standard rate of about 4–5 ml/kg/h is generally adequate. If the patient is normovolaemic, the rate should be slower (2.5–5 ml/kg/h) to prevent circulatory overload. In patients with pre-existing cardiac disease, the rate may need to be further decreased to 0.5–1 ml/kg/h. At the other extreme, 5–15 ml/kg/h is recommended to treat acutely hypovolaemic animals and, in a life-threatening emergency, rates up to 40–60 ml/kg/h may be required (bolus technique).

Transfusion monitoring

In this instance, monitoring means evaluating the response to therapy and looking for signs of acute transfusion reactions such as a change in attitude, vomiting, pruritus, altered capillary refill time, fever, tachycardia, dyspnoea or erratic respirations, peripheral oedema, disseminated intravascular coagulation, urticaria, hypotension, icterus or haemoglobinaemia. Blood pressure, heart rate, body temperature, urine output and haematocrit measurements, evaluation of serum colour and electrocardiography are recommended to monitor a blood transfusion during anaesthesia. Acute haemolysis is supportive of direct incompatibility. If even mild hypothermia occurs, up to 4–5 hours after transfusion, the most likely cause is an incompatibility between the donor white blood cells and recipient antigens. For any reaction, treatment involves stopping the blood transfusion immediately and providing supportive care. If the reaction is mild, the transfusion can be reinitiated at a slower rate. Although corticosteroids (dexamethasone sodium phosphate at 2 mg/kg i.v. or hydrocortisone at 10 mg/kg i.v.) and diphenhydramine (Benadryl, 0.5 mg/kg i.m.) are often used to prevent or lessen the signs of an acute haemolytic transfusion reaction, there is currently no objective evidence to support this practice. Donor antibodies reacting to recipient white blood cell antigens may cause white blood cell aggregates or emboli in the recipient's lungs. This may result in pulmonary oedema or hyperthermia and has been termed transfusion-induced acute lung injury. Serial arterial blood gas analysis and pulse oximetry may detect this complication in an anaesthetized patient.

Some adverse reactions may not be due to incompatible blood types, but instead to improper handling or administration of the blood. Dark brown or black blood units should be discarded, as they may be colonized by bacteria, which can lead to sepsis. Bleeding can occur if large volumes of factor-free blood components are administered. In patients affected with coagulopathies, monitoring the platelet number, activated clotting time, partial thromboplastin time, prothrombin time and buccal mucosal bleeding time may be beneficial. Lung microemboli can cause respiratory insufficiency if the blood product is not filtered properly. Circulatory overload can occur if blood is administered in excess or too rapidly, particularly in patients with pre-existing cardiac or renal disease. These patients should be monitored for classic signs of vascular overload such as an increase in central venous pressure, dyspnoea, vomiting, chemosis or pulmonary oedema. Citrate toxicity can occur if large volumes of blood are administered rapidly and the liver's ability to metabolize the compound is transiently overwhelmed. Citrate binds calcium, causing signs of transient hypocalcaemia with hypotension, a narrow pulse pressure and, rarely, cardiac dysrhythmias. Usually this complication is self limiting but calcium supplementation may be necessary in some cases. Ionized calcium concentrations should be measured during transfusions of critically ill patients and whenever massive transfusions are administered rapidly.

Solutions carrying oxygen

The inability to readily obtain blood products or a cross match can have life-threatening consequences. Safe and effective blood substitutes are becoming available commercially, after over 50 years of research and development. Three categories of acellular, oxygen-carrying and plasma volume expanders exist. First are the free

Category	Whole blood	Liposome-encapsulated haemoglobin	Stroma-free polymerized haemoglobin	Fluorocarbon
Haemoglobin (g/dl)	14–16	16	13	–
Osmolarity (mOsm/l)	280–310	290	280	–
Oncotic pressure (mmHg)	25	0	25–30	20–25
Half-life (hours)	Varies	15 (rats)	30–40 (mice)	13 (humans)
P_{50} (mmHg)	26	18	34	–
Methaemogolobin (%)	<2	13	<3	–

Figure 11.12: Comparison of whole blood to three different categories of red cell-free oxygen-carrying solutions.

haemoglobin-based solutions. There are at least four different ways to solubilize haemoglobin: by intra-molecular cross linking, by producing polymers, by conjugating haemoglobin or by producing haemoglobin microspheres. To date, the haemoglobin for these solutions has been of bovine or human origin. Alternatively, human or ovine haemoglobin has been synthesized by bacteria. The second category are liposome-encapsulated haemoglobin solutions, with the haemoglobin being surrounded by a synthetic membrane. The third category are the perfluorocarbons; organic solutions with high oxygen solubility (Figure 11.12).

Several haemoglobin solutions have reached phase I trials and one, Oxyglobin Solution (Biopure, Boston, Massachusetts), was introduced in 1998 to the veterinary market in the United States. The solution is a polyionic colloidal fluid (130 mmol/l sodium, 4 mmol/l potassium and 110 mmol/l chloride) with a pH of 7.8. It has been administered under a number of experimental and a few clinical conditions to over a dozen different species. The recommended dosage is 15–30 ml/kg i.v. at a rate not to exceed 10 ml/kg/h. If administered more rapidly, circulatory overload may occur because of its oncotic pressure (see Figure 11.12) and the increase in vascular resistance that it may cause. To date, the primary concern is the potential for renal toxicity, as serum creatinine concentrations transiently increased in rats when they were administered a high dose (Lee *et al.*, 1989). Transient haemoglobinuria has also been observed in healthy Beagles.

Perfluorocarbons may be an ideal fluid to deliver oxygen in situations of poor microcirculation. Twenty per cent Fluosol-DA (Green Cross, Osaka, Japan) has been infused into coronary vessels during cardiac procedures to prevent myocardial ischaemia. Another perfluorocarbon, polyfluoro-octobromide (Perflubon) may also become available soon. Additional experience with all of these solutions is necessary to determine their exact indications, contraindications and adverse effects.

REFERENCES AND FURTHER READING

Auer L and Bell K (1981) The AB blood group system of cats. *Animal Blood Groups and Biochemical Genetics* **12**, 287–297

Bland RD, *et al.* (1985) Hemodynamic and oxygen transport patterns in surviving and nonsurviving postoperative patients. *Critical Care Medicine* **13**, 85–90

Concannon KT, Haskins SC and Feldman BF (1992) Hemostatic defects associated with two infusion rates of dextran 70 in dogs. *American Journal of Veterinary Research* **53(8)**, 1369–1375

Conroy JM, *et al.* (1996) The effects of desmopressin and 6% hydroxyethyl starch on Factor VIII-C. *Anesthesia and Analgesia* **83**, 804–807

Cornelius LM, Finco DR and Culver EH (1978) Physiologic effects of rapid infusion of Ringer's lactate solution into dogs. *American Journal of Veterinary Research* **39**, 1185–1190

Davies MJ (1990) The role of colloids in blood conservation. *Internal Anesthesiology Clinics* **28(4)**, 205–209

Dietz NM (1996) Blood substitutes: fluids, drugs or miracle solutions? *Anesthesia and Analgesia* **82**, 390–405

Giesecke AH and Egbert LD (1985) Perioperative fluid therapy-crystalloids. In: *Anesthesia*, ed. R Miller, pp. 1313–1328. Churchill Livingstone, New York

Giger U and Bücheler J (1991) Transfusion of type-A and type-B blood to cats. *Journal of the American Veterinary Medical Association* **198**, 411–418

Giger U, Gelens CJ, Callan MB and Oakley DA (1995) An acute hemolytic transfusion reaction caused by dog erythrocyte antigen 1.1 incompatibility in a previously sensitized dog. *Journal of the American Veterinary Medical Association* **206(9)**, 1358–1362

Giger U, Kilrain CG, Filippich LJ and Bell K (1989) Frequencies of feline blood groups in the United States. *Journal of the American Veterinary Medical Association* **195**, 1230–1232

Giger U and Oakley D (1998) Current feline transfusion therapy: unique issues in cats. In: *Proceedings of the VI International Veterinary Emergency and Critical Care Symposium*, pp. 207–210

Griot-Wenk ME, Callan MB, Casal ML, Chisholm-Chait A, Spilalnik SL, Patterson DF and Giger U (1996) Blood type AB in the feline AB blood group system. *American Journal of Veterinary Research* **57**, 1438–1442

Hurst TS, Turrentine MA and Johnson GS (1987) Evaluation of microwave-thawed canine plasma for transfusion. *Journal of the American Veterinary Medical Association* **190(7)**, 863–865

Jones JA (1995) Red blood cell substitutes: current status. *British Journal of Anaesthesia* **74**, 697–703

Kirk RW and Bistner SI, eds (1985) Blood transfusions. In: *The Handbook of Veterinary Procedures and Emergency Treatment, 4th edn*, pp. 624–625. WB Saunders, Philadelphia

Krausz MM, David M and Amstislavsky T (1994) Hypertonic saline treatment of hemorrhagic shock in awake rats. *Shock* **2(4)**, 267–270

Lanier WL, Stangland KJ, Scheithauer BW, Milde JH and Michenfelder JD (1987) The effects of dextrose infusion and head position on neurologic outcome after complete cerebral ischemia in primates: examination of a model. *Anesthesiology* **66**, 39–48

Lee R, Atsumi N, Jacobs EE Jr, Austen WG and Vlahakes GJ (1989) Ultrapure, stroma-free, polymerized bovine hemoglobin solution: evaluation of renal toxicity. *Journal of Surgical Research* **47**, 407–411

Lundy EF, Kuhn JE, Kwon JM, Zelenock GB and D'Alecy LG (1987) Infusion of five percent dextrose increases mortality and morbidity following six minutes of cardiac arrest in resuscitated dogs. *Journal of Critical Care* **2**, 4–14

Malcolm DS, Friedland M, Moore T, Beauregard J, Hufnagel H and Wiesmann WP (1993) Hypertonic saline resuscitation detrimentally affects renal function and survival in dehydrated rats. *Circulatory Shock* **40**, 69–74

Matthew CB (1994) Treatment of hyperthermia and dehydration with hypertonic saline in dextran. *Shock* **2(3)**, 216–221

Mathews KA (1996) Blood/Plasma transfusion. In: *Veterinary Emergency and Critical Care Manual*. pp. 10–11. Life Learn, Guelph

Mazzoni MC, Borgstrom P, Arfors KE and Intaglietta M (1990) The efficacy of iso- and hyperosmotic fluids as volume expanders in fixed-volume and uncontrolled hemorrhage. *Annals of Emergency Medicine* **19(4)**, 350–358

Miller RD (1990) Transfusion therapy. In: *Anesthesia, 3rd edn*, ed. RD Miller, p. 1483. Churchill Livingstone, New York

Moon PF and Kramer GC (1995) Hypertonic saline-dextran resuscitation from hemorrhagic shock induces transient mixed acidosis. *Critical Care Medicine* **23(2)**, 323–331

Moon PF, Gabor L, Gleed RD and Erb HN (1997) Acid-base, metabolic, and hemodynamic effects of sodium bicarbonate or tromethamine administration in anesthetized dogs with experimentally induced metabolic acidosis. *American Journal of Veterinary Research* **58(7)**, 771–776

Moon PF, Hollyfield-Gilbert MA, Myers TL, Uchida T and Kramer GC (1996) Fluid compartments in hemorrhaged rats after hyperosmotic crystalloid and hyperoncotic colloid resuscitation. *American Journal of Physiology* **207**, F1–F8

Nguyen TT, Zwischenberger JB, Watson WC, Traber DL, Prough DS, Herndon DN and Kramer GC (1995) Hypertonic acetate dextran achieves high-flow-low-pressure resuscitation of hemorrhagic shock. *Journal of Trauma: Injury, Infection and Critical Care* **38(4)**, 602–608

Niebauer GW (1991) Autotransfusion for intraoperative blood salvage: a new technique. *Compendium: Small Animal* **13**, 1105–1116

Norsworthy GD (1977) Blood transfusion in the cat. *Feline Practice* **7**, 29

Rentko VT (1992) Red blood cell substitutes. *Problems in Veterinary Medicine* **4(4)**, 647–651

Ring J, *et al.* (1977) Frequency of anaphylactoid reactions following infusion of colloid volume expanders. *Langenbecks Arch Chirurgie* Supplement, 31–35

Strauss RG, Stansfield C, Henriksen RA and Villhauer PJ (1988) Pentastarch may cause fewer effects on coagulation than hetastarch. *Transfusion* **28**, 257–260

Turrentine MA, Kraus KH and Johnson GS (1988) Plasma from donor dogs, pretreated with DDAVP, transfused into a German Shorthair Pointer with type II von Willebrand's disease. *Veterinary Clinics of North America* **18**, 275

PART THREE

Anaesthetic Management

CHAPTER TWELVE

Ophthalmic Surgery

Jacqueline C. Brearley

INTRODUCTION

Anaesthesia for ophthalmic surgery provides several challenges. These include regulation of intraocular pressure, prevention of the oculocardiac reflex, restricted anaesthetist access to the patient's head and the need to avoid trauma to the surgical site on recovery from anaesthesia. Many patients presenting for cataract surgery are also suffering from diabetes mellitus.

GENERAL CONSIDERATIONS

Vascular access

Hindlimb venous catheterization is preferable, as it allows maximal access without disruption to the surgeon or surgical site. The lateral saphenous or femoral veins may be used. A T-port extension attached to the catheter improves access while minimizing the risk of dislodging the catheter.

Endotracheal intubation

The endotracheal tube (ETT) should be secured to the bottom jaw or around the back of the head to avoid distortion of the area around the eye, which may occur if the tube is tied to the maxilla. Care should be taken to avoid kinking or other occlusion of the tube during positioning, draping and surgery. Occlusion can be difficult to detect, particularly if it is partial. Careful monitoring of the respiratory character, oxygenation and, if available, end-tidal carbon dioxide tension, should aid in this. A guarded ETT that contains a supporting coil embedded in the wall should be used to prevent tube kinking if the operative procedure requires flexion of the neck.

Anaesthetic breathing system

Any system which minimizes the amount of tubing and valves near the head of the animal is suitable. Thus the most commonly used systems for ophthalmic anaesthesia are co-axial arrangements (Bain, Lack or Circle) for animals weighing over 10 kg. In animals weighing under 10 kg an Ayre's T-piece with a Jackson–Rees modification may be used.

Influence of ophthalmic drugs on anaesthesia

Most drugs used in the treatment of ophthalmic conditions are applied topically to the conjunctival sac and may be given either intermittently or by continuous infusion. Subconjunctival injection of some drugs allows a slow release into the tear film. Topically administered drugs include steroids, non-steroidal anti-inflammatory drugs (NSAIDs), antibiotics, carbonic anhydrase inhibitors, β-adrenoceptor antagonists, miotics and mydriatics. In general, these have a limited systemic effect, but in susceptible individuals or those with severe conjunctivitis and/or uveitis, the possibility of systemic effects should be considered.

Drugs administered systemically include steroids, antibiotics, analgesics and diuretics (diuretics acutely decrease intraocular pressure in cases of glaucoma).

Diuretics act either by providing a solute load, e.g. mannitol (0.5 g/kg i.v.), or by carbonic anhydrase inhibition, e.g. acetazolamide (2–10 mg orally). Mannitol is the most frequently used drug for reducing intraocular pressure before surgery. Hydration status and serum electrolyte concentrations should be assessed before their administration.

Recovery

Because surgery is generally fairly delicate, using fine suture material, the animal's recovery from anaesthesia needs to be as smooth as possible to avoid damage to the surgical site. Good analgesia during and after surgery will aid this. This is generally provided by systemic analgesics although local anaesthetic blockade may be a useful adjunct (see later). Sedation in the recovery period may be required. Although Elizabethan collars may prevent self-trauma, they often cause the animal to panic initially, and cause distress. This may in turn cause the animal to damage itself. Paw bandages in conjunction with good analgesia are usually more successful.

PHYSIOLOGY RELATED TO OPHTHALMIC ANAESTHESIA

Control of intraocular pressure

The pressure within the eye is determined by the external pressure of the periocular structures (e.g.

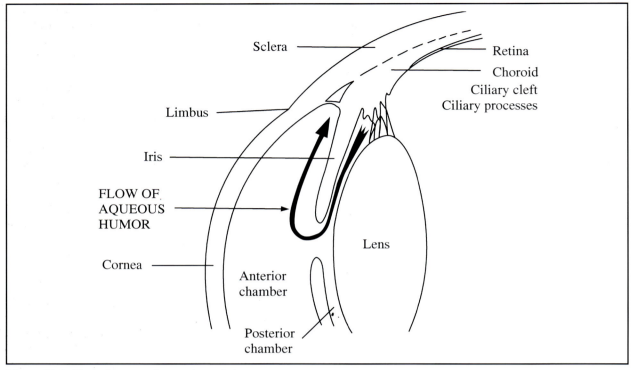

Figure 12.1: Flow of aqueous humor through the eye.

extrinsic muscles) on the globe and its internal structures. The most variable of the internal structures are the volume of the aqueous humor (which is dependent on the rates of production and removal) and the choroidal vascular volume, both of which can be influenced by anaesthesia.

The normal intraocular pressure in dogs is 10–25 mmHg above atmospheric pressure. The aqueous humor is formed by two mechanisms. The most important is by ultrafiltration of plasma from the fenestrated capillaries in the ciliary body processes. This is an active enzymatic process involving carbonic anhydrase. The second mechanism involves secretion of solutes from the ciliary epithelium, with accompanying water. The fluid is secreted into the posterior chamber and then flows into the anterior chamber through the pupil. From the anterior chamber the aqueous humor drains into the uveal veins through the trabecular meshwork of Fontana at the angle between the iris and the cornea (Figure 12.1), finally reaching the jugular veins.

It is within the power of the anaesthetist to control intraocular pressure to some extent by controlling arterial blood pressure, central venous pressure and end-tidal carbon dioxide tension. These factors generally influence the rate of aqueous production (rather than rate of removal) and the choroidal vascular volume. A fuller list of factors that influence intraocular pressure is shown in Figure 12.2.

The aim of the anaesthetist should be to maintain intraocular pressure within normal limits. Too high a pressure at worst may risk the evisceration of the globe and at best can make surgery very difficult. It may result in a rupture of the globe, converting a relatively simple conjunctival flap procedure for a deep ulcer into a more complex procedure to salvage an open globe. Too low a pressure may result in distortion of the globe during intraocular surgery, again hindering surgery and making placement of sutures difficult.

Increase intraocular pressure
Increased venous pressure (increases blood volume in eye) caused by coughing, vomiting, retching and 'bucking' on endotracheal tube
Increased arterial pressure
Hypercapnia
Hypoxia
Increased pressure on globe (blepharospasm, orbital tumours)
Drugs (atropine, suxamethonium)

Decrease intraocular pressure
Decreased venous pressure
Decreased arterial pressure
Hypocapnia
High arterial oxygen tension
Majority of anaesthetic agents
Osmotic diuretics
Carbonic anhydrase inhibitors

Figure 12.2: Factors influencing intraocular pressure.

The oculocardiac reflex

It has been known for many years that traction on the extrinsic muscles of the eye can result in slowing of the heart and the development of bradydysrhythmias, e.g. asystole, atrioventricular block and pulsus bigeminus. This reflex is mediated on the afferent side by branches of the ciliary nerves (which in turn are branches of the trigeminal nerve) and on the efferent side by the cardiac branches of the vagus nerve (Figure 12.3). This reflex is relatively rare in adult dogs and cats, to the extent that prophylactic vagal blockade by an anticholinergic drug is unwarranted. However, in animals with high vagal tone (e.g. very young animals), consideration should be given to preventing or blocking this reflex. This can be achieved by gentle handling of the globe, the use of local anaesthetic blockade (with its inherent problems) or pretreatment with an anticholinergic drug approximately 30 minutes before surgery. Atropine (0.04 mg/kg) or glycopyrrolate (0.02 mg/kg) by intramuscular or subcutaneous injection is said to be effective. However, routine premedication with these drugs is not advocated for ophthalmic surgery.

Central eye position

The production of a central eye to ease surgical access for ocular and intraocular surgery is generally in the hands of the anaesthetist. In the dog under a light plane of anaesthesia, the eye is central, but surgical stimulation at this point will cause retraction of the eye into the socket. At a plane of surgical anaesthesia, the eye rotates down causing the cornea to be obscured under the nictitating membrane and the lower eyelid. Deeper planes of anaesthesia, while giving a central eye, are associated with excessive physiological depression, increasing the risks of respiratory arrest (without ventilatory support) and cardiac arrest.

Traditionally, a central pupil has been produced during a plane of surgical anaesthesia by traction on the globe either by stay sutures or by manipulation with a pair of forceps on the conjunctiva. These methods cause trauma to the eye and can interfere with surgical access.

The most reliable method is to use a non-depolarizing muscle relaxant e.g. vecuronium (0.1 mg/kg) or atracurium (0.2–0.5 mg/kg). This produces a central immobile eye, which will not vary its position with depth of anaesthesia. The disadvantage of this method is that intermittent positive-pressure ventilation is mandatory as the respiratory muscles will be paralysed, in addition to the extrinsic eye muscles. The duration of action of vecuronium at the above dose is approximately 20 minutes and that of atracurium 40 minutes. An acetylcholinesterase blocking agent (e.g. neostigmine or edrophonium) should be administered at the end of surgery to increase acetylcholine concentrations at the neuromuscular junction. The muscarinic effects of these drugs (bradycardia, salivation, etc.) should be blocked by the concurrent use of an anticholinergic, e.g. atropine (0.04 mg/kg) or glycopyrrolate (0.02 mg/kg) (see Chapter 10).

A central eye position may also be achieved using local anaesthetic techniques. Regional anaesthesia of the eye and orbit may be produced either by blocking the ophthalmic branch of the trigeminal nerve, or by retrobulbar deposition of local anaesthetic.

Ophthalmic nerve block requires deposition of approximately 1–2 ml of local anaesthetic solution (either 2% lignocaine (lidocaine) or 0.5% bupivacaine) close to the orbital fissure. Because of the close proximity of this nerve to the abducens, oculomotor and trochlear nerves, akinesis of the globe also results.

A 2.5 cm, 22 gauge needle is introduced ventral to the zygomatic process, approximately 0.5 cm cranial to the rostral border of the vertical ramus of the mandible. The needle is advanced in a medial, dorsal and caudal direction so that its tip is close to the orbital fissure. Close inspection of a skull is recommended before this technique is attempted.

Retrobulbar anaesthesia is associated with a higher morbidity than ophthalmic block. Complications include subarachnoid injection of local anaesthetic, intravascular injection and puncture of the globe. Needle insertion can be either at the lateral canthus (directing the needle towards the opposite temporomandibular joint), or at the most dorsal point on the curvature of the orbit and following the orbit around ventrally.

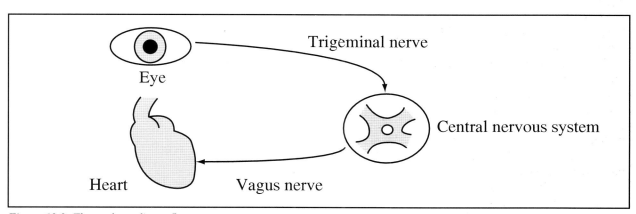

Figure 12.3: The oculocardiac reflex.

FACTORS INFLUENCING THE CHOICE OF ANAESTHETIC REGIMEN

Choice of anaesthetic regimen depends on the surgical procedure proposed, the temperament of the animal and the envisaged length of hospital stay. Obviously the surgical procedure takes precedence, but other factors are also important.

Day case or inpatient

If all other factors are equal, the length of hospital stay envisaged will generally depend on the subsequent treatment for the ophthalmological condition or other concerns with the eye. For example, intraocular surgical patients are often hospitalized for more than 24 hours postoperatively in case extensive uveitis develops or the aqueous humor starts to leak. Patients may be hospitalized to ensure regular postoperative medication e.g. two-hourly eye drops, which may be impossible for the owner to administer, or to keep the animal quiet and away from its home surroundings, which may excite it. In such cases a longer-acting agent or combination of agents may be chosen, as a rapid recovery is neither desirable nor necessary. Therefore, thiopentone may be chosen over propofol, or halothane over isoflurane. Longer postoperative stay will also allow the administration of opioid analgesics for postoperative analgesia, which would not be possible if the animal was treated as a day case.

Temperament of the animal

The treatment of cats differs slightly from dogs. Because of their temperament, and often because of the degree of socialization that the animals have previously experienced, cats may not adapt well to the hospital environment. This frequently makes the anaesthetic and analgesic treatment of cats for ophthalmological conditions a challenge.

Questions which should be asked regarding the temperament include:

- Is the animal safe to be nursed, or is it too aggressive in the hospital environment? If the latter is the case, then regardless of the medical/surgical condition, the animal may be treated on a day-case basis with a premedication that allows safe handling before anaesthesia but sufficient return of consciousness postoperatively to go home soon after surgery. Thus medetomidine in combination with an opioid could be used as the premedicant, with the α_2-agonist being reversed at the end of surgery to give a more rapid recovery but leaving the opioid to act as an analgesic in the immediate postoperative period
- Is the animal likely to inflict postoperative self-trauma and therefore require postoperative sedation to safeguard the surgical site?

- Will acepromazine alone be sufficient in low doses? If the self-mutilation is due to discomfort, analgesia will also be required. If opioids are used, a smaller dose of acepromazine should be needed
- Is the animal very nervous?

These are examples of the types of questions that should be considered and that play a role in determining the drugs used in a particular case.

EXAMPLES OF PROTOCOLS FOR SPECIFIC PROCEDURES

Surgical conditions can be divided in terms of anatomical sites. These are:

- Periocular surgery
- Ocular surgery
- Intraocular surgery.

Anaesthesia for periocular surgery

Types of procedure

- Eyelid surgery, e.g. entropion, ectopic cilia, distichiasis
- Parotid duct transposition
- 'Face lift' procedures for severe entropion
- Nasolacrimal duct/puncta surgery.

Surgical considerations

- Chronic painful conditions
- Surgical site often subject to swelling
- Inflammatory process can disrupt surgical site
- Surgery often relieves discomfort to some extent immediately after anaesthesia
- Often a day case.

Premedication

Systemic analgesics are very useful preoperatively as pain, lacrimation and blepharospasm are often presenting signs of chronic eyelash irritation of the cornea. Keratoconjuctivitis sicca (dry eye) can cause the dog discomfort, but this is most effectively relieved by the application of artificial tears rather than a systemic analgesic.

The partial opioid agonists are generally adequate, e.g. buprenorphine at 0.01 mg/kg or butorphanol at 0.2 mg/kg. Buprenorphine, with its relatively long duration of action, may have a particular role in these procedures as it is a potent analgesic that will provide good immediate postoperative analgesia and will allow a smooth transition to an NSAID for more prolonged postoperative analgesia if required. The problem with these cases is that the animals have often been in discomfort for some time and so may be sensitized to irritants around the eye, making the control of pain more difficult in some cases.

The NSAIDs have a particular role to play in periocular surgery for the control of postoperative swelling and thereby limiting distortion of the surgical site.

Induction of anaesthesia

Most of the common induction agents, e.g. propofol and thiopentone, are suitable. The choice will often depend on whether the animal is a day patient or not. Propofol confers the advantages of a smooth complete recovery, with no 'hangover' effect. This makes it ideal for day-case surgery.

Maintenance of anaesthesia

While many of the procedures under this heading are relatively minor, they are not necessarily short, e.g. complex entropion/ectropion corrections. For short procedures, intravenous maintenance with propofol may suffice, but inhalational anaesthesia is preferable for more prolonged (>20 minutes) surgery. Isoflurane may have a slight advantage over halothane as a maintenance agent, due to the more rapid recovery. If intravenous maintenance is chosen, oxygen supplementation should be provided either by nasal tube or via an orotracheal tube, as respiratory depression is common with propofol. Whichever maintenance technique is chosen, routine monitoring of anaesthesia should be undertaken, however short the procedure.

Anaesthesia for ocular surgery

Types of procedure

- Foreign body removal
- Keratectomy
- Peribulbar sampling
- Enucleation
- Conjunctival flap
- Laser treatment for glaucoma.

Surgical requirements

- Central eye if corneal surgery is contemplated
- Relaxed eye without retraction into orbit
- Minimization of haemorrhage – particularly with enucleations
- Preservation of an intact eye, particularly with deep corneal ulcers or foreign bodies.

Premedication and preparation

Careful preoperative handling is required to avoid rupture of an eye with a deep corneal ulcer, and to avoid movement of corneal foreign bodies. This will be aided by adequate sedation and analgesia. Premedicants which may induce emesis (e.g. morphine, medetomidine, xylazine) should not be given because vomiting will increase intraocular pressure and may result in disruption of the eye.

Catheterization of the lateral saphenous vein should be practised in positions other than lateral recumbency, because many animals may resent this position but be perfectly happy when standing, or lying in sternal recumbency. The use of a T-port extension attached to the catheter allows injection of the induction agent with minimal restraint or support of the animal.

Induction of anaesthesia

Choice of induction agent is more dependent on considerations other than the surgical procedure proposed (see above). However, an injectable agent is recommended rather than an inhalational technique. A smooth induction is very important in these cases as any struggling or excitement will increase intraocular pressure.

Endotracheal intubation should only be attempted when the animal is sufficiently deep to allow this procedure without 'bucking' on the ETT. Such bucking will increase intraocular pressure and again may cause globe disruption. The use of suxamethonium (succinylcholine) to facilitate endotracheal intubation of cats is contraindicated in cases with deep corneal ulcers because it increases intraocular pressure.

Maintenance of anaesthesia

Methods of maintenance of anaesthesia are again dependent on factors other than the surgery, but a central eye may be required (see section on central eye position).

Anaesthesia for intraocular surgery

Types of procedure

- Intraocular foreign body removal
- Extracapsular cataract extraction
- Phacoemulsification of cataracts
- Luxated lens extraction
- Intraocular tissue sampling.

Surgical requirements

- Central eye
- Controlled intraocular pressure
- Neutral pupil which can be controlled topically
- Control of perioperative uveitis.

Premedication and preparation

Many patients with cataracts also have diabetes mellitus. Assessment of blood glucose levels should be part of the preoperative examination of all animals with cataracts. (See Chapter 19 for details on anaesthetizing diabetic patients.)

Topical treatment with anti-inflammatory agents (e.g. flurbiprofen or prednisolone) for several hours before surgery is thought to decrease postoperative uveitis. If a dilated pupil is required, this can be achieved with topical atropine (or tropicamide) before surgery. The animal should be premedicated with a systemic opioid and sedative to ensure a calm animal for induction of anaesthesia. A systemic NSAID is also thought to help in the control of postoperative uveitis. Unless blood pressure is measured during surgery, the administration of the majority of this class of drugs is best left to the recovery period because intraoperative hypotension in conjunction with an NSAID may lead to subsequent renal damage. Some ophthalmologists use a steroid, e.g. dexamethasone, to aid in the control of postoperative uveitis.

Premedication with either high-dose pure opioid agonists (which induce miosis) or anticholinergics (which induce mydriasis) should be avoided, as topical control of the pupil size provides the surgeon with much more flexibility.

Induction of anaesthesia
Choice of agent depends on the anaesthetist and factors other than the procedure, as discussed above.

Maintenance of anaesthesia
A central eye is necessary for most of the procedures in this group, and details may be found in the section on central eye position.

CHAPTER THIRTEEN

Dental and Maxillofacial Surgery

Tanya Duke

INTRODUCTION

The type of patient presented for dental or maxillofacial surgery can vary, but many will be geriatric or have brachycephalic anatomy. In such patients, anaesthesia can pose a great risk. The type of surgical procedure may also influence the course of anaesthesia by introducing risks to airway security or the possibility of haemorrhage.

PRINCIPLES AND POTENTIAL PROBLEMS

Airway security
During surgery for dental and maxillofacial conditions, the airway should be adequately secured by endotracheal intubation, as debris, blood and irrigation fluids from the oral cavity can enter unprotected airways and cause aspiration pneumonia. This condition, which can be fatal, is easier to prevent than cure.

Endotracheal tubes
Endotracheal tubes (ETTs) should be checked for defective cuffs and obstructed lumens before use. The tubing should be cut to fit the patient from mid neck to the level of the incisor teeth. A properly positioned ETT reduces apparatus dead space and the risk of endobronchial intubation. Excessively long ETTs that protrude from the oral cavity are prone to kinking and are difficult to secure to the jaw with gauze bandage. Knots placed around the ETT can become sodden by irrigation fluids and saliva, and may loosen and increase the risk of accidental extubation. Knots should be tied around the ETT connector for greater security and not around the ETT itself.

Pharyngeal packing
Pharyngeal packing can be used for greater airway security, but it is imperative that it is removed before extubation. A length of damp gauze bandage is superior to individual surgical swabs since bandage can be packed tightly around the ETT, and is less likely to be forgotten if the free end is left visible.

Possible problems during manipulations of the head include kinking of the ETT, extubation and circuit disconnections. These problems are common during diagnostic imaging as the patient has to be positioned for radiography in a darkened room. In spontaneously breathing patients, inadvertent disconnection allows air breathing, reduced inspired anaesthetic concentrations and decreased depth of anaesthesia. Surgical drapes can conceal circuit disconnections unless sudden emptying of the rebreathing bag is observed. Apnoea alarms and capnograms are useful for detecting accidental disconnection. Inspiration against an obstructed airway caused by a kinked ETT may lead to pulmonary oedema. Guarded endotracheal tubes (see Chapter 4) may be used in patients at high risk of endotracheal tube kinking.

Long anaesthetic periods
Close attention to life support is needed during lengthy surgical procedures that require prolonged anaesthesia. Oxygen should be delivered at an inspired concentration of at least 33% to compensate for the deterioration in pulmonary function that accompanies anaesthesia (hypoventilation, reduced functional residual capacity (FRC), atelectasis and ventilation/perfusion mismatch), even in healthy young patients.

Reduced cardiac output and arterial blood pressure produced by anaesthesia should be offset by intravenous fluid therapy. Intravenous Hartmann's (lactated Ringer's) solution should be given at a rate of 10 ml/kg/h. Before inducing anaesthesia, a catheter should be aseptically placed into an appropriate superficial vein. Catheters ensure that irritant injectable agents are not given perivascularly, and they also allow immediate venous access in an emergency. Catheters should not be removed until the patient is fully conscious after anaesthesia.

Hypothermia can result from lengthy anaesthesia and the use of cool irrigation fluids. It can cause anticholinergic resistant bradycardia, reduced cardiac output and haemoconcentration, and cardiac fibrillation can occur at a body temperature of about 28°C. Requirements for anaesthetic agents are reduced during hypothermia, and care should be taken to avoid a relative overdose of anaesthetic agent. External heat can be supplied with heating blankets and warmed intravenous and irrigation fluids. Thermal injuries due to 'hot spots' are rarely produced by circulating warm water blankets, but occur more often with electrical heating mats. Patients can be insulated with towels, bubble packing or aluminium foil. Hyperthermia can occasionally occur in large heavy coated dogs connected to rebreathing circuits for long periods. In such cases, active cooling should be initiated before damage occurs to vital organs.

Haemorrhage

Blood loss and hypovolaemia may occur during some dental and maxillofacial procedures. Blood loss should be estimated either by weighing blood soaked swabs or by measuring the amount of blood collected in a suction jar. As a rough guide, a fully soaked 3 x 3 inch swab contains about 7 ml of blood, and a 4 x 4 inch swab contains about 10 ml of blood. The normal patient can tolerate blood loss of up to 20% of circulating volume through compensatory mechanisms, but these mechanisms are not as efficient when the patient is anaesthetized. Rates of intravenous isotonic crystalloid fluid infusion should be increased to 30–40 ml/kg/h to compensate for hypotension. As the blood loss approaches 20% of circulating volume, fluid replacement therapy with blood should begin. Colloids such as gelatins, dextrans or starches can be used at a dose of up to 20 ml/kg, but while they support tissue perfusion they are not a replacement for red blood cells. If haemorrhage is anticipated during the procedure, patients should be cross matched beforehand with a healthy donor. Donor blood should be given at the same rate that the patient's blood is lost.

An alternative to cross matching with a donor is autologous transfusion. A week before surgery, 10% of the patient's blood volume is removed and replaced with intravenous fluids. The blood is stored at 4°C in acid-citrate-dextrose or citrate-phosphate-dextrose transfusion packs until required. In any case, before potentially haemorrhagic procedures, the patient must have a full haematological examination and clotting profile performed. See Chapter 11 for further information.

Haemostasis

Vasoconstrictors such as topically applied adrenaline should not be used for haemostasis if the patient is anaesthetized with halothane. A few drops can be used with caution in a 1:20,000 dilution if the patient is anaesthetized with isoflurane, and monitored by electrocardiography. Phenylephrine at the same dilution is less arrhythmogenic, but even a few drops of this drug can be absorbed sufficiently to increase systemic vascular resistance through adrenergic receptor stimulation.

Analgesia

Some dental and maxillofacial procedures produce strong surgical stimulation, resulting in a variable plane of anaesthesia. A widely varying plane is often the result of poor analgesia. Opioids should be provided at the time of premedication, and local nerve blocks should be considered before surgery (see below). Further increments of injectable opioids can be provided intraoperatively, or nitrous oxide can be given. Analgesics should be continued into the recovery period.

PATIENTS REQUIRING DENTAL PROCEDURES

Geriatric patients

Dental procedures range from simple extractions of deciduous teeth in young healthy patients to lengthy complicated procedures in older systemically compromised patients. Most patients requiring anaesthesia for dental procedures are considered to be geriatric (i.e. 75–80% of the animal's anticipated life span is completed). Even clinically healthy geriatric patients have physiological changes that can influence the course of anaesthesia. Elderly patients are often distressed and confused by a change in routine and require constant reassurance. Age-related changes in the cardiopulmonary system include:

- Decreased ability to compensate for blood pressure and circulating volume changes
- 30% decrease in cardiac output
- Decreased lung compliance
- High small airway closing volume
- Decreased partial pressure of oxygen in arterial blood (PaO_2).

A noticeable decrease in circulation time is seen during induction, and further increments of injectable anaesthetic agents should not be given too soon. See Chapter 23 for further information on anaesthesia for the geriatric patient.

Brachycephalic patients

Many brachycephalic patients require dental or maxillofacial procedures, and these patients pose an anaesthetic challenge. Upper airway obstruction from stenotic nares, an elongated soft palate, laryngeal saccule eversion, laryngeal collapse, laryngeal oedema and hypoplastic trachea should be anticipated. The degree of obstruction may be assessed from the clinical history and a physical examination before surgery.

Problems of the upper airway may benefit from surgical correction at the time of planned dental procedures. Severe upper airway obstruction eventually results in cor pulmonale, and evidence for this should be checked. Induction of anaesthesia causes relaxation of pharyngeal musculature, and the degree of upper airway obstruction is increased until endotracheal intubation is performed. Potent sedative agents such as xylazine should be avoided during premedication as these exacerbate upper airway obstruction.

Mild sedation with low doses of acepromazine and buprenorphine or pethidine (meperidine) is adequate in dogs. Boxers are prone to vasovagal syncope with acepromazine and either should receive an anticholinergic or phenothiazine should be avoided. Fractious dogs should not be muzzled, but an Elizabethan collar can prevent handlers from being injured. Preoxygenation by mask for 5 minutes will help prevent hypoxia during induction, but mask induction using an inhalational agent should be avoided where possible. A rapid reliable induction technique should be used with drugs such as methohexitone, thiopentone or propofol and endotracheal intubation expertly performed.

Airway obstruction is possible during recovery. There are two methods of dealing with airway support in the recovery period. Firstly, opioids with potent anti-tussive action, such as butorphanol, morphine or oxymorphone, can be given to dogs to allow toleration of the ETT for as long as possible, even until they are sternal. A disadvantage is that complete recovery may be lengthy. Secondly, induction drugs with relatively short plasma half-lives, such as methohexitone, propofol or a benzodiazepine/ketamine combination, ensure a rapid recovery and return of the patient's ability to maintain its own airway. Isoflurane provides more rapid recoveries than halothane.

Even after taking these precautions, once the ETT is removed there is still a risk of obstruction until the patient is fully awake. Obstruction can be alleviated by pulling the patient's tongue forwards and keeping the mouth open to encourage mouth breathing. Hypoxia can be alleviated by giving oxygen. Placing the patient in sternal recumbency allows more uniform expansion of the lungs and may promote a more rapid return to consciousness. If recovery is delayed because the patient has been given a potent μ-agonist, such as morphine, methadone or oxymorphone for analgesia, and the patient has been extubated, an alternative to reintubation may be to reverse the μ-agonist. If naloxone is used for this purpose to reverse sedation, analgesia is also reversed. To avoid this unintended scenario, butorphanol (0.2 mg/kg slowly intravenously) or buprenorphine (0.006 mg/kg i.v.) can be used for reversal. Butorphanol produces reversal 1–2 minutes after injection, but buprenorphine can take 10–15 minutes. It is wise to be prepared to perform tracheostomy on patients that present with upper airway obstruction.

ANAESTHESIA FOR ROUTINE DENTAL PROCEDURES

Preanaesthetic preparation
It is important to ensure that a thorough clinical examination has been performed on the patient before giving an anaesthetic. Many procedures are

considered to be routine, and clients may believe that anaesthetizing their pet will be straightforward. In elderly patients there is increasing likelihood of systemic disease that may have gone unnoticed by the client. A thorough examination helps to eliminate problems in the perioperative period. Elective procedures can be delayed until the patient is stable, and urgent procedures can be undertaken with the clinician (and client) cognisant of problems that may occur. Further information regarding systemic disease and anaesthesia may be found in other chapters on anaesthetic management.

Premedication
Many geriatric patients are likely to be distressed by the upheaval in their routine and being with strangers in unfamiliar surroundings. Premedication provides a calming effect and makes the patient more manageable. Important considerations for dental anaesthesia include the provision of intraoperative analgesia with an opioid, the ability to reduce the amount of major depressant anaesthetic agents and the reduction of undesirable side effects. Combinations of acepromazine and opioid are suitable in most cases. Alpha$_2$-adrenoceptor agonists should only be used in young healthy patients, and only when there is a full appreciation of the side effects. Oxygen and ventilatory support must be available when these drugs are used.

Anticholinergics can reduce undesirable parasympathetic effects such as salivation and bradycardia. Glycopyrrolate has a duration of action of 2–3 hours and is a more potent anti-sialagogue than atropine. For further information see Chapter 7.

Induction
The passage from consciousness to unconsciousness should be as smooth and excitement-free as possible. In healthy patients methohexitone, thiopentone, propofol and alphaxolone/alphadolone are recommended as they produce a reliable rapid induction. In patients with cardiopulmonary compromise or severe hepatic or renal disease, they should be used with caution (see Chapter 14). Xylazine/ketamine or medetomidine/ketamine combinations for induction of anaesthesia should not be used in geriatric or debilitated patients. See Chapter 8 for further details regarding injectable drugs.

Maintenance
For short procedures of less than 15 minutes, incremental boluses of short-acting injectable anaesthetics such as methohexitone, thiopentone, propofol, benzodiazepine/ketamine and alphaxolone/alphadolone can be used. Dental procedures, however, can be lengthy and this increases the risks of deterioration in physiological status, especially in elderly compromised patients, and anaesthesia is best maintained with

an inhalational technique. Inhaled anaesthetics are usually administered in an oxygen-enriched mixture and this greatly improves oxygen delivery to tissues.

MAXILLOFACIAL TRAUMA AND ELECTIVE MAXILLOFACIAL SURGERY

Patients requiring elective procedures such as hemimandibulectomy need to be thoroughly examined and any concurrent disease stabilized before anaesthesia is induced. Any consequences of the surgical procedure (e.g. haemorrhage) should be anticipated. The upper airway should be examined for potential difficulties in intubation. Patients with traumatic injuries must be stabilized and other potential injuries addressed before anaesthesia. See Chapter 21 for further information regarding patients with trauma. Most procedures can be managed with conventional orotracheal intubation, but occasionally passing the ETT through a pharyngotomy site or a tracheotomy may be necessary.

Preoxygenation should be performed in case there are difficulties in intubation. Once the patient is stable, rapid sequence induction techniques after light premedication can be used to establish an airway. Maintenance of anaesthesia can be provided by inhalational techniques. Positioning for surgery is important and the ETT must be securely tied to prevent accidental disconnections. Right-angled adaptors can be attached to the ETT adaptor to enable breathing circuits to be diverted away from the surgical site. Breathing circuits such as Bain, Lack, Ayre's T-piece and circle systems are useful because they do not have heavy valves at the patient end of the circuit, which could place drag on the ETT.

Monitoring aids are useful, because surgical drapes may make examination of eye position impossible. Cats should be closely watched during recovery, as they are prone to upper airway obstruction if the nasal passages are occluded with blood and debris. Until cats are fully recovered from the effects of the anaesthetic, they seem reluctant to mouth breathe during the critical time from extubation. Anaesthetic agents providing rapid recovery are useful to decrease the time from extubation until the cat is fully aware of its surroundings. Analgesics without major sedative effects, such as buprenorphine or butorphanol, can be used without delaying recovery. Oxygen can be provided through a preplaced nasal catheter, mask or head tent (see Chapter 21).

RECOVERY AND ANALGESIA

Good nursing, analgesics, warmth, fluids and continuous observation help to eliminate postoperative problems. Before extubation, the pharyngeal area should be inspected for fluids, blood clots and foreign objects and any removed. Suction apparatus is useful to ensure that the pharynx is dry.

Delirious recoveries may be the result of pain, excitatory anaesthetic agents or hypoxia. Patients recovering from oral surgery often try to rub their faces, and sedatives, analgesics or an Elizabethan collar may help prevent self-inflicted trauma. For restless patients, acepromazine can be given at a low dose (0.02 mg/kg i.v.). Some patients greatly benefit from oxygen given during recovery. Oxygen can be supplied by mask or by a nasal catheter placed before recovery.

Analgesics should be provided pre- or intraoperatively, but may require supplementation (see Chapter 6). Opioids are the analgesics of choice for the perioperative period. Local anaesthesia can be provided by using mandibular and maxillary nerve blocks with 2% lignocaine (lidocaine) or 0.5% bupivacaine. Bupivacaine provides longer analgesia than lignocaine. Aspiration should be attempted before injection to ensure that the analgesic drug is not injected into a blood vessel. Nerve blocks can be performed before or after surgery, but placing the local anaesthetic beforehand can decrease the amount of other anaesthetic drugs needed and lower the postoperative requirement for analgesics.

Maxillary nerve block
This desensitizes the maxilla, upper teeth, nose and upper lip.

For this nerve block, a needle (A, Figure 13.1) is inserted at an angle of 90 degrees medially, ventral to the border of the zygomatic process, and approximately 0.5 cm caudal to the lateral canthus of the eye. The local anaesthetic (0.25-1.0 ml) is deposited around the maxillary nerve as it crosses the palatine bone, between the maxillary foramen and foramen rotundum.

Mandibular nerve block (inferior alveolar branch)
This desensitizes the lower teeth and lower lip.

For this nerve block, a needle (22 or 25 gauge, 1.9 cm or 2.5 cm) is inserted at the lower angle of the jaw approximately 1.5 cm rostral to the angular process. The needle (B, Figure 13.1) is passed dorsally along the medial surface of the mandibular ramus. The mandibular foramen can be palpated within the oral cavity and the needle point guided accurately to the nerve. Cats require 0.25 ml of local anaesthetic and dogs require 0.5-1.0 ml.

SPECIAL TECHNIQUES

Placement of a nasal oxygen catheter
After instilling a few drops of 2% lignocaine (without adrenaline) on to the nasal mucosa, a lubricated 3.5-6 Fr polyvinyl infant feeding tube is advanced into the

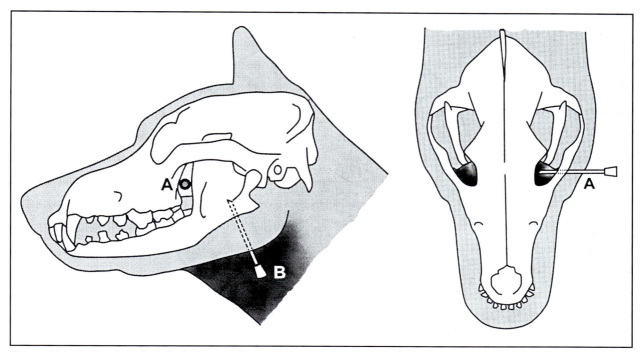

Figure 13.1: *Positioning of needle during maxillary (A) and mandibular (B) nerve block in the dog. Similar positioning is used in the cat.*

Reproduced from Muir and Hubbell (1995) with permission of Mosby Inc.

ventral nasal meatus to the level of the carnassial teeth. The tube is secured to the head by butterfly tapes and sutures. A drop of cyanoacrylate glue deposited between the tube and nostril helps to secure the tube where it makes a tight turn caudally (Figure 13.2). Extension tubing connects the nasal tube to an oxygen flowmeter, and oxygen is insufflated at a flow rate of 50–150 ml/kg/min. If oxygen insufflation is to be used for more than a few hours, the gas should be humidified by bubbling it through sterile water.

Pharyngotomy for diversion of the ETT

Occasionally, the ETT may be required to pass from the trachea through a temporary pharyngotomy to connect with the breathing circuit. This allows the surgeon access to the oral cavity without the hindrance of an ETT. Once the ETT is in place, a pharyngotomy can be performed and the proximal end of the ETT removed from its adaptor and passed mediolaterally through the pharyngotomy site, and the adaptor reconnected allowing anaesthesia to continue with an inhalational technique. Injectable anaesthetic drugs may be required to maintain anaesthesia during movement of the ETT. Propofol is useful for this as it does not accumulate with repeat boluses, but thiopentone can also be used for one or two incremental boluses.

After surgical preparation of the cervical area and angle of the mandible, an index finger is introduced into the oral cavity. The finger is used to locate the pyriform sinus rostral to the epihyoid bone (Figure 13.3). The tissues are incised and dissected through to the oral cavity. Forceps may be thrust through the mucosa and then used to grasp and pull the proximal end of the ETT laterally. The incision can be closed in a routine manner once it is not required.

Elective tracheotomy

A patient that can otherwise breathe normally but cannot open the mouth, should be induced and maintained with incremental boluses of a non-cumulative anaesthetic agent such as propofol until the jaws are opened or a tracheotomy is performed.

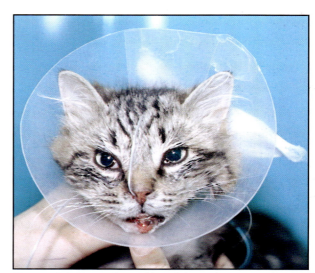

Figure 13.2: *Cat with nasal line delivering oxygen. The nasal line is secured in place with tissue glue, and butterfly strips are sutured to the head.*

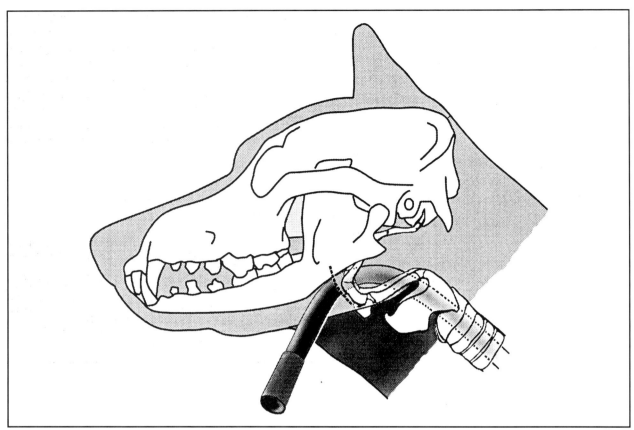

Figure 13.3: *Placement of endotracheal tube through pharyngotomy site.*

Reproduced from Muir and Hubbell (1995) with permission of Mosby Inc.

Elective tracheotomies can be performed under aseptic conditions while there is an orotracheal tube in place. The ventral surface of the trachea at the level of the second, third or fourth tracheal rings is exposed by a midline incision and the sternohyoideus muscles retracted. Two stabilizing sutures are placed around the tracheal rings at the site of tracheal incision to facilitate apposition later. A transverse incision between the rings is made through the annular ligament and mucosa up to 65% of the circumference of the trachea. Alternatively, a U-shaped ventral tracheal flap is created based on the second tracheal ring and extending two rings distally. The flap is raised as a hinge to allow placement of the ETT. This flap is used for long-term intubation as it prevents excessive pressure of the tube on the surrounding tissue. Postoperatively, the incision should be left to granulate, but this does require intensive care to allow cleaning of the tracheotomy site, and constant observation of the patient. Some clinicians prefer to close the incision postoperatively, but there may be a risk of subcutaneous emphysema, localized swelling and subsequent risk of airway obstruction.

Feeding tubes

In patients that cannot feed and drink normally, a nasogastric, pharyngostomy, oesophagostomy or gas-

trostomy tube offers an alternative method of providing nutrition and fluids (Crowe, 1986).

Indwelling nasogastric intubation

After desensitizing the nasal mucosa, a lubricated 5 or 6 Fr polyvinyl infant feeding tube is passed into the ventral nasal meatus. Placement into the oesophagus is easy in the tracheally intubated anaesthetized patient. In conscious patients the head should be held with the nose pointing down while the tube is advanced as this helps prevent accidental insertion into the trachea. The tube should be advanced until the distal end is positioned in the distal oesophagus (preferred location) or in the stomach. The stylette, if used, should then be removed. Placement should be verified by radiography or by auscultation of bubbles when air or sterile saline is instilled through the tube. The tube should then be capped and sutured in place with butterflies made from sticky tape. An Elizabethan collar will be necessary in some patients to prevent them from removing the tube. Although this technique is easy to perform, it is limited to short periods of feeding with liquidized foods.

Pharyngostomy tube

A technique similar to that described for a pharyngotomy tube can be used, but long-term maintenance can result in dysfunction of the larynx and aspiration. The technique of placement is therefore modified slightly so that the tube exits as caudodorsally as possible, close to the entrance to the oesophagus. In the modified technique, the incision is made in the lateral wall of the pharynx, caudodorsal to the hyoid apparatus.

Oesophagostomy tube

This site is currently the preferred position for placement of a feeding tube. It avoids the complications of peritonitis from gastrotomy tubes, and the risks of aspiration and damage to mucosa from the previously described sites. Under anaesthesia, the lateral cervical region is clipped and prepared for surgery; the left side is commonly used, but the right side can be used if necessary. Curved forceps are inserted into the proximal cervical oesophagus via the pharynx. The tips of the forceps are then turned laterally and pressure applied so the instrument can be palpated. A skin incision large enough to accommodate the feeding tube is made over the tips of the forceps. The forceps can be pushed through the oesophagus or, in large

dogs, an incision can be made. The feeding tube is premeasured and marked from stomach or distal oesophagus to incision site. The distal end is grasped by the forceps and pulled through the oesophagus out of the mouth. With the aid of forceps the distal end is then turned on itself to pass back into the oesophagus until the loop disappears. The distal tip is correctly positioned using the mark on the tube. This method helps to straighten the tube and limit kinks (Crowe and Devey, 1997).

REFERENCES AND FURTHER READING

Crowe DT (1986) Enteral nutrition for critically ill or injured patients. Parts I, II and III. *Compendium of Continuing Education. Small Animal* **8**, 603-826

Crowe DT and Devey JJ (1997) Esophagostomy tubes for feeding and decompression: clinical experience in 29 small animal patients. *Journal of the American Animal Hospital Association* **33**, 393-403

Hartsfield SM (1990) Anaesthetic problems of the geriatric dental patient. *Problems in Veterinary Medicine* **2**, 24-45

Muir WW III and Hubbell JAE (1995) *Handbook of Veterinary Anesthesia, 2nd edn.* Mosby, St Louis

CHAPTER FOURTEEN

Cardiopulmonary Disease

R. Eddie Clutton

INTRODUCTION

Cardiopulmonary disease is frequently encountered in companion animal practice; congenital cardiac anomalies are not uncommon while diminished cardiopulmonary function is a hallmark of the ageing process. Acquired cardiac disease is common in dogs and cats. Infectious respiratory diseases are also common and elderly animals living in urban environments may suffer from the effects of air pollution. The lungs are a common target for metastatic disease. Conditions characterized by chronic vomiting are associated with low-grade aspiration pneumonia. It may be necessary to anaesthetize animals with cardiopulmonary disease for diagnosis, for surgical correction of the condition or for incidental operations.

As the term 'cardiopulmonary disease' encompasses so many conditions it is meaningless. The cardiopulmonary system functions to ensure that the rate of delivery of oxygenated blood (DO_2) meets or exceeds the requirements of that of the whole body ($\dot{V}O_2$). These processes involve the combined activity of the lungs, heart and blood, and elements of the autonomic and somatic nervous systems that are responsible for the control of blood pressure and ventilation respectively. Thus cardiopulmonary disease can be taken to mean any disease that limits DO_2 to peripheral tissue, and this can involve any condition affecting the heart, the lungs and the oxygen-carrying capacity and flow characteristics of blood, and the nervous elements that control these processes. In this chapter, cardiovascular disease refers to conditions affecting the heart and blood vessels, and pulmonary disease refers to conditions affecting the airways and lung.

CARDIOVASCULAR DISEASE

Problems
Cardiovascular disease increases the risks from anaesthesia because:

- It increases the likelihood of cardiopulmonary failure and death caused by anaesthetics
- It adversely affects other organ systems (the most important secondary effects are on the heart: chronic myocardial overwork results in changes such as hypertrophy, which impairs myocardial oxygenation)
- It alters drug disposition (Figure 14.1)
- Drugs used in its treatment may interact with anaesthetics.

Risks from anaesthesia are reduced if:

- An accurate diagnosis is obtained, so that the primary (haemodynamic) and secondary effects of the condition are completely understood
- There is adequate preoperative preparation, i.e. the cardiovascular reserve is recruited
- The anaesthetics used offset, rather than aggravate, the haemodynamic effects of the condition
- The adverse haemodynamic effects of surgery are understood and minimized
- Problems of secondary complications, altered drug behaviour and drug interactions are recognized
- A range of adjunct drugs is available to treat both the autonomic nervous system and cardiovascular system
- There is adequate preoperative physiological monitoring.

Preoperative management

Preoperative examination
Preoperative examination aims to establish a diagnosis and to predict the capacity of the cardiopulmonary system to withstand anaesthesia and surgery. These steps form the basis of preoperative preparation of the animal and the selection of appropriate anaesthetics.

No single test predicts an animal's capacity to tolerate anaesthesia and surgery; an overall picture must take into account both the haemodynamic derangement and the significance of secondary changes. However, the most useful index of cardiopulmonary fitness – at least in dogs – is exercise tolerance.

A thorough review of the animal's medical history and a physical examination may establish a diagnosis.

Effect of disease	Pharmacological significance
Reduced drug volume of distribution	Greater sensitivity to *injectable** anaesthetics; reduced doses and/or infusion rates required
Slower circulation time	Slower response after intravenous injection; longer wait necessary between incremental injections
Poor peripheral perfusion	Lower drug bioavailability after intramuscular, subcutaneous or oral drug administration
Reduced cardiac output	More rapid rate of rise of alveolar concentration of inhalation anaesthetic. Accelerated rate of induction. More rapid response to altered vaporizer settings. Greater attention required to vaporizer settings
Reduced renal perfusion	Reduced renal clearance of drugs. Metabolic acidosis increases sensitivity to weak acidic drugs, e.g. thiopentone. Hypoalbuminaemia increases unbound:bound drug fraction; increased sensitivity to albumin-bound compounds
Reduced hepatic blood flow	Diminished extraction of drugs undergoing extensive hepatic metabolism; prolonged effect
Increased ventilation/perfusion inequality and venous admixture	Slower onset and response to altered inspired concentrations of inhalation anaesthetic

Figure 14.1: *Effects of cardiopulmonary disease on drug behaviour.*

Effect greatest with drugs given by intravenous rather than intramuscular or subcutaneous injection.

Often, more complex procedures such as radiography, electrocardiography, arterial blood gas analysis, ultrasonography or cardiac catheterization are required. These procedures may upset conscious animals and affect the test results or, worse, they may precipitate the animal's deterioration. In trying to establish a diagnosis it may be necessary to consult a veterinary cardiologist.

Thoracic radiographs provide information on cardiac chamber enlargement and they assist in identifying pulmonary changes. Animals in *extremis* should be examined in the lateral decubital position while being supplied with oxygen.

Electrocardiography should be performed on most animals with cardiopulmonary disease (certainly all dogs) especially when pulse irregularities are detected. A cursory examination of the ECG suffices for risk assessment because arrhythmias are more important in anaesthesia than signs of chamber enlargement or axis deviation. A single lead ECG can be taken with the animal standing or resting if enforced recumbency proves stressful. Many sedatives are arrhythmogenic although some, e.g. acepromazine, are anti-arrhythmic.

Arterial blood gas analysis quantifies the ability of the lungs to oxygenate blood, eliminate carbon dioxide (CO_2) and influence acid-base status. Although equipment for blood gas analysis is rare in veterinary practices, samples (collected anaerobically and placed on ice) can usually be analysed at local hospital laboratories. Arterial puncture can be stressful and may affect results by lowering CO_2 and increasing or decreasing oxygen (O_2) tension. Sedatives usually increase the partial pressure of CO_2 in arterial blood ($PaCO_2$) and may lower the partial pressure of O_2 in arterial blood (PaO_2).

When tricuspid valve disease, low cardiac output or passive venous congestion are present, venous blood samples should be taken to evaluate hepatic and renal function. The haematocrit, plasma haemoglobin concentration ([Hb]), serum protein concentrations and plasma electrolyte concentrations (sodium [Na^+], potassium [K^+] and chloride [Cl^-]) should also be examined.

Preoperative preparation

Preoperative preparation aims to lower risk by reversing the effects of pre-existing disease. The amount of preoperative preparation depends on the extent of dysfunction and the operation intended, but must be balanced against the needs for immediate surgery. Elective operations must be postponed until treatment has achieved a 'plateau' effect and undesirable drug effects have been controlled. The primary condition is treated first because many secondary complications resolve as cardiopulmonary function improves.

Primary condition

Uncontrolled cardiac failure is a contraindication to anaesthesia and so must be treated. Ventricular function is improved by:

- Using diuretics, a sodium-free diet and interventions such as pericardiocentesis to eliminate retained fluids (Figure 14.2)

Drug	Indications	Dose	Side effects
Digoxin	Heart failure Atrial premature complexes Atrial tachycardia Atrial fibrillation Sinus tachycardia due to heart failure	**Rapid i.v.:** Using 250 μg/ml injectable solution, prepare 10-20 μg/kg. Inject 50% i.v. and wait 30-60 minutes. Give 25% dose i.v. and wait another 30-60 minutes before giving the final aliquot, if necessary. **Rapid oral:** Using tablets, 10-30 μg/kg is given at presentation and again at 12 hours. **Maintenance:** 10-20 μg/kg divided bid	Perioperative arrhythmias: sinus block*, AV block*, atrioventricular junctional rhythm, atrial and ventricular ectopic beats and ventricular tachycardia. Anorexia. Vomiting. Diarrhoea. Lethargy. Ataxia. Toxic signs occur at lower concentrations in presence of hypokalaemia. Toxicity enhanced by hyperkalaemia, alkalosis, hypoxaemia, hypercalcaemia and hypomagnesaemia. Monitor electrocardiogram throughout rapid digitalization. Any possibility that preoperative bradycardia/bradyarrhythmias result from digoxin toxicity should prompt administration of a test dose of atropine 20 μg/kg to ensure that intraoperative heart rate increases are possible
Diuretics Loop	Rapid elimination of excessive fluid	Frusemide (2-5 mg/kg every hour) i.v. rapid onset and effective in dogs and cats, then 1-4 mg/kg i.m. or orally sid to tid thereafter	Should be used only with vasodilators, i.e. angiotensin-converting enzyme inhibitors. Hypovolaemia. Hypotension. Hypokalaemia aggravates digoxin toxicity. Metabolic alkalosis. Hypochloraemia. Use carefully in conditions in which cardiac output relies on ventricular filling pressures. Monitor effect by weight loss
Thiazides	Slow elimination of excessive fluid	Hydrochlorothiazide 2-4 mg/kg orally bid	As above
Potassium-sparing	Slow elimination of excessive fluid	Spironolactone 1-2 mg/kg orally sid or bid	Plasma potassium levels unchanged
Phosphodiesterase inhibitors	See below		
Potassium	Hypokalaemia following prolonged diuretic therapy and/or cachexia	Cats 2-6 mmol/day orally Dogs 0.2-0.5 mmol/kg orally tid	Hyperkalaemia and dysrhythmias when plasma levels exceed 7 mmol/l. Potassium-sparing diuretics - spironolactone, amiloride and triamterene do not warrant potassium supplementation

Figure 14.2: *Drugs for preoperative preparation of animals in heart failure.*

*Sodium intake should be restricted to 10–40 mg/kg (0.1–0.4%) diet dry matter. If possible, cases should receive a formulated low-sodium diet or a prescription diet.

- Using digoxin, dopamine, dobutamine or phosphodiesterase inhibitors to improve myocardial contraction (see Figure 14.2)
- Using vasodilators, cage rest and anxiolytic drugs to reduce cardiac work (Figure 14.3)
- Controlling residual arrhythmias (Figure 14.4).

Some arrhythmias, e.g. third degree atrioventricular block, arise *de novo*, i.e. are not secondary to cardiovascular disease, and are solely responsible for inadequate cardiac output. These are treated with suitable anti-arrhythmic drugs or by implanting a pacemaker.

Cardiac failure may result from non-cardiac disease, e.g. hyperthyroidism, phaeochromocytoma, in which case treatment must be aimed at the inciting condition.

Secondary complications

Secondary effects of cardiopulmonary disease that are life threatening, e.g. ventricular arrhythmias, need immediate treatment. Other secondary effects may persist after the primary condition is treated because of irreversible damage.

Arrhythmias

Arrhythmias are the most important secondary complication because:

Drug	Indications	Dose	Side effects
Glyceryl trinitrate	Emergency venodilation/ afterload reduction, e.g. pulmonary oedema	Glyceryl trinitrate 2% 0.25-2.0″ (0.6-5 cm) (dogs), 0.25-0.5″ (0.6-1.2 cm) (cats) bid to qid to medial pinna	Hypotension, tachycardia, azotaemia
Nitroprusside	Rapid afterload reduction	Sodium nitroprusside infusion: 1-15 μg/kg/min (dogs)	Hypotension, tachycardia, azotaemia. Rapid effects; monitor blood pressure
Hydralazine	Reduce afterload (arteriolar dilation) e.g. acute mitral valve regurgitation	Hydralazine 0.5-3.0 mg/kg orally bid (dogs)	Acute: hypotension, tachycardia. Chronic: hypernatraemia, hypokalaemia
α_1-Antagonists	Reduce afterload	Prazosin (dogs <15 kg) 1 mg orally bid or tid, (dogs >15 kg) 2 mg orally bid or tid, 0.25-1 mg orally (cats) bid or tid Phenoxybenzamine 0.2-1.5 mg/kg orally bid (dogs) 0.5-1 mg/kg orally bid cats	Hypotension, tachycardia, depression, weakness. Effects wane with constant use
Angiotensin-converting enzyme inhibitors	Non-emergency afterload control	Captopril 3-6 mg/kg orally bid or tid (cats) Enalapril 0.5-1 mg orally sid or bid (dogs) 0.25-0.5 mg/kg orally (cats) Benazepril 0.25-0.5 mg/kg orally sid (dogs and cats)	Hypovolaemia, hypotension, tachycardia, hyperkalaemia May aggravate hypotensive effects of acepromazine (use lower acepromazine dose and prepare for crystalloid infusion)
Phosphodiesterase inhibitors	Mixed effects: inotropy, chronotropy, diuresis, vasodilation	Propentophylline 2.5-3 mg/kg orally bid (dogs)	

Figure 14.3: *Vasodilators for preoperative preparation of animals in heart failure. Vasodilators must not be used in: hypotension, hypovolaemia, pre-renal failure, fixed or dynamic obstruction of ventricular function, poor diastolic function.*

- Some reduce cardiac output and cause hypotension. The haemodynamic significance of benign arrhythmias may be increased in cardiac diseases
- Untreated, benign arrhythmias may degenerate into lethal rhythms like ventricular fibrillation (VF), asystole or electromechanical dissociation during surgery. Anaesthetists must be able to differentiate malign and benign arrhythmias from artefacts and be able to treat the arrhythmias
- Spontaneously arising intraoperative arrhythmias indicate a deterioration in the environment of the myocardium as a result of poor anaesthetic management, i.e. deranged blood gases, pH, temperature and electrolyte values.

Some arrhythmias disappear as cardiac function improves. If they do persist, an alternative cause must be investigated and/or non-specific anti-arrhythmic treatment instituted (see Figure 14.4). For simplicity, preoperative arrhythmias are categorized here as bradyarrhythmias (slow heart rates (HRs)) and tachyarrhythmias (fast HRs).

Bradyarrhythmias: Preoperative bradycardia may be secondary to hypoglycaemia (insulinomata), hyperkalaemia (Addison's disease), hypertension or hypothyroidism. It may be iatrogenic (digoxin and β_1- antagonist) or idiopathic, e.g. canine sick sinus syndrome. Bradyarrhythmias deserve investigation because further slowing of the HR is likely under anaesthesia. At very slow HRs, myocardial blood flow is reduced and the heart fails.

If emergency surgery is needed, the heart is tested first with atropine and then with isoprenaline to assess whether HR increases (see Figure 14.4). A reaction to either drug indicates the appropriate chronotropic treatment for controlling intraoperative

Drug	Indications	Dose	Side effects
Type 1a	Ventricular arrhythmias and ventricular tachycardia Malignant ventricular arrhythmias, refractory supraventricular tachycardias, acute atrial fibrillation	Procainamide 4-8 mg/kg over 5 minutes then 25-50 µg/kg/min Quinidine 6-10 mg/kg i.m. or 6-20 mg/kg orally tid or qid (dogs)	Procainamide causes myocardial depression, hypotension and electrocardiographic abnormalities if given rapidly Hypotension, arrhythmias
Type 1b	Malignant ventricular arrhythmias	Lignocaine 2-4 mg/kg i.v. then 25-75 µg/kg/min	
Type 2	Tachyarrhythmias	Propranolol 50 µg/kg i.v. every 2 minutes to effect; maintenance 0.25-1 mg/kg orally tid (dogs and cats)	Hypotension, bradycardia, bronchospasm, obtunded sympathetic responses to hypovolaemia, hypercapnia, hypoxaemia, etc., acute aggravation of congestive failure
Type 3	Ventricular arrhythmias	Bretylium; effects undetermined	
Type 4 Calcium channel blockers	Supraventricular tachycardia, ventricular tachycardia, atrial fibrillation	Diltiazem 0.5-1.5 mg/kg orally tid (dogs); 1.75-2.5 mg/kg orally bid or tid (cats)	Bradycardia, other arrhythmias, hypotension, acute aggravation of congestive failure
Antimuscarinics	Bradyarrhythmias	Atropine 20-40 µg/kg i.m. or s.c. Glycopyrrolate 5-10 µg/kg i.m. or s.c. Isopropamide 2.5-5 mg/kg orally bid or tid Propantheline 3.75-7.5 mg/kg orally bid or tid	
β_1-Agonists	Bradyarrhythmias	Isoprenaline 5-10 mg orally tid or qid (dogs) Terbutaline 1.25-5 mg/dog orally bid or tid; 300 µg-1.25 mg/cat orally bid or tid	

Figure 14.4: Anti-arrhythmic drugs for preoperative preparation of animals in heart failure.

bradyarrhythmias. If neither drug increases HR, surgery should be postponed or a means of artificial ventricular pacing found.

Tachyarrhythmias: Preoperative tachyarrhythmias should be investigated as they compromise myocardial O_2 balance (m$(D-V)O_2$) (see Figure 14.6). Unremedied myocardial hypoxia will result in ventricular arrhythmias and eventually cardiac arrest. This is likely when catecholamines are released (see Figure 14.7). Vagal manoeuvres, e.g. carotid sinus massage and ocular pressure, are said to convert atrial tachycardia to

sinus rhythm, but rarely do. Digoxin, with or without β_1-antagonist drugs, is nearly always required.

Pulmonary oedema
Pulmonary oedema often indicates left heart failure and occurs in several conditions, such as mitral valve incompetence, mitral stenosis and aortic stenosis. The condition must be treated before anaesthesia because it decreases lung compliance (increases lung 'stiffness'), increases work of breathing and impairs oxygenation. It is most likely to occur when plasma oncotic pressure is low, e.g. in hypoalbuminaemia.

Drug class	Indications	Drug	Precautions
Type 1a	Ventricular arrhythmias and ventricular tachycardia	Procainamide 4-8 mg/kg over 5 minutes then 25-50 µg/kg/min	Procainamide causes myocardial depression, hypotension and electrocardiographic abnormalities if given rapidly
Type 1b	Malignant ventricular arrhythmias	Lignocaine 2-4 mg/kg i.v. then 25-75 µg/kg/min	
Type 2	Tachyarrhythmias	Propranolol 50 µg/kg i.v. every 2 minutes to effect Maintenance 0.25-1 mg/kg orally tid (dogs and cats)	Hypotension, bradycardia, bronchospasm, obtunded sympathetic responses to hypovolaemia, hypercapnia, hypoxaemia, etc., acute aggravation of congestive failure
Type 3	Ventricular arrhythmias	Bretylium; effects undetermined	
Antimuscarinics	Hypotension due to slow heart rate, bradycardia, bradyarrhythmias	Atropine 20-40 µg/kg i.v. Glycopyrrolate 5-10 µg/kg i.v.	
Negative chronotropes	Idiopathic tachycardia, tachyarrhythmias	Morphine 0.25-0.5 mg/kg i.v. Alfentanil 1-5 µg/kg every 5 minutes i.v. Fentanyl 1-2.5 µg/kg i.v. repeated every 20 minutes or so Digoxin 5-10 µg/kg i.v. Neostigmine 25-50 µg/kg i.v. Edrophonium 1 mg/kg i.v.	Monitor heart rate and electrocardiogram; severe bradycardia and hypotension in overdose

Figure 14.5: Anti-arrhythmic drugs used for rapid control of haemodynamic variables during anaesthesia.

Changes in blood pH

Blood gas abnormalities caused by cardiopulmonary disease may in turn exacerbate the primary condition and create self-reinforcing cycles. For example, low cardiac output causes tissue hypoperfusion and metabolic acidosis. Metabolic acidosis further depresses cardiac contractility. Treatment should be directed at the primary lesion, e.g. hypoperfusion, renal failure or inadequate pulmonary perfusion.

Polycythaemia

Polycythaemia (haematocrit > 0.55) results from any condition that causes hypoxia, e.g. right to left intrapulmonary shunts (neoplasm, bronchitis) or extrapulmonary shunts (ventricular septal defect). Polycythaemia increases blood viscosity and mimics an increased systemic vascular resistance (SVR). Increased SVR increases ventricular wall tension during systole which restricts coronary blood flow and eventually leads to ventricular failure. In peripheral tissue, viscous blood 'sludges' in capillaries and limits oxygen delivery. High haematocrit values are lowered preoperatively by normovolaemic haemodilution – the simultaneous removal of blood and infusion of plasma, colloids or crystalloid solutions.

Right heart failure

Right ventricular (RV) failure raises central venous pressure (CVP) and favours capillary transudation throughout the body, resulting in pleural and/or pericardial effusion, ascites, hepatomegaly, splenomegaly and/or peripheral oedema. Pleural and pericardial effusions may restrict ventilation, and accumulation of pericardial fluid impedes cardiac filling (cardiac tamponade).

Renal dysfunction

Hyperkalaemia: Increased potassium concentrations are arrhythmogenic; patients should be treated with sodium bicarbonate solutions, calcium gluconate, insulin–glucose solutions or cation exchange resins. In extreme cases, peritoneal dialysis may be required.

Azotaemia: The presence of compounds containing nitrogen in the blood, along with other effects of renal failure (acidaemia, hyperkalaemia), causes

Factors reducing mDO_2	Factors increasing $m\dot{V}O_2$
Low blood oxygen tension (PaO_2) Low haemoglobin concentration Coronary vasospasm (severe hypocapnia) Low arterial blood pressure Decreased heart rate	Increased heart rate Systolic wall tension, afterload Contractility Increased basal metabolic rate

Figure 14.6: *Factors affecting myocardial oxygen balance ($m(D-\dot{V})O_2$).*

Conditions increasing plasma catecholamine levels
Noxious surgical stimulation ± inadequate anaesthesia/analgesia Endotracheal intubation under 'light' anaesthesia Hypotension Hypoxaemia Hypercapnia Hypoglycaemia Hyperthermia Severe hypothermia Postoperative pain
Endocrine disease
Hyperthyroidism Phaeochromocytoma
Drugs
Antimuscarinics β-Agonists Thyroxine Phosphodiesterase inhibitors

Figure 14.7: *Factors causing perioperative 'sympathomimesis'.*

bradyarrhythmias and increases myocardial sensitivity to anaesthetics. Treatment depends on whether failure is predominantly renal or prerenal.

Hypoalbuminaemia: Low concentrations of serum albumin render animals sensitive to albumin-bound drugs like thiopentone. Low plasma oncotic pressure facilitates the formation of pulmonary oedema. In conjunction with high CVP, hypoalbuminaemia contributes to peritoneal, pleural and pericardial effusions.

Liver dysfunction

Coagulation abnormalities: If there is any suspicion of impaired clotting, a coagulation test must be performed. Coagulopathies are treated by the preoperative infusion of fresh blood – even before minor operations, such as dentistry.

Hypoglycaemia: Glucose concentrations of 4.1–14.75 mmol/l (70–250 mg/dl) must be established perioperatively with intravenous dextrose solutions because impaired delivery of glucose to the brain, which is more likely with cardiovascular disease, will result in severe neuronal damage.

Delayed drug metabolism: Hepatic dysfunction may impair the rate of elimination of long-acting drugs like pentobarbitone and acepromazine.

Other considerations

Effective circulating blood volume (ECBV): Pre-existing fluid deficits must be rectified and the over zealous use of diuretics avoided in those conditions in which cardiac output depends on preload.

Anaemia: A haemoglobin concentration of 12–15 g/dl is considered necessary for optimal arterial blood O_2 content (CaO_2). Below this concentration, cardiac output increases to compensate for the anaemia. This increases myocardial work which, with the reduced CaO_2, leads to myocardial hypoxia. Low haemoglobin concentration is resolved preoperatively by blood transfusion with fresh whole blood after acute haemorrhagic losses, or by packed cells (haematocrit >0.65) in chronic normovolaemic anaemia. Stored blood should be transfused 24 hours before anaesthesia to allow any abnormalities that may have occurred during storage to resolve *in vivo*. Over transfusion must be avoided as this increases ventricular afterload and promotes pulmonary oedema.

Hypokalaemia: Low serum potassium concentrations (caused by loop diuretics) should be increased to normal before surgery because hypokalaemia prevents the conversion of ventricular tachycardia to sinus rhythm by anti-arrhythmic drugs. Treatment is by potassium supplementation, either orally or by the infusion of crystalloid solutions 'spiked' with potassium chloride. The infusion rate of potassium should not exceed 0.5 mmol/kg/h (see Figure 14.2).

Pyrexia: Pyrexia increases cardiopulmonary activity by raising the metabolic rate (O_2 and glucose consumption and CO_2 production increase). Mild hypermetabolism causes few problems, but the cause must be identified. Considerable risk occurs when pyrexia results from endocarditis or meningitis. Some antibiotics, e.g. aminoglycosides and chloramphenicol, may interact adversely with anaesthetics.

Drugs

Drugs used to treat heart failure may produce undesirable side effects, which complicate anaesthesia. For example, digoxin causes arrhythmias, and so opinions differ over preoperative digitalization. Some recommend that animals in cardiac failure facing elective operations should be digitalized, but that the morning dose should be withheld on the day of surgery. Digitalized animals facing emergency operations, however, should not have the drug withdrawn. In non-digitalized animals facing emergency operations the infusion of inotropes like dobutamine may be as effective (and less hazardous) than rapid intravenous digitalization.

As a rule, attempting to limit potential interactions by withdrawing drugs before anaesthesia may cause more problems than it solves. The fear of interactions should not be used as an excuse for inadequate preparation. Ideally, surgery should be postponed until treatment has achieved a maximal effect, and drug side effects have been minimized.

Anaesthetic techniques

Options

Major surgery can be performed under sedation (which keeps the animal still) and local anaesthesia, providing the surgical site is amenable to local techniques. Sedation or anaesthesia may be required for some tests. The assumption that sedatives are safer than general anaesthesia seems intuitive, and administration more straightforward. However, sedatives may be unpredictable, provide an inadequate duration of effect, cause adverse physiological effects and fail to provide conditions for both invasive physiological measurement and the support of ventilation. In contrast, general anaesthesia allows tracheal intubation so that intermittent positive-pressure ventilation (IPPV) is possible. The level of anaesthesia can be adjusted to suit the investigation at any moment. General anaesthesia with volatile agents provides rapid recoveries after prolonged investigations because their elimination is independent of cardiac, hepatic and renal function.

Local anaesthetic injected into the spinal or extradural space can, under certain circumstances, cause catastrophic haemodynamic effects.

Pre-anaesthetic medication with a neuroleptanalgesic combination such as acepromazine and butorphanol, induction with an ultra-short-acting injectable anaesthetic such as propofol, and light general anaesthesia produced with halothane (and possibly nitrous oxide (N_2O)) provide adequate conditions for minor operations in animals with modest cardiac disease, providing attention is paid to ventilation, temperature, circulating blood volume and perioperative analgesia. This technique is, however, inadequate in animals with advanced disease undergoing major operations because it does not prevent the autonomic nervous responses to noxious (surgical) stimulation which adversely affect cardiovascular function.

Balanced anaesthesia is more appropriate in such cases and involves using the lowest dose of anaesthetic capable of producing unconsciousness (which minimizes myocardial depression) with a potent analgesic (to obtund reflex responses to surgery) and a muscle relaxant (to improve surgical conditions). Nitrous oxide is frequently included because it has modest cardiovascular effects and reduces the delivered concentration of inhalant drug required to produce a given level of anaesthesia. Balanced anaesthesia is not without complications; neuromuscular blocking agents eliminate both respiration and the most obvious sign of inadequate anaesthesia – movement.

Drug selection

Selecting the most appropriate anaesthetic for a particular animal is simplified by categorizing acquired cardiovascular diseases (see Figure 14.8). As a rule, the anaesthetics chosen should have minimal effect on myocardial contractility and peripheral venous tone. In addition to providing adequate conditions for surgery (analgesia and muscle relaxation), the anaesthetic chosen should:

* Reverse the haemodynamic disorder by mimicking the effects of medical treatment (this requires a knowledge of drug effects, which are summarized in Figure 14.9)
* Be compatible with drugs used perioperatively to improve cardiovascular function
* Be suitable in the presence of secondary cerebral, myocardial, hepatic or renal complications
* Be minimally affected by altered pharmacokinetics.

Identifying an ideal technique is difficult because of a paucity of data on anaesthetic behaviour in companion animals with cardiopulmonary disease. The data summarized in Figure 14.9 are simplistic and imply that drug behaviour is independent of other variables. It is not, and an obsession with drug suitability based on theoretical haemodynamic effects diverts attention from other perioperative factors exacerbating cardiopulmonary derangement. In any case, the adverse haemodynamic effect of an anaesthetic can easily be negated. For example, the myocardial depressant effect of halothane is reversed by infusing fluids and/or infusing inotropes.

The assumption that new anaesthetics are safer than the older agents for animals with cardiopulmonary disease is misconceived and dangerous. Drugs often behave differently in animals with cardiovascular disease, and so when using unfamiliar drugs it is difficult to determine if an undesirable effect is normal or indicates deteriorating conditions. Allegedly safer anaesthetics provide a temptation to anaesthetize those animals that would previously have been regarded as unacceptable risks. Under these circumstances the use of unfamiliar drugs (which are unlikely to be safer) in susceptible animals may have dire consequences. Ultimately, anaesthetic risk depends as much on the anaesthetist's experience with an agent as it does on the drug's calculated lethality (therapeutic index), and so it is better to choose any fundamentally safe, and familiar, technique over one that may in theory be more appropriate but which is unfamiliar.

Pre-anaesthetic medication

Pre-anaesthetic medication should alleviate an animal's anxiety and pain, and enable venous catheterization, venepuncture or mask induction to be conducted without stress to the animal. Neuroleptanalgesic combinations based on low-dose acepromazine and opioids are useful in dogs and cats. The opioid chosen depends on several factors including its haemodynamic effects. For example, the author favours morphine, except when bradycardia is undesirable, when pentazocine or pethidine are used instead. Neuroleptanalgesic combinations are safe in cats: morphine 0.1–0.25 mg/kg does not produce undesirable neurological effects provided it is injected intramuscularly with acepromazine 0.05–0.1 mg/kg.

Category	Example	Problems	Management goals
High cardiac output	Secondary to hypermetabolic conditions: hyperthyroidism; phaeochromocytoma; hypercapnia	Slow induction to anaesthesia with volatile agents. Increased risk of myocardial hypoxia, arrhythmias. High output failure in response to catecholamines	Avoid increases in heart rate Suppress myocardial contractility Suppress afterload Avoid catecholamine release
Low cardiac output Fixed Obstructive (valvular) Cardiac tamponade Fixed heart rate Ventricular	Mitral and aortic regurgitation and stenosis, pulmonary hypertension Canine sick sinus syndrome Cardiomyopathy 'End stage' heart disease	Heart rate unable to increase output in response to challenge. Intolerant of **any** changes affecting cardiac output. Increased systemic vascular resistance (SVR) causes hypertension; more importantly, reduced systemic vascular resistance, venomotor tone or heart rate causes marked hypotension	Maintain or increase heart rate (not >20% resting) Maintain sinus rhythm Avoid falls in systemic vascular resistance Avoid myocardial depression/ maintain contractility Avoid myocardial ischaemia Maintain preload
Variable Inefficient heart rate	Ventricular tachycardia Hypothyroidism	Myocardial hypoxia, hypotension Myocardial hypoxia, hypotension	Reduce heart rate and variables decreasing myocardial oxygen balance (m(D-$\dot{V}$)O$_2$) Increase heart rate
Inadequate contractility	Cardiomyopathy 'End stage' heart disease	Myocardial hypoxia, hypotension	Maintain contractility Minimize variables decreasing myocardial oxygen balance (m(D-$\dot{V}$)O$_2$)
Inadequate preload	Hypovolaemia, septicaemia	Hypotension	Maintain preload Increase systemic vascular resistance Avoid high inflation pressures during positive-pressure ventilation
Excessive afterload	Polycythaemia, hypertension, cor pulmonale	Myocardial hypoxia, arrhythmias, end organ damage in brain, eyes, heart, kidney and arteries	Decrease systemic vascular resistance

Figure 14.8: Classification of cardiac failure.

Drug	Cardiac output ($\dot{Q}_t$)	Inotropy	Heart rate	Systemic vascular resistance	Mean arterial pressure	Pulmonary vascular resistance	Central venous pressure	Electrocardiogram
Acepromazine	↔↓	↔	↔↓	↓↓	↓	?	↓	Type 1b anti-arrhythmic effect, may cause some slowing, first degree atrioventricular block
Diazepam	↔	↔	↔	↔↓	↔	?	↔	
Midazolam	↔↓	↔↓	↔↑	?	↔↓	?	?	
Morphine*	↔	↔	↓	↓	↔	?	↓↓	Bradycardia, bradyarrhythmias, though tachycardia/hypotension (histamine release) may follow rapid i.v. injection of *any* opioid
Pethidine	↔↓	↔↓	↑	↔↓	↓	?	↑	
Butorphanol	↔	↔	↔↓	↔	↔↓	?	?	
Buprenorphine	↔	↔	↔↓	↔	↔↓	?	?	
Atropine	↑	↔	↑↑↑	↔	↔↑	?	?	Tachycardia, ventricular arrhythmias
α_2-Agonists	↓	↔	↓↓↓	↑–↓	↑–↓	?	?	Bradycardia, first or second degree atrioventricular block. Xylazine may 'sensitize' myocardium to catecholamines
Thiopentone	↓	↔↓	↑↑	↔↓	↓	?	↓	Occasionally causes transient ventricular arrhythmias
Alphaxalone/ alphadolone	↓	↓	↑↑	↓	↓	↑	↓	
Ketamine	↑↑	↑↑	↑	↑	↑↑	?	?	
Propofol	↓	↓	↔↓	?	↓	?	?	
Halothane	↓↓	↓↓	↔↓	↔	↓	↔↓	↑	'Sensitizes' myocardium to catecholamines
Isoflurane	↔↑	↔↓	↑	↓↓	↓↓	↔↓	↑	
Nitrous oxide	↔↑	↓	↑	↔	↔↑	↑	↔	
Desflurane	↑	↔↓	↑	↓↓	↓↓	↔↓	↑	
Sevoflurane	↔↑	↔↓	↔	↓	↓	↓	?	
Fentanyl	↔↓	↔	↓↓	↔	↔↓	?	↔	Bradycardia, bradyarrhythmias (negated by co-injection of atropine)
Alfentanil	↔↓	↔	↓↓	↔	↔↓	?	↔	Bradycardia, bradyarrhythmias (negated by co-injection of atropine)

Figure 14.9: *Summary of the haemodynamic effects of sedatives and anaesthetics. Data have been derived from several species and sources. Drug effects will be influenced by physiological, pathological and pharmacological factors unique to individual patients, so under certain conditions minimal or even opposite changes to those described may be seen.*

* Non-steroidal anti-inflammatory drugs e.g. carprofen, ketoprofen, have not been included in this list because of minimal direct haemodynamic effects.
↑, increased; ↓, decreased; ↔, no change; ↔↓, none, OR, slightly decreased effect; ↑–↓, biphasic effect; ?, no information found.

Diazepam- or midazolam-based combinations offer theoretical benefits because benzodiazepines are largely devoid of cardiovascular effect. They are, however, unreliable sedatives and often cause stimulation even in depressed animals. They are useful in cats when combined with ketamine and/or acepromazine.

Medetomidine should not be used for pre-anaesthetic medication in ill animals. The availability of an antagonist does not justify the use of medetomidine or other α_2-agonists in high risk cases given the widespread cardiovascular disturbances they cause.

Antimuscarinic drugs (atropine and glycopyrrolate) may be required if bradycardia is present or likely to develop. They should not be used routinely as they can cause arrhythmias, especially in animals whose myocardial oxygen balance is precarious. There seems to be little evidence for the belief that glycopyrrolate is safer than atropine in this respect.

Severely debilitated animals should not be left unattended once pre-anaesthetic medication has been given, and there are advantages in applying the ECG and other physiological monitors, which the patient will tolerate, at this stage. In very poorly animals, the insertion of central venous and/or arterial catheters under local anaesthesia may be possible. Enriching inspired air with O_2 will rarely do harm at this stage. This can be achieved in several ways if the direct application of a mask is resented.

Induction

Induction of anaesthesia must be stress free and not unduly compromise haemodynamic function. Induction enables atraumatic intubation of the trachea using a minimum effective dose (MED) of anaesthetic. Anaesthesia must, however, be adequate for tracheal intubation otherwise ventricular arrhythmias may arise – at least in dogs. Bucking against the endotracheal tube (ETT) promotes lung collapse. Failing to intubate the airway of animals with cardiopulmonary disease is indefensible.

There are no ideal induction techniques. Some favour ketamine and diazepam combinations, etomidate or high-dose neuroleptanalgesic combinations for high-risk cases, although these have their own specific disadvantages and offer few advantages over properly administered thiopentone, propofol, alphaxolone/ alphadolone or methohexitone. Problems with intravenous anaesthetics usually arise from a failure to appreciate abnormal pharmacokinetics (see Figure 14.1) rather than from drug effects *per se*. Any ultra-short-acting injectable anaesthetic is suitable providing the MED is given carefully, i.e. a normal dose is prepared but a lower than normal dose given initially and at a slow rate. A sufficient interval must be left between deciding that intubation conditions are inadequate and giving further injections.

In severely compromised sedated animals the author uses halothane delivered in a 1:2 O_2:N_2O mixture by mask (halothane is better tolerated than isoflurane). At the first sign of resistance to the mask a hypnotic dose of thiopentone (1–3 mg/kg) or propofol (1 mg/kg) is injected intravenously. These doses eliminate reaction but do not cause apnoea, so induction continues. Despite causing atmospheric contamination, the technique allows for rapid recovery if problems arise.

Induction by mask or by the combination of mask with subanaesthetic doses of intravenous agents (including alphaxolone/alphadolone 3 mg/kg) is feasible in well sedated cats. Providing the animal is sedated, induction by chamber is preferable because it avoids the stress of restraint.

Transient ventricular arrhythmias are not uncommon during induction. The incidence seems to be reduced if intravenous anaesthetic solutions are diluted, e.g. 1.25% thiopentone, and injected slowly. Nevertheless, syringes prefilled with rapidly acting anti-arrhythmic drugs, such as lignocaine (lidocaine) and atropine, should be available and the ECG monitored throughout.

Postinduction apnoea is normal with intravenous anaesthetics, especially propofol, and may cause haemoglobin desaturation. Apnoea after normal doses, however, is inconsequential providing the trachea is intubated promptly and the lungs inflated thereafter with O_2-enriched gas, at a rate of 2–3 breaths per minute.

Maintenance

Anaesthesia should provide surgical conditions using drugs that are non-cumulative and that preserve cardiopulmonary function. Volatile anaesthetics have a profoundly depressant effect on haemodynamic function and so the MED (just preventing any autonomic nervous response to surgery) must always be used. The MED is lowered (and haemodynamic function preserved) by other drugs, notably N_2O, opioid analgesics and benzodiazepines. By relieving volatile anaesthetics from the task of relaxing skeletal muscle, neuromuscular blocking agents also lower the requirement for volatile anaesthetics. In veterinary anaesthesia, inhalant anaesthesia still offers considerable advantages over total intravenous techniques. Other factors to consider during the maintenance period are discussed below.

Body position: Extreme head-up body positions impair venous return, while extreme head-down positions impair breathing, reduce functional residual capacity (FRC) and lower cerebral perfusion pressure; both positions must be avoided. Excessive fixation of the forelimbs with ropes may lower chest wall compliance and increase the work of breathing in spontaneously breathing animals.

Depth of anaesthesia: Anaesthetic overdose and inadequate anaesthesia are equally undesirable in animals with unstable cardiopulmonary function. Sympathoadrenal responses include catecholamine release which, by increasing the oxygen demand of the whole body, HR , cardiac contractility and afterload, threaten $m(D-\dot{V})O_2$. They also create conditions for oedema formation. Inadequate anaesthesia produced with theoretically appropriate drugs is more hazardous than adequate conditions provided by inappropriate agents. In one study, increasing the inspired concentration of halothane – a well known arrhythmogen – was effective at suppressing ventricular arrhythmias in both dogs and cats (Muir *et al.,* 1988). Pre-emptive and polymodal pain treatment are very desirable in animals with cardiovascular disease.

Anaesthetic overdose depresses cardiopulmonary function, and so close attention must be paid to the depth of anaesthesia. This should be altered to meet variations in noxious stimulation and should be maintained using the MED. Autonomic nervous responses to surgery are best controlled with potent analgesics, e.g. alfentanil or fentanyl given intravenously, rather than intravenous or inhalational anaesthetics.

Surgical manipulation: During operations involving thoracic viscera, unavoidable manipulation of the heart and great vessels may limit cardiac output, e.g. rotating the heart kinks the great veins and impairs ventricular filling. Accidental epicardial stimulation with surgical instruments produces ventricular ectopic beats, while the use of cold irrigation fluids impairs contractility.

Ventilatory mode: Cardiovascular disease frequently affects pulmonary function. Ventilatory inadequacy causes hypoxia, hypercapnia or both, which are poorly tolerated by animals with cardiovascular disease. Both are potent arrhythmogens because they simultaneously promote sympathetic nervous activity (and solicit an increase in cardiac work) while impairing myocardial contractility.

During surgery, spontaneously breathing animals normally hypoventilate and retain CO_2. The thoracolumbar pump is, however, preserved and, provided respiratory depression is not severe, cardiac output is not unduly depressed. Severe hypoventilation may occur in animals with chest wall and neural lesions (see below).

Controlled ventilation is required whenever spontaneous efforts fail to maintain normal arterial blood gas values. However, by raising the mean intrathoracic pressure, it inhibits the thoracolumbar pump, reduces venous return and causes hypotension. Pulmonary vascular impedance increases during inspiration and momentarily lowers RV stroke volume. This may be hazardous when pulmonary blood flow is reduced, e.g. in pulmonary embolism, severe pulmonic stenosis or pulmonary hypertension, in which injudicious IPPV critically lowers pulmonary blood flow.

Careful IPPV, which is advantageous in most animals with cardiopulmonary disease, achieves an adequate minute volume of ventilation with minimal elevation of the mean intrathoracic pressure. This requires that the inspiratory:expiratory (I:E) time ratio is short (about 1:3), that peak airway pressures are kept to a minimum (ideally 15–20 cm H_2O) and that there is no positive end-expiratory pressure.

High inflation pressures are beneficial in conditions characterized by left to right shunts, e.g. patent ductus arteriosus, because they limit volume loading of the left ventricle. Higher inflation pressures also oppose pulmonary transudative forces and should be used if pulmonary oedema is likely.

Fluid balance: Fluid loss, haemorrhage or venodilation are poorly tolerated in conditions that rely on ventricular filling pressures to maintain cardiac output, e.g. cardiac tamponade. In these cases, one or more large bore catheters should be dedicated to fluid administration. Ideally, fluids are replaced as they are lost, and on a like-for-like basis. Body fluids are lost as blood (haemorrhage), urine, water vapour, evaporation from the respiratory tree and surgical site and as transudate into a third space created by surgery (third space losses). Only haemorrhage and urinary loss are easy to quantify. Blood loss is measured by weighing blood-soaked swabs (1 ml blood weighs 1.3 g) and for each millilitre of blood shed, 1 ml blood or colloid solution or 3 ml of crystalloid solution should be given. Third space losses into damaged tissue are impossible to quantify, but it is widely accepted that the infusion of crystalloid solution at 5, 10 or 15 ml/kg/h compensates for the effects of mild, moderate and major operations respectively. Concessions are necessary when ideal fluids are unavailable. The common statement that sodium-containing solutions should not be used in animals with cardiac disease is a counsel of perfection and when critical perioperative hypovolaemia arises, the rapid administration of any isotonic fluid will be life saving (a sodium load can be dealt with later using loop diuretics).

Over transfusion with blood and colloidal solutions (and to a lesser extent crystalloid solutions) increases ventricular afterload and reduces pulmonary compliance, and must be avoided in cases with left heart failure as it may lead to pulmonary oedema. Haemorrhage during corrective cardiovascular surgery is usually not excessive, but the aorta or pulmonary artery can be inadvertently damaged, with critical results. The means of rapidly transfusing large volumes of blood or colloid, e.g. adequate fluid stores and a pressurising device, should be available.

Body temperature: Accidental hypothermia is likely in young animals undergoing operations for the correction of cardiac anomalies in which viscera are exposed for prolonged periods. This is undesirable because hypothermia impairs cardiopulmonary function: it depresses ventilation, increases blood viscosity and shifts the oxyhaemoglobin dissociation curve to the left. Arrhythmias may arise spontaneously in the chilled heart, with fibrillation becoming increasingly likely as temperatures approach 28°C. It also initiates shivering during recovery, which increases whole body VO_2 fourfold. The core temperature should be preserved throughout the perioperative period using prophylactic, rather than active, measures. Irrigation fluids should be warmed to 37°C before use.

Deliberate hypothermia involves actively cooling cerebral and myocardial tissue to 16–20°C to reduce VO_2 during periods of deliberate circulatory arrest. The technique is frequently used in conjunction with cardiopulmonary bypass and so is beyond the scope of this chapter.

Monitoring: During anaesthesia there is no single indicator of adequate cardiovascular function, and so the overall picture can only be determined by the measurement and interpretation of many variables. In cases with modest cardiovascular disease undergoing incidental surgery, a minimum acceptable level of monitoring would include the continuous surveillance of consciousness, pulse rate and quality (by palpation), mucous membrane colour, capillary refill time, respiratory rate, depth and rhythm, core (oesophageal) temperatures, absolute blood loss, rate of bleeding and the colour of blood at the surgical site. If skin temperature is measured simultaneously the core–peripheral temperature gradient, which many believe reflects tissue perfusion, may be calculated (see Chapter 5). Normally the gradient is less than 6°C. Heart and lung sounds are most easily monitored using an oesophageal stethoscope. The high incidence of cardiac arrhythmia in companion animal anaesthesia warrants routine ECG monitoring, while simplicity and the value of information justify the measurement of urine output. Central venous pressure measurement is useful in cases where cardiac output depends on ventricular preload. Pulse oximetry is easy to perform and gives useful information, providing the probe allows accurate measurement. Devices with a bouncing plethysmograph are most useful because they display pulsatile blood flow and indicate mechanical cardiac activity. In high-risk cases, arterial blood pressure should be monitored directly. The major advantages of capnometry and pulse oximetry over serial arterial blood gas analysis in general practice is that they are economically feasible. However, the inexperienced are advised against the indiscriminate use of complicated electronic monitors in high-risk cases as these may, by producing excessive information of varying quality, detract from the appraisal of vital signs. In any case, monitoring a given variable can only be fully justified if the anaesthetist can interpret its significance and make an appropriate response.

Neuromuscular blockade
Neuromuscular blocking agents may be useful in animals where severe cardiovascular disease complicates management; their use is best avoided by the inex-

perienced. Atracurium and vecuronium are devoid of significant cardiovascular effects and may be used to improve surgical conditions and facilitate IPPV. Overdose, which may prolong recoveries, is avoided if drug administration is based on continuous monitoring of neuromuscular transmission. Postoperative hypoventilation is prevented if neuromuscular block is antagonized; an edrophonium (1 mg/kg) atropine (40 µg/kg) mixture injected over 2 minutes does not produce autonomic nervous or electrocardiographic changes in dogs (Clutton, 1994).

Cardiovascular adjunct drugs
Many drugs used for preoperative preparation can be used during surgery to offset adverse haemodynamic events. However, the formulations used must be rapid in onset and short acting and should be safe when given intravenously. Haemodynamic problems encountered during anaesthesia in animals with cardiovascular disease and their treatment are shown in Figure 14.10. The control of intraoperative arrhythmias is detailed in Figure 14.5.

Recovery
Risk is greatest during the recovery of animals that have not undergone corrective surgery; the cardiovascular system has to contend with pain, hypoventilation and hypothermia. Intraoperative monitoring and medications should continue until urine output is adequate, the ECG is stable and the extremities are warm and perfused. Pain must be aggressively relieved in a polymodal approach; after high laparotomy or thoracotomy, pain from the incision site can discourage deep breathing and promote lung collapse. Frequent repositioning may be necessary in animals that do not breathe deeply. Inspired gases should be enriched with O_2 until the animal can maintain adequately saturated haemoglobin (SpO_2 >90%) while breathing room air. This is especially important if the animal shivers.

Acquired conditions
In veterinary practice, it is common for acquired cardiovascular diseases to complicate anaesthesia in elderly animals presented for straightforward operations. Further problems arise with advancing age. Given the unfeasibility of discussing anaesthetic management for all cardiovascular conditions affecting companion animals, this section concentrates on those which are common examples of conditions categorized in Figure 14.8.

Feline hyperthyroidism
Cats with hyperthyroidism require anaesthesia for thyroidectomy but are at risk of high output cardiac failure and ventricular arrhythmias. Preoperative management aims to restore euthyroidism and a normal

Drug class	Indications	Drug	Precautions
β_1-Agonists	Hypotension due to poor myocardial contractility and/or bradycardia	Dobutamine 1-20 µg/kg/min Dopamine 1-20 µg/kg/min Isoprenaline 10-50 ng/kg/min Adrenaline 22-33 µg/kg i.v. then 10-100 ng/kg/min	Monitor heart rate and electrocardiogram (ECG); severe tachycardia, hypertension and ventricular arrhythmias in overdose
β_1-Antagonists	Tachycardia, tachyarrhythmias, arrhythmias associated with myocardial hypoxia. Hypotension due to reduced cardiac output in hypertrophic cardiomyopathy. Hypotension due to excessive heart rate	Propranolol 50 µg/kg every 2 minutes Esmolol	Monitor heart rate and ECG; severe bradycardia and hypotension in overdose
α_1-Agonists	Hypotension due to α_1-antagonists and/or inadequate systemic vascular resistance	Methoxamine 50-100 µg/kg every 5-15 minutes i.v. Phenylephrine 10 µg/kg every 5-15 minutes i.v. Noradrenaline 10-50 ng/kg/min i.v.	Monitor heart rate and urine output; bradycardia and oliguria in overdose
α_1-Antagonists	Hypertension due to excessive α_1-agonist activity, myocardial hypoxia due to high afterload	Phentolamine 25-100 µg/kg i.v.	Monitor heart rate and blood pressure; hypotension in overdose
Vasodilators	Severe hypertension rapid afterload reduction Emergency venodilation/ afterload reduction (pulmonary oedema)	Sodium nitroprusside i.v. infusion: 1-15 µg/kg/min (dogs) Glyceryl trinitrate 2% 0.25-2.0" (0.6-5 cm) (dogs), 0.25-0.5" (0.6-1.2 cm) (cats) bid to qid to medial pinna	Hypotension, tachycardia, azotaemia. Rapid effects; monitor blood pressure Hypotension, tachycardia, azotaemia. Rapid effects; monitor blood pressure

Figure 14.10: Adjunct drugs used for rapid control of haemodynamic variables during anaesthesia.

cardiac output by controlling thyroid hormone concentrations with carbimazole (5 mg/animal tid). This may take several weeks. Emergency (non-thyroid) surgery may be necessary in unprepared animals. In these, preinduction stress, caused by overzealous restraint, an unsympathetic environment, pain etc., must be minimized. For this reason, O_2, which may be needed to alleviate dyspnoea, should be given by chamber rather than by mask. Preoperative and intraoperative cardiac hyperactivity and arrhythmias may require treatment; β_1-antagonist drugs like propranolol are suitable. The goals of anaesthesia are to:

- Avoid all factors reducing m(D-$\dot{V}$)O_2 (see Figure 14.6)
- Suppress ventricular arrhythmias.

Pre-anaesthetic medication should include acepromazine for its anti-arrhythmic and sedative effects. If sedation is not achieved then induction in a chamber, using halothane (in preference to isoflurane), may prove less stressful than an intravenous technique. Drugs increasing or maintaining HR and/or contractility, e.g. atropine, ketamine and isoflurane, are probably less safe than those with a depressant effect, e.g. halothane. Drugs increasing afterload and ventricular wall tension, e.g. α_2- agonists, should not be used, while anything that increases plasma catecholamine concentrations must be avoided (see Figure 14.7). The other effects of elevated metabolic rate (increased O_2 consumption and increased CO_2 production) indicate that attention should be paid to the breathing system and that the lungs should be moderately hyperventilated. For further details see Chapter 19.

Hypertrophic cardiomyopathy

Hypertrophic cardiomyopathy (HCM) is not uncommon in young to middle-aged male cats and may occur secondary to hyperthyroidism; it is rare in dogs. Hypertrophic cardiomyopathy is often asymptomatic and its first signs may be pulmonary oedema or sudden death during anaesthesia. In this condition a muscular subaortic stenosis forms during systole, which momentarily restricts left ventricular (LV) outflow and may cause mitral regurgitation. The obstruction is worsened by increased HR and myocardial contractility and by decreased LV diastolic volume and ventricular afterload, all of which lower cardiac output.

Cats with HCM must not be stressed preoperatively (see feline hyperthyroidism) but should receive supplemental O_2. Pulmonary oedema, if present, is treated with O_2, frusemide, cage rest and glyceryl trinitrate ointment. Pleural effusions are relieved by thoracentesis. Heart failure, if present, is controlled with frusemide and vasodilators: glyceryl trinitrate ointment, captopril or enalapril. Digoxin may be given but is not always required; systolic function is usually normal. Digoxin-resistant tachycardia may respond to propranolol or diltiazem. The goals of anaesthesia are to:

- Suppress HR
- Suppress contractility
- Suppress ventricular arrhythmias
- Maintain filling pressures
- Maintain or increase SVR
- Avoid all factors reducing m$(D-V)O_2$.

Halothane may have advantages over isoflurane in this condition. Intraoperative hypotension should be treated with α_1-agonists like methoxamine, rather than β_1-agonists, while hypertension should be controlled by increasing the delivered concentration of halothane; vasodilators are unsuitable. Tachycardia arising from surgical stimulation should be controlled with analgesics like alfentanil; β_1-antagonists may be used if the cause is non-physiological.

Mitral valve incompetence

Initially, mitral valvular incompetence represents a fixed low cardiac output condition because, during systole, a proportion of the stroke volume (which depends on the size of the valve orifice) regurgitates into the left atrium. Later, ventricular failure becomes more important. Complications include atrial fibrillation and pulmonary oedema. Atrial fibrillation must be converted to sinus rhythm because the contribution of the atrium to ventricular filling is more important when cardiac output is reduced by disease. Atrial fibrillation usually resolves as vasodilator drugs reduce the volume of blood regurgitating into, and dilating, the left atrium. In time, high back-pressure from the pulmonary veins leads to RV and congestive failure.

If congestive failure is present and time allows, the animal should be prepared and anaesthesia managed as for fixed low output conditions. In unprepared animals facing emergency operations, however, the problem is one of low cardiac output/poor contractility, as occurs with dilated cardiomyopathy (see below). In addition to the haemodynamic objectives listed in Figure 14.8, anaesthesia in animals with leaking mitral valves should aim to:

- Produce mild reductions in SVR
- Produce modest increases (<10% preoperative values) in HR
- Avoid bradycardia and hypertension.

A reduction in SVR promotes forward flow, while modest increases in HR reduce the regurgitant fraction and prevent falls in diastolic pressure, which compromises coronary perfusion. Low doses of acepromazine are useful, although high doses may cause severe hypotension, especially if angiotensin-converting enzyme (ACE) inhibitors have been given. Additional sedation may be achieved by the coinjection of an opioid agonist drug with chronotropic activities, e.g. pethidine. Ultra-short-acting intravenous anaesthetics are suitable for induction in animals with mild to moderate disease, although care should be taken. In advanced cases, a venous catheter should be placed before induction, and fluids infused in case venodilation (as occurs with thiopentone) reduces ventricular filling. In severely affected animals, a combined mask/intravenous technique is suitable. Bradycardia and hypertension must be avoided during anaesthesia as both increase valvular regurgitation. Thus, isoflurane has some advantage over halothane. Nitrous oxide increases SVR but the benefits from its inclusion usually outweigh the disadvantages. Ventricular preload should be maintained using intravenous fluids, while IPPV is of value when there are signs of pulmonary oedema.

Aortic valve regurgitation

The haemodynamic consequences of aortic and mitral valve regurgitation are similar and so, therefore, are the goals of management.

Mitral valve stenosis

Mitral valve stenosis fixes cardiac output by limiting LV filling during diastole and presents a considerably greater challenge than mitral valve regurgitation. Coincidental increases in left atrial and pulmonary venous pressures lead to atrial fibrillation and pulmonary oedema respectively. Cardiac output depends on the adequate transfer of blood across the stenotic valve, which in turn depends on slow HRs (increased diastolic filling time) and sinus rhythm, rather than atrial fibrillation. The left ventricle is small so any slowing of HR causes hypotension. As in any fixed low output condition, anaesthesia must:

· Maintain cardiac output
· Maintain or produce modest increases in HR
· Maintain SVR
· Maintain sinus rhythm
· Avoid injudicious IPPV.

The dilemma here is that cardiac output must be maintained without provoking pulmonary oedema by overtransfusion or by increasing RV output. Inotropes should only be used when signs of RV failure are present, while fluids are given on a strict 'as needs' basis. Cardiac output relies on the maintenance of HR and SVR. The latter should be maintained with α_1-agonist drugs; peripheral vasodilators must be avoided. Positive pressure ventilation must be imposed very judiciously because while it retards pulmonary fluid transudation, it increases RV afterload. Furthermore, the lungs may have limited compliance, being engorged with extra blood, and so higher inflation pressures are necessary.

The fact that N_2O increases pulmonary vascular resistance (PVR) has led many to condemn its use in cases with pulmonary hypertension. Volatile anaesthetics, however, reduce PVR to a great extent and so compensate for this.

Cardiac tamponade

As the pericardium is only slightly distensible, space-occupying masses or effusions within the pericardial sac raise intrapericardial pressure and limit filling of the atria and right ventricle. This reduces LV stroke volume so cardiac output becomes heart-rate dependent, while arterial and venous constriction maintain blood pressure. When the elastic limits of the pericardial sac are reached, a small volume increment causes a disproportionate increase in intrapericardial pressure and a critical reduction in cardiac output.

Some causes of cardiac tamponade, e.g. congenital peritoneopericardial diaphragmatic hernia, are amenable to surgical treatment. Pericardial effusions must be relieved (pericardiocentesis) preoperatively. Diuretics must be used carefully in animals with signs of oedema: over use may reduce right-sided filling pressure. Anaesthesia should aim to:

· Avoid any reduction in SVR
· Avoid any reduction in HR.

Slowing of the HR critically decreases cardiac output, and so positive chronotropes must be available and ready for use. Adequate cardiac output also depends on adequate ventricular filling pressure: hypovolaemia and other factors limiting venous return must be avoided. If IPPV is necessary, low tidal volumes should be imposed at high rates to minimize the increase in intrathoracic pressure. Central venous pressure reflects RV filling pressures and should fall dramatically after pericardectomy. Drugs causing marked arteriolar or venular dilation must not be used.

Cor pulmonale

Cor pulmonale describes RV changes resulting from pulmonary hypertension. Pulmonary hypertension results from lung diseases like chronic bronchitis and bronchiectasis. Chronic hypoxia, arising from lung disease, causes pulmonary hypoxic vasoconstriction and aggravates the condition. Pulmonary hypertension eventually leads to right-sided congestive heart failure. Risks from anaesthesia are high in cor pulmonale: the complications of RV failure are aggravated by lung disease.

Elective operations should be postponed until all reversible elements of pulmonary disease have been treated and pulmonary arterial pressure lowered. Lowering of pulmonary arterial pressure is achieved most simply with O_2, which reverses hypoxic pulmonary vasoconstriction. In chronic conditions, bronchodilators and antibiotics may be beneficial (see below). If right-sided failure is present, cage rest, low-salt diets and short-term diuretic treatment should be imposed. Digoxin should only be used if signs of congestive failure are obvious. Polycythaemia may necessitate normovolaemic haemodilution. In treating pulmonary hypertension, vasodilators may cause more problems than they solve and so should be used carefully, if at all. Anaesthesia should aim to:

· Maintain or reduce PVR
· Avoid excessive lung inflation pressures.

Volatile anaesthetics alone, or with N_2O, are suitable because all relax vascular smooth muscle, reduce PVR and attenuate airway responsiveness to endotracheal intubation. Airway pressures imposed during IPPV must be the lowest required for adequate lung inflation.

Traumatic myocarditis

In dogs, if the epicardium is damaged by blunt trauma to the thoracic wall, ventricular arrhythmias frequently develop 12–24 hours later. The ventricular arrhythmias, combined with other effects of injury, e.g. pain and anxiety, result in an inefficiently high HR that threatens $m(D-\dot{V})O_2$. Treatment is aimed at reducing plasma catecholamine concentrations and involves sedation and analgesia, cage rest, the administration of O_2 and the restoration of ECBV. In some cases, low-dose acepromazine with morphine given intramuscularly eliminates arrhythmias. In others, lignocaine injection followed by infusion may be required. Procainamide is used on the rare occasions that lignocaine fails. The haemodynamic effects of anaesthesia should:

- Reduce HR
- Avoid all factors reducing m(D-$\dot{V}$)O_2
- Suppress arrhythmias.

Neuroleptanalgesic combinations are suitable for pre-anaesthetic medication. Anaesthetics slowing or reducing myocardial O_2 demand, e.g. halothane, may be more suitable than those that maintain cardiac output, e.g. isoflurane. Preoperative anti-arrhythmic treatment, e.g. lignocaine infusion, should be continued throughout the operative period and into recovery if necessary. Further details may be found in Chapter 21.

Canine sick sinus syndrome
The implantation of an artificial pacemaker is required when cardiac pacemaker activity fails to initiate a mechanical response consistent with adequate cardiac output. The most frequent reason for pacemaker implantation in dogs is high-grade second degree heart block, third degree heart block, persistent atrial standstill and canine sick sinus syndrome. Before surgery, an attempt is made to increase HR with positive dromotropes like atropine, glycopyrrolate or isoprenaline. When medical treatment is partly successful, the animal may be given isopropamide, propantheline, isoprenaline or terbutaline before surgery.

The operation usually takes place in two stages. First, a temporary pacing wire is passed via the external jugular vein into the right ventricle. This may be performed under deep sedation, i.e. neuroleptanalgesia, with overlying tissue infiltrated with local anaesthetic. Once the electrode tip of the pacemaker wire is located at the RV apex (under fluoroscopy) and the heart 'captured', i.e. it responds to the pacemaker unit, then general anaesthesia can be induced with little risk, and the permanent pacemaker implanted in the soft tissue of the neck or abdomen (this approach, which involves passing the permanent pacing wire through the diaphragm before its insertion in the ventricular epicardium, requires thoracotomy).

In some animals it is more convenient to position the temporary pacing wire under general anaesthesia, although this incurs a real risk of cardiac arrest. Several steps may minimize the risk of fatal outcome. First, pre-anaesthetic medication should either have no effect on or, preferably, increase HR. Second, drugs which have shown some chronotropic effect in the subject, should be made available, e.g. atropine or isoprenaline. Third, the ECG should be monitored as soon as pre-anaesthetic medication is given. Fourth, endotracheal intubation should only be attempted once the animal is adequately anaesthetized (any ultra-short-acting intravenous anaesthetic is suitable) and, finally, provisions must be available for emergency transvenous pacing and direct current (DC) defibrillation.

Dilated (congestive) cardiomyopathy
Dilated (congestive) cardiomyopathy is common in large-breed male dogs and characterized by severe myocardial failure. The left ventricle is thin walled flabby and dilated. Both atrial (atrial premature depolarizations, atrial fibrillation) and ventricular arrhythmias (premature ventricular depolarizations (PVDs)) are common and most dogs eventually develop both left and right heart failure. While some dogs respond to treatment, others die suddenly. In cats, dilated cardiomyopathy results from taurine deficiency. It produces characteristic signs of right, not left failure, and responds to dietary taurine supplementation (250 mg bid).

Animals with dilated cardiomyopathy can die suddenly under anaesthesia, so preoperative preparation is conducted until clinical signs are minimal. Treatment involves management of heart failure with digoxin, frusemide and vasodilators like prazosin, hydralazine or captopril. This is particularly important when atrial fibrillation is present. The haemodynamic goals of anaesthesia are to:

- Maintain cardiac output
- Avoid factors reducing m(D-$\dot{V}$)O_2.

Preoperative HR should be preserved and arrhythmias treated as they arise. Isoflurane offers advantages over halothane, although inotropes and chronotropes may still be required. Venous return must be maintained using fluids.

Hypovolaemia: absolute and relative
A low variable cardiac output state exists when inadequate ECBV limits ventricular preload. This arises when intravascular volume losses exceed gains, e.g. haemorrhage, polyuria, vomiting, diarrhoea and extensive burns, but can occur when a normal volume circulates within an expanded vascular bed, e.g. in severe dilation caused by Gram-negative septicaemia. The restoration of an ECBV reduces most of the problems associated with this condition, and so elective surgery must be postponed until this is so. The challenge lies in the emergency case in whom fluid resuscitation is inadequate. In such cases the anaesthetist must:

- Maintain ventricular filling pressures
- Maintain SVR
- Avoid high lung inflation pressures.

Great care must be taken with dosing of all injectable drugs as the volume of distribution is smaller. Perioperative fluid balance should be monitored by careful record keeping of infused volume (volume in), urine output measurement (volume out) and CVP. Systemic vascular resistance is preserved by avoiding vasodilatory drugs and/or giving α_1-agonists. Acepromazine should not be used at doses >12.5 µg/kg, if at all. Thiopentone, a potent venodilator, must be used with care. The production of surgical anaesthesia should rely more on high doses of opioid analgesics rather than inhaled anaesthetics. Both halothane and isoflurane lower blood pressure, and their delivered concentration should be minimized by the co-administration of N_2O. High intrathoracic pressures must be avoided if IPPV is imposed, as these reduce venous return.

Canine hypertension

Problems with anaesthesia in hypertensive dogs are unexamined because the condition itself is rarely diagnosed (Dukes, 1992). However, there are at least four risk factors. First, increased LV afterload and mass jeopardizes m$(D-\dot{V})O_2$. Second, hypertension occurs in diseases which themselves elevate risk, e.g. polycythaemia and primary renal disease. Third, chronic hypertension damages the brain, eyes, heart, kidneys and peripheral vessels. Finally, chronic hypertension shifts the autoregulation curve for renal and cerebral perfusion to the right, which means that blood flow in these organs becomes pressure dependent at relatively high values. Blood pressure values that would ensure adequate perfusion in normotensive animals are inadequate in hypertensive cases.

If surgery allows, anaesthesia in an animal with chronic hypertension should be delayed until normal arterial pressure is restored with low-sodium diets, diuretics, β_1-antagonists, α_1-antagonists and vasodilators, which may take several weeks. With non-elective operations, anaesthesia must:

- Maintain or modestly increase blood pressure
- Maintain or modestly reduce SVR
- Avoid factors reducing m$(D-\dot{V})O_2$.

It is, however, impossible to achieve these haemodynamic goals simultaneously. Management therefore depends on extensive monitoring and the judicious use of both inotropes and vasoactive adjunct drugs. Preoperative HR should be preserved and arrhythmias treated as they arise. Isoflurane offers some advantages over halothane, although inotropes and chronotropes may still be required. Venous return must be maintained using fluids.

Congenital conditions

Many anomalies may be asymptomatic and, in young animals requiring incidental operations, present little challenge beyond the haemodynamic effects of the lesion itself. In some cases, however, the anomaly causes rapid deterioration in cardiovascular function. In such cases, additional problems arise during anaesthesia because of the subject's immaturity, corrective surgical manipulations and advanced techniques that may be necessary for operation.

Anaesthesia and surgery performed on very young subjects is technically difficult because of their size. Physiological immaturity is another consideration. However, the advantages of postponing surgery are less than the disadvantage – a disproportionately increasing anaesthetic risk. It is safer to perform surgery on an animal when it is young rather than wait until the subject is larger and more mature.

Accidental hypothermia is likely during surgical correction of cardiac anomalies in small subjects as they have a high surface area:volume ratio, are physiologically immature, require longer surgery time, have a large visceral surface exposed during thoracotomy and are deeply anaesthetized. Also, the lungs are ventilated extensively with medical gases, which may be inadequately warmed and humidified.

Special techniques that are often required during cardiovascular surgery, e.g. thoracotomy, deliberate hypotension, cardiopulmonary bypass (CPBP) and induced hypothermia complicate anaesthesia, influence drug disposition and, if performed improperly, increase morbidity and mortality.

The classification of acquired disorders applies to congenital conditions but requires elaboration. Many developmental anomalies are characterized by abnormal left-to-right, or right-to-left conduits through which blood shunts between the left (systemic arterial) and right (pulmonary arterial) circulation. These are of considerable significance.

Left-to-right shunts, exemplified by the more common form of patent ductus arteriosus (PDA), atrial septal defects (ASD) and ventricular septal defects (VSD), are associated with massive increases in pulmonary blood flow and volume overload of either the left (PDA), right (ASD) or both (VSD) ventricles.

Right-to-left shunts are characterized by cyanosis (unresponsive to oxygen administration) and polycythaemia and are more dangerous. They occur in PDAs complicated by persistent pulmonary hypertension. In all types, pulmonary flow is reduced so response to inhaled anaesthetics is sluggish. However, forelimb–brain circulation time is rapid, permitting fast induction with intravenous agents.

Patent ductus arteriosus

The most common type of PDA involves a left-to-right shunt. A proportion of LV output enters the pulmonary artery and recirculates through the lung. The reduced blood volume entering the descending aorta causes hypotension in the absence of compensatory changes. The increased LV volume load and RV pressure load often leads to biventricular hypertrophy. Treatment involves surgical ligation of the ductus arteriosus.

In some cases, postparturient PVR remains high and exceeds SVR, causing blood to flow in a right-to-left direction, and eventually leading to RV failure. In addition, mucosal membranes in the lower half of the body, e.g. the penis, are cyanosed, while cranial structures are normal because oxygenated blood still flows down the brachiocephalic trunk and left subclavian artery. Surgery is inadvisable in these cases because the ductus arteriosus functions as a relief valve; ligation precipitates right heart failure.

Anaesthesia and surgery in young asymptomatic dogs carries low risk and the outcome is rewarding. Risk increases if surgery is delayed: left atrial dilation may precede fibrillation. When signs of heart failure are present, the animal should be stabilized. Treatment should continue until there is little radiographic evidence of cardiomegaly, pulmonary congestion and pulmonary oedema. During surgery the haemodynamic objectives are to minimize, and yet maintain, a left-to-right pressure gradient. This is achieved by anaesthetics which:

- Maintain cardiac output
- Avoid profound decreases in SVR
- Avoid marked increases in PVR

Cardiac output is best maintained with fluids, and inotropes given to maintain, or produce slight rises in, HR. A modest drug-induced reduction in SVR is also desirable as this increases systemic blood flow, reduces RV afterload and may reduce left-to-right blood flow before ligation. Increasing PVR over SVR with excessive lung inflation pressures could cause right-to-left shunting during parts of the cardiac cycle and lower SpO_2. Increased pulmonary blood flow means the level of unconsciousness changes sluggishly after vaporizer settings are changed. Most of these haemodynamic effects are achieved with isoflurane.

Ligation raises diastolic pressure and may initiate a transient reflex bradycardia known as Bramham's sign. The ligature must be slackened and retightened more slowly if this persists, or if hypotension or bradyarrhythmias develop. There is little justification for atropine.

The surgical correction of a right-to-left PDA is imprudent, but on occasion it may be necessary to anaesthetize affected animals for incidental operations. These animals are at considerable risk from anaesthesia because they are usually hypoxic (PaO_2 <7.9 kPa (60 mmHg)) and polycythaemic. Attempts should be made to reverse the shunt, by the judicious use of α_1-agonists, i.e. drugs increasing SVR, and α_2-antagonists, like tolazoline, which lower PVR.

Pulmonic stenosis

A stenotic pulmonary valve limits RV outflow. In response, RV systolic pressure increases, which may render the tricuspid valve insufficient and cause right atrial enlargement. Given time, the right ventricle hypertrophies, and then fails. The condition may be corrected by surgery or balloon valvuloplasty. The latter involves passing a balloon-tipped catheter via the jugular vein, the right atrium and the right ventricle,

up the pulmonary outflow tract and into the stenosis. The balloon is then inflated and should physically dilate the stenosis (Martin *et al.*, 1992).

Signs of RV failure must be treated before operation because the ventricle will be sensitive to the depressant effects of anaesthetics and IPPV. The haemodynamic goals of anaesthesia are to:

- Maintain myocardial contractility
- Maintain or reduce HR
- Maintain RV preload
- Avoid excessive lung inflation pressures.

Volatile anaesthetics are suitable for this operation. Isoflurane maintains contractility but halothane reduces HR and so improves RV filling. Dobutamine may be used to increase RV contractility providing it does not increase HR. Adequate preload should be maintained by infusing fluids.

Aortic stenosis

In aortic stenosis, a constricted outflow tract restricts LV output and initiates hypertrophy and greater contractility, which threatens $m(D-\dot{V})O_2$. This is particularly hazardous because reduced diastolic arterial pressure, characteristic of aortic stenosis, leads to a critical reduction in coronary blood flow and sudden death. The condition can be treated by valvotomy (which necessitates cardiopulmonary bypass) or balloon valvuloplasty (which does not). Animals with this condition may require incidental operations.

Severe cases with congestive failure respond poorly to diuretics, low-salt diets and rest, although β-adrenergic antagonists may be beneficial in long-term management of increased intraventricular pressures and hypertrophy. The haemodynamic goals of anaesthesia are to:

- Avoid hypotension by maintaining SVR, not increasing cardiac output
- Maintain HR within 20% of preoperative values
- Avoid factors reducing $m(D-\dot{V})O_2$.

Modest falls in blood pressure will cause disproportionately large reductions in coronary arterial filling pressure and myocardial DO_2. Preservation of sinus rhythm is important as the left ventricle depends on a synchronized atrial contraction to assure LV filling (junctional or escape rhythms must be controlled as they arise). Intravascular fluid volume must be maintained. Providing HR and rhythm are maintained, the myocardium is not overly depressed and ECBV is maintained, the most likely cause of intraoperative hypotension is drug-induced vasodilation. This should be remedied with α_1-agonists.

Ventricular septal defect

The haemodynamic effect of a VSD depends on its size and shunt direction. The latter depends on the right–

left ventricular pressure differential, which depends on PVR and SVR respectively. Blood normally flows left to right, because pressures in the left ventricle exceed those in the right. However, chronic hypoxia causes pulmonary hypertension, which may increase PVR to the point where shunt flow ceases or reverses direction.

Anaesthesia for surgical correction requires cardiotomy and CPBP. However, dogs with VSD may require anaesthesia for other operations. Cardiac failure must be treated if present. The haemodynamic goals of anaesthesia are to maintain a left-to-right shunt. This occurs if anaesthetics:

- Maintain SVR above PVR.

Blood pressure should be maintained with α_1-agonists while high lung inflation pressures should be avoided.

Management of intraoperative arrhythmias

The possibility of intraoperative arrhythmias is high in animals with cardiopulmonary disease. For the sake of simplicity these are divided into bradyarrhythmias and tachyarrhythmias

Bradyarrhythmias

The HR may slow during anaesthesia due to any of the causes listed in Figure 14.11, causing significant hypotension and coronary hypoperfusion.

Cause	Response
Inadequately treated/recurring preoperative causes	See Figures 14.2, 14.3 and 14.4
Anaesthetics	Establish causative agent; consider positive chronotropes*
Anaesthetic overdose	Reduce delivered concentration of inhaled drug and ventilate lungs*
Hypothermia	End surgery and re-warm; consider gastric or colonic lavage with warm water
Hypertension	Consider vasodilators and/or β_1-antagonists
Vagal stimulation	Check surgery†
Hyperkalaemia	Hyperventilate with oxygen, give bicarbonate (HCO_3) (1 mmol/kg over 10 minutes)
Severe acidosis	Hyperventilate lungs with oxygen and give HCO_3 (as above)
Severe hypoglycaemia	50% dextrose
Severe hypoxia	Ventilate lungs with 100% oxygen
Terminal myocardial hypoxia	Initiate cerebrocardiopulmonary resuscitation

Figure 14.11: *Causes of intraoperative bradyarrhythmias and suggested treatment.*

* 'Lightening' anaesthesia or starting surgery, if it has not already begun, is the simplest treatment for drug-induced bradycardia. Antimuscarinic drugs safely reverse opioid-induced bradycardia but their use with α_2-agonists is controversial. † If bradycardia, bradyarrhythmias or atrioventricular conduction blocks arise during a specific surgical manipulation, surgery must be suspended and the level of anaesthesia assessed. Lightly anaesthetized animals should be more deeply anaesthetized and surgery continued more gently. If the problem persists then atropine, glycopyrrolate or isoprenaline should be given.

Cause	Response
Inadequate anaesthesia or analgesia	Increase inspired concentration, give low dose of i.v. anaesthetic (alfentanil or fentanyl), (see Figure 14.5)
Hypercapnia	Intermittent positive-pressure ventilation (IPPV)
Hypoxaemia	Provide 100% oxygen IPPV
Hypotension, shock, septicaemia	Give i.v. fluids rapidly
Drugs	Discontinue β_1-agonists, if given (see Figure 14.5)
Hyperthermia	Consider abdominal lavage with ice-cold fluids
Hypokalaemia	Give potassium chloride; 0.05 mmol/kg over 1 minute, repeat if necessary
'Idiopathic' tachycardia	Consider non-specific negative chronotropes (see Figure 14.5)
Hyperthyroidism	Consider non-specific negative chronotropes (see Figure 14.5)

Figure 14.12: *Causes of intraoperative tachycardia and suggested treatment.*

Tachyarrhythmias

Increases in HR may indicate undetected hypovolaemia or another physiological derangement (Figure 14.12). Severe tachycardia is hazardous as it reduces cardiac output and threatens myocardial O_2 balance. Diagnosis is assisted by noting the rate of onset. Sudden increases in HR indicate inadequate anaesthesia, while insidious changes result from slowly worsening blood gas derangements and hypovolaemia. Three responses are appropriate whenever tachycardia or tachyarrhythmias arise. First, the level of unconsciousness is evaluated, and a possible link between surgery and rhythm disturbance examined. If such a link exists the level of anaesthesia is deepened and surgery continued with gentler manipulation. If this is unsuccessful, a short-acting vagomimetic opioid drug like alfentanil, oxymorphone or morphine should be given. Second, several lung inflations with O_2-enriched gas will usually suppress arrhythmias resulting from hypercapnia and/or hypoxaemia. Third, the rapid infusion of fluids often slows increased HRs due to hypovolaemia or hypotension, although the response may be slow and slight.

Intraoperative ventricular arrhythmias

Tachyarrhythmias often deteriorate, becoming more dangerous rhythms. For example, untreated pleomorphic PVDs in time coalesce and become ventricular tachycardia. This in turn leads to ventricular fibrillation and death. Tachyarrhythmias must be treated aggressively using the three responses described above followed by intravenous lignocaine. The beneficial effects may be short lived and, although repeated injections can be given, it is preferable to infuse a lignocaine and saline mixture. If lignocaine is ineffective, intravenous procainamide may be used. If PVDs persist and deteriorate into ventricular tachycardia then cardioversion with an externally synchronized DC non-phasic defibrillator in conjunction with lignocaine should be attempted. If lethal rhythms arise then cardiopulmonary resuscitation must be attempted (see Chapter 24).

Note: the appearance of intraoperative PVDs in digitalized animals may point to relative digoxin overdose caused by hypokalaemia. The latter commonly follows respiratory alkalosis, i.e. excessive ventilation. In minor cases a reduction in alveolar ventilation may effect a cure, otherwise potassium chloride (up to 0.05 mmol/kg) should be given intravenously over 1 minute. A repeated dose may be necessary.

PULMONARY DISEASE

Problems

The principal function of the pulmonary system is gas exchange, i.e. to replenish venous blood with O_2 and to remove CO_2. This depends on ventilation - the bulk flow of fresh gas into the alveoli. In turn, ventilation depends on an unobstructed airway and an effective respiratory muscle effort, and is controlled by centres in the medulla oblongata. These increase ventilation in response to high plasma CO_2 concentrations (>5.3 kPa (40 mmHg)) and/or low O_2 tensions. Efficient gas exchange also depends on processes within the lung that match alveolar ventilation ($\dot{V}$) with alveolar perfusion ($\dot{Q}$). On this basis, pulmonary disease can be defined broadly as any process threatening gas exchange, i.e. any condition:

- Obstructing the airway
- Impairing respiratory muscle effort
- Depressing the neural control of breathing
- Impairing ventilation/perfusion ($\dot{V}/\dot{Q}$) ratios.

In this chapter, respiratory disease is categorized as:

- Difficult orotracheal intubation
- Upper airway obstruction
- Hypoventilation caused by abnormal chest wall and neural function
- Impaired oxygenation caused by:
    V/Q discrepancies
    Chronic obstructive pulmonary disease
    Asthma/bronchoconstriction.

Pulmonary disease increases risk from anaesthesia because:

- Anaesthetics suppress protective upper airway reflexes, impair mucociliary function, depress ventilation and derange processes ensuring $\dot{V}/\dot{Q}$ matching
- The disease affects other organ systems in ways that further increase risk: blood gas derangements cause arrhythmias; chronic hypoxia leads to polycythaemia
- Its management may involve drugs that affect anaesthesia
- The disease alters the uptake of inhalation anaesthetics
- Conditions severely restricting gas movement into the alveolar space are life threatening and demand immediate treatment.

Risk during anaesthesia is reduced if:

- An accurate diagnosis is established
- The underlying pathophysiological processes are understood
- Pulmonary function is improved preoperatively
- The anaesthetic offsets, rather than aggravates, the effects of underlying pathophysiological processes
- Perioperative physiological monitoring is adequate.

Difficult orotracheal intubation
Conditions that can prevent mouth opening and orotracheal intubation are not usually associated with other respiratory disease, and affected animals breathe normally when conscious. However, after induction of anaesthesia, it may be impossible to secure the airway, which is then at risk from soft tissue obstruction and regurgitation/aspiration. Conditions causing problems with orotracheal intubation include:

· Eosinophilic myositis
· Movement-limiting pathology of the temporomandibular joint (TMJ)
· Jaw fractures
· Painful, or space-occupying, periocular lesions.

When these problems are identified preoperatively they can be circumvented by performing tracheotomy under deep sedation and local anaesthesia. In many cases, however, the significance of the condition may not be appreciated until the animal is unconscious and attempted intubation proves difficult or impossible.

If tracheotomy under sedation is unfeasible the animal must be rendered unconscious, the mouth forcibly opened and the trachea intubated as rapidly as possible. A means of transtracheal oxygenation and IPPV (tracheostomy) must be available in case this is impossible. Steps must be taken to lower the risk of regurgitation/aspiration by depriving the animal of food and avoiding morphine and α_2-agonists. Before induction, O_2 by mask may prove advantageous.

The ideal induction technique, which would provide analgesia yet preserve breathing, does not exist, but benzodiazepine/ketamine combinations are preferred over thiopentone, propofol or alphaxolone/alphadolone. Once the animal is unconscious (and in sternal recumbency) strong gauze straps should be passed over the mandible and maxilla and sufficient force exerted until the mouth can be opened and the glottis identified. If painful TMJ disease is present, profound analgesia or deep general anaesthesia should be provided to prevent reactions to articulation of the TMJ. If the mouth cannot be opened, so that direct laryngoscopy is impossible, a blind intubation technique must be attempted (as in the horse). Non-steroidal or steroidal anti-inflammatory drugs should be given before the animal recovers from anaesthesia, when many show signs of severe discomfort.

Upper airway obstruction
Endotracheal intubation provides an unobstructed airway in unconscious animals and protects the respiratory tree from vomitus. In brachycephalic breeds, dislodgement of the soft palate or other pharyngeal tissue into the airway may occur after sedation, during anaesthesia and at recovery when the loss of pharyngeal reflex control, combined with laryngeal hypoplasia, lateral ventricular eversion and collapsing arytenoid cartilages, may result in severe obstruction. Airway patency is similarly threatened in non-brachycephalic breeds in conditions like:

· Laryngeal hemiparalysis
· Subepiglottic cyst
· Intermandibular masses
· Laryngospasm
· Pharyngeal and retropharyngeal:
    Neoplasia
    Abcessation
    Oedema
    Haemorrhage
    Air (often with pneumomediastinum)
· Collapsing trachea.

Upper airway obstruction is managed by introducing an adequately sized cannula beyond the obstruction site, so that O_2 may be delivered and the lungs inflated until airway patency is restored. Tracheal intubation may not be possible if space-occupying pharyngeal lesions obstruct the view of the rima glottidis and make blind intubation impossible. For these reasons, facilities for emergency tracheotomy should be available.

Life-threatening obstruction
Animals with obstructive upper airway lesions may present *in extremis*. Such animals should be preoxygenated (for as long as it takes to prepare them for tracheo-stomy) using a large-bore needle introduced into the tracheal lumen downstream from the obstruction or as close to the thoracic inlet as possible. An emergency tracheotomy is then performed with or without local anaesthetic. A more permanent tracheostomy can be performed later under general anaesthesia.

Less severe obstruction
These cases present as semi-emergencies requiring airway reconstruction under general anaesthesia, but there is usually adequate time to determine the cause of obstruction. This is important because dyspnoea arising from tracheal collapse or laryngeal paralysis is alleviated by sedative pre-anaesthetic medication, while in other cases, e.g. brachycephalic syndrome, it is aggravated. The oropharynx and upper respiratory tract should be examined by direct vision using a bright light source and a long-bladed laryngoscope. The retropharyngeal area and trachea should be palpated for unusual structures that may compress the airway.

Whether pre-anaesthetic medication is given or not, the animal should be preoxygenated. Induction of anaesthesia may be performed with any ultra-short-acting intravenous agent and the trachea intubated as swiftly as possible. A laryngoscope may be useful. When tracheal collapse is present, the tip of the ETT must extend beyond the site of obstruction.

General approach to 'chest wall/neural' and pulmonary conditions

Conditions affecting the lower airway, chest wall and the control of breathing are rarely emergencies and so preoperative preparation is possible. Planning anaesthesia in animals with pulmonary disease is straightforward, providing the underlying pathophysiology is understood and reversed.

Preoperative examination

A thorough review of the medical history, and physical examination, may establish a diagnosis although more complex procedures such as radiography, electrocardiography, arterial blood gas analysis, ultrasonography, primitive lung function tests and bronchoscopy may be required.

Haematology: An elevated haematocrit provides supporting evidence for significant cardiopulmonary diseases because chronic hypoxia causes secondary polycythaemia. It should be appreciated that a polycythaemic animal may appear cyanotic even when O_2 saturation is normal.

Arterial blood gas analysis: Arterial blood gas analysis provides useful quantitative information on the lungs' ability to oxygenate blood, eliminate CO_2 and influence acid-base status. Venous samples are less useful as they do not reflect pulmonary function.

Radiography: Radiographs are valuable in examining intrathoracic lesions. For animals with respiratory embarrassment, inappropriate positioning in the lateral and/or dorsal position may cause distress and struggling and is potentially hazardous. Dyspnoea related to body position (orthopnoea) is avoided by using lateral decubitus and dorsoventral projections.

Pulse oximetry: Pulse oximetry is well tolerated and may be applied in the conscious animal breathing air. However, an SpO_2 <90% may be due to factors other than pulmonary disease.

Bronchoscopy: The introduction of flexible bronchoscopes, which can be passed through gas-tight grommets on suitable endotracheal swivel connectors, has greatly facilitated bronchoscopy although in very small animals, effective ventilation ceases if the endoscope obstructs the airway.

Chest wall and neural disorders

Figure 14.13 lists conditions in which bulk gas flow into the alveoli is inadequate for the maintenance of normal CO_2 concentrations (oxygenation may not be impaired). Animals with these conditions develop severe hypercapnia, respiratory acidosis and possibly hypoxaemia when sedated or anaesthetized, unless the lungs are periodically inflated with at least 20% O_2.

Before surgery, an attempt should be made to address the cause (Figure 14.13) as in many cases this will limit the adverse haemodynamic effects of IPPV. Pre-anaesthetic medication must not impair spontaneous breathing and the animal should not be left unattended until anaesthesia is induced. During this interval, inspired gas should be enriched with O_2. Anaesthesia can be induced with any ultra-short-acting intravenous agent providing the trachea is intubated without unnecessary delay. When restrictive chest wall changes and/or impaired neural control are the only contributors to respiratory depression, the risk of anaesthesia effectively disappears once the trachea is intubated and periodic lung inflation begun. However, some conditions also involve pulmonary disease compromising blood oxygenation, in which case additional measures are required.

When painful chest wall lesions, e.g. pleurisy, prevent adequate ventilation, the administration of analgesics, including those with respiratory depressant effects, improves breathing.

Pulmonary conditions

In some conditions blood oxygenation improves by simply enriching inspired gas with O_2. In others, endotracheal intubation and periodic lung inflation with O_2 (rather than air) is necessary. Specific therapies are required when chronic obstructive pulmonary disease (COPD), or bronchospasm, are present.

Inadequate oxygenation

Many conditions altering V/Q ratios and/or retarding gas diffusion across the alveolar-capillary membrane are associated with a diminished ability to oxygenate blood. These include:

- Neoplasia
- Pneumonia
- Pulmonary contusion
- Embolism
- Chronic bronchitis
- Chronic emphysema
- Heart–lung anomalies
- Pulmonary oedema.

Preoperative preparation with drugs that produce a wide, dry and clean airway aims to relieve reversible disease and optimize pulmonary function (Figure 14.14). Attempts to improve ventricular function may be appropriate in conditions characterized by chronic pulmonary hypertension. When disease is severe, the option of using local anaesthetic techniques and sedation should be considered.

Aetiology	Location	Response
Neural factors	Overdose with depressant drugs Intracranial tumours Severe hypothermia or hyperthermia Infection: meningitis or encephalitis Head trauma Status epilepticus	Antagonism Methods reducing intracranial pressure (ICP) Restore normal temperature Antibiotics Methods reducing ICP Anticonvulsant therapy
Pleural resistance	Pleuropericardial herniation Diaphragmatic herniation Pleuritis (pain)* Hydrothorax, pyothorax, pneumothorax, chylothorax Haemothorax	No immediate treatment; impose head-up position No immediate treatment; impose head-up position Analgesics Thoracentesis†; drain Thoracentesis†; drain, autotransfuse
Abdominal resistance	Pancreatitis (pain)* Tympany Haemoperitoneum Pregnancy Pyometra Ascites	Analgesics Gastric decompression Paracentesis abdominis†, autotransfusion Impose head-up position Impose head-up position Paracentesis abdominis†; slow drainage
Thoracic wall resistance	Obesity Restrictive bandaging Flail chest Injury (pain)* Skeletal abnormalities e.g. kyphosis, lordosis, pectus excavatum Myasthenia gravis	Weight reduction programme if possible Remove if possible Apply bandages; analgesics Analgesics No treatment Physostigmine, corticosteroids
Lower airway obstruction	Collapsing trachea Foreign body Neoplasia Oedema Cardiomegaly	Sedation, endotracheal intubation Bronchoscopy None See cardiac failure Diuretics, see cardiac failure
Pulmonary resistance	Pulmonary oedema Extensive fibrosis Pulmonary hypertension	See cardiac failure No treatment Oxygen therapy

Figure 14.13: *Causes and preoperative treatment of chest wall/neural conditions.*

* Hypoventilation caused by pain may disappear once consciousness is lost.
† Risk of vasculogenic 'shock' if large volumes of fluid are withdrawn and so haemodynamic variables should be monitored during aspiration and preparations made for the rapid administration of crystalloid solution, plasma substitute solution or whole blood.

Pre-anaesthetic medication using drugs with profound respiratory depressant effects should not be used. Animals should be preoxygenated. Ventilation should be controlled during anaesthesia; spontaneous ventilation tends to cause hypoventilation which leads to further atelectasis and further 'shunting'. Clearly, 100% O_2 should be given throughout to maximize the diffusion gradient across the abnormally large diffusion path. Low inflation pressures must be used in any condition in which pulmonary damage is likely, e.g. trauma.

Chronic obstructive pulmonary disease
Chronic obstructive pulmonary disease refers to conditions in which irreversible airflow limitations result from chronic bronchitis and emphysema.

Chronic bronchitis
Chronic bronchitis is common in elderly dogs from urban environments. The term describes any condition in which the production of mucoid bronchial secretion is increased. Chronic hypoxaemia results in polycythaemia and cor pulmonale. Hypoventilation results

Drugs	Indication	Dose	Side effects
Antibiotics	Bacterial infection of the respiratory tree Increased airway secretions	Lipid-soluble antibiotics are recommended for bronchial infections: Chloramphenicol 15-30 mg/kg i.v., s.c., i.m., orally bid (cats); dogs 25-60 mg/kg i.v., s.c., i.m., orally bid Trimethoprim/sulphadiazine 15 mg/kg s.c , orally tid for 14 days (cats and dogs)	Potential for adverse interactions with anaesthetics. Chloramphenicol retards metabolism of barbiturates
Diuretics	Pulmonary oedema and viral pneumonias These have obstructive and restrictive component and enhance V/Q discrepancies Conditions with increased lung water	See Figure 14.2	May aggravate purulent conditions by increasing the viscosity of airway secretions
Bronchodilators			May produce intrapulmonary 'steal' when gas flow is restricted by external airway compression. Airway dilation in healthy lung diverts inspired gas from affected region whose $\dot{V}/\dot{Q}$ ratio is then further lowered
Antimuscarinics	Bronchoconstriction	Atropine 40 μg/kg	Viscidification of airway secretion
β$_2$-Agonists	Bronchoconstriction	Terbutaline 1.25-5 mg/dog orally bid or tid; 0.3-1.25 mg/cat orally bid or tid	
Phosphodiesterase inhibitors	Bronchoconstriction	Aminophylline 10 mg/kg i.v. tid or qid (dogs); 6.6 mg/kg orally bid or 2-5 mg/kg slow i.v. (cats) Etamiphylline 70-140 mg/kg i.m., s.c., or 100 mg orally tid (cats and dogs <10 kg); 140-420 mg/kg i.m., s.c. or 100-300 mg orally tid (dogs 10-30 kg) 420-700 mg i.m., s.c. or 300-400 mg orally tid (dogs >30 kg) Theophylline 10-20 mg/kg orally sid or bid or 2-5 mg/kg slow i.v. in emergencies (cats); 10 mg/kg i.v. tid or qid, or 20 mg/kg orally sid or bid	
Glucocorticoids	To suppress tissue reaction associated with pulmonary contusion, smoke inhalation injury and barotrauma	Prednisolone sodium succinate Dexamethasone phosphate	Hypothalamic-pituitary axis depression
Antihistamines	Bronchoconstriction	Chlorpheniramine 2-4 mg orally bid or tid (small dogs); 4-8 mg/kg orally bid or tid (large dogs); 2 mg/cat orally bid	Sedation; potentiation of sedatives
Antitussives	Non-productive and exhausting coughing	Codeine 0.5-2 mg/kg orally bid (dogs) Butorphanol 50-100 μg/kg i.m., s.c. or 0.5-1 mg/kg orally bid or qid (dogs) 50-500 μg/kg i.m., s.c. tid or qid (cats)	Respiratory depression, sedation, potentiation of sedatives Respiratory depression, sedation, potentiation of sedatives
Mucolytics	To facilitate clearance of viscid secretion	Bromhexine 3-15 mg/dog i.m. bid; 2-2.5 mg/kg orally bid (dogs); 3 mg/cat i.m. sid 1 mg/kg orally sid (cats) Acetylcysteine. Nebulize 50 mg as a 2% saline solution over 30-60 minutes or instil 1-2 ml of a 20% solution into the trachea	

Figure 14.14: Drugs used for preoperative preparation of animals with pulmonary diseases.

in a chronic hypercapnia which desensitizes the respiratory centres. Chronic bronchitis is characterized by:

- Hypersensitive respiratory reflexes (bucking, bronchospasm)
- Hypoxic respiratory drive. This is nearly abolished by anaesthetics and if animals breathe an O_2-rich mixture in recovery, hypercapnia and even CO_2 narcosis may occur
- Increased sensitivity to respiratory depressants
- High airway pressures for IPPV.

Emphysema

In emphysema, there are abnormally large air spaces distal to the terminal bronchioles and destruction of alveolar walls. Lung elastic recoil is lost, resulting in over expansion, early closure of airways during expiration and gas trapping. Ventilation is usually well maintained, albeit by an exaggerated effort. In emphysema, expiration is prolonged.

When COPD is severe, the option of using local anaesthetic techniques and sedation should be considered. When general anaesthesia is required, some degree of preparation is necessary. The objective of preoperative treatment is to make the pulmonary tree clean, dry and wide using antispasmodics, mucolytics, steroids and bronchodilators. Drugs may be used to soften secretions, while coupage (thumping the chest wall to dislodge viscid airway secretions) may prove beneficial. Other drugs used preoperatively to improve pulmonary function are described in Figure 14.14. Antibacterial treatment should also render the animal non-pyrexic. Anti-tussive drugs should not be given unless chronic coughing is unproductive and exhausting. Inspired gas enriched with O_2 is desirable, although gases should be warmed and humidified using heated humidifiers or nebulizers.

For pre-anaesthetic medication, anti-sialagogues should be avoided because secretions may become inspissated; atropine also inhibits the mucociliary carpet. Potent opioids, or high doses of other opioids, are not used for pre-anaesthetic medication because they can precipitate bronchospasm and depress respiration. Butorphanol should be considered when an anti-tussive effect, but not profound analgesia, is desired. After pre-anaesthetic medication and throughout the perioperative period, animals must be positioned so that purulent material from infected lung cannot drain to healthy tissue. Induction should be smooth and a deep level of anaesthesia present after induction, so that tracheal intubation does not stimulate hyperactive laryngeal and cough reflexes and bronchospasm.

During anaesthesia, ventilation should be controlled because airway turbulence may critically increase the work of breathing and impair lung expansion. The ventilatory pattern should provide a long expiratory pause. Minute volume of ventilation should be increased to accommodate the increased alveolar dead space volume. If N_2O is chosen, an inspired concentration of 50% is appropriate. Airway suction should be applied before recovery in bronchitic cases.

Dry cold medical gases further viscidify airway secretions, while many drugs and anaesthetics impair the function of the mucociliary carpet. Therefore, gases should be humidified and warmed. Tracheobronchial suction should be performed as often as possible. Oesophageal stethoscopy is a useful guide to the progression of accumulated secretion.

During recovery, the ETT should be left *in situ* for as long as possible to continue endobronchial suctioning. Perioperative anti-tussive drugs should not be given indiscriminately as these will favour accumulation of secretions. Postoperative pulse oximetry is useful as it indicates when O_2 supplementation can be withdrawn. (If O_2 is not humidified it will impair expectoration.)

When the possibility exists that respiratory disease is caused by infective agents, breathing systems and ETTs must be sterilized or discarded.

Bronchoconstriction

In some conditions, including asthma in cats, bronchoconstriction occurs because of local chemical mediators initiating bronchospasm. Bronchoconstriction can also result from proliferative changes in the airway (chronic bronchitis). Bronchodilators may improve gas flow in any condition in which the airway is narrowed by bronchoconstriction and so improve ventilation. Severe bronchospasm may critically limit bulk gas flow, while even minor disturbances will affect the distribution of gas to well perfused lung units.

Preoperative preparation aims to restore airway flow, using antispasmodics, steroids, antihistamines and β_2-agonists (see Figure 14.14). Handling must be conducted carefully as stress may precipitate bronchospasm. Animals that have been receiving glucocorticoids for prolonged periods may have suppressed adrenal function and require additional steroid cover perioperatively.

Pre-anaesthetic medication with acepromazine and/or low-dose ketamine is satisfactory in cats; the former has antihistaminic properties, while the latter is a bronchodilator. Opioids have a propensity to release histamine and should probably be avoided. Atropine may be useful in some types of obstructive disorders because it causes bronchodilation and, as a drying agent, it may reduce airway secretions.

Thiopentone or alphaxolone/alphadolone should probably not be used for induction as both can provoke bronchospasm. In sedated cats, induction in a chamber with halothane is probably ideal because there is little stress and halothane is a potent bronchodilator.

If asthmatic problems arise during operation, aminophylline or another phosphodiesterase inhibitor should be given intravenously. In emergencies, adrenaline at 0.22 mg/kg may be required. Beta$_1$-antagonists should not be used in animals prone to asthma.

REFERENCES AND FURTHER READING

Clutton RE (1994) Edrophonium for neuromuscular blockade antagonism in the dog. *Veterinary Record* **134,** 674–678

Dukes J (1992) Hypertension: a review of the mechanisms, manifestations and management. *Journal of Small Animal Practice* **33,** 119–129

Luis-Fuentes V (1993) Cardiomyopathy in cats. *In Practice* November, 301–308

Martin MWS, Godman M, Luis-Fuentes V, Clutton RE, Haigh A and Darke PGG (1992) Assessment of balloon pulmonary valvuloplasty in six dogs. *Journal of Small Animal Practice* **33,** 443–449

Muir WW, Hubbell JAE and Flaherty S (1988) Increasing halothane concentration abolishes anesthesia-associated arrhythmias in cats and dogs. *Journal of the American Veterinary Medical Association* **192,** 1730–1735

CHAPTER FIFTEEN

Thoracic Surgery

Peter J. Pascoe and Rachel C. Bennett

INTRODUCTION

While opening the thoracic cavity is still required for many procedures, there are many techniques being developed to make 'thoracic' surgery less invasive. The recent introduction of implantable coils may make surgery for a patent ductus arteriosus a thing of the past. The development of more sophisticated instruments for thoracoscopy and the advancement of stapling techniques may allow more procedures to be carried out without a large intercostal or sternal incision. While these advances will provide less surgical morbidity for the patients, the anaesthetist must still be cognizant of the underlying pathophysiology of the condition and the planned procedure and use appropriate drugs and monitoring techniques to ensure a successful outcome.

PREOPERATIVE EVALUATION

Whenever the thoracic wall is breached this has significant effects on the pulmonary system, and so it is important to perform a careful evaluation of the thoracic wall before embarking on thoracic surgery. Preoperative evaluation is also covered in Chapters 2 and 14, but repetition here will help to reinforce the importance of thorough patient assessment before thoracic surgery.

Patient history

Historical information about the patient is as important in the evaluation of respiratory disease as it is in any condition to aid in an accurate diagnosis. Chronic illnesses may imply a slowly changing condition, but often with pulmonary disease the physiological reserve is such that a chronically progressive disease may present acutely because the animal may show very few signs with small lesions in the lung or thoracic cavity. A question that is often not asked about small animal patients relates to exercise tolerance – this can give important information about the likely risk of anaesthetizing the animal. The patient with poor exercise tolerance (due to some intrathoracic lesion) is at greater risk than the animal with normal tolerance. Another question that may provide some useful insight is whether the animal adopts any strange postures when it sleeps – an animal with a bilateral pleural effusion may have learned to sleep in a relatively upright position while an animal with unilateral changes may always sleep on one side.

Pulmonary function

When presented with a patient with a respiratory complaint, careful observation can help to establish the type of lesion. Patients with poor compliance of the lung (restrictive diseases such as pulmonary oedema, pneumonia, fibrosis or pleural effusion) tend to adopt a rapid shallow ventilatory pattern, whereas patients with obstructive diseases (laryngeal paralysis, collapsing trachea, small airway disease) tend to adopt a slower pattern with increased respiratory effort. In these cases trying to differentiate an inspiratory dyspnoea (usually extrathoracic causes) from an expiratory dyspnoea (intrathoracic lesions) may help to direct the clinician to the site of the lesion. Observing the movement of the chest and diaphragm may help to differentiate a problem with motor function from a pulmonary lesion. Dysrhythmias of the diaphragm and intercostal muscles can lead to paradoxical breathing where the thoracic wall collapses on inspiration as the diaphragm moves caudally and the abdomen expands. This pattern could be associated with severe respiratory obstruction, paralysis of the intercostal muscles or a lesion of the central nervous system (CNS) which has altered normal respiratory rhythm generation.

Examination of the mucous membranes for signs of cyanosis, flushing or slow capillary refill time may help to direct further examination. Mucous membrane colour has limitations for the diagnosis of hypoxaemia. Cyanosis, if present, is a strong predictor for hypoxaemia, although studies in humans have shown that clinicians are not very good at detecting cyanosis, even in patients with significant desaturation (Comroe and Botelho, 1947; Morgan-Hughes, 1968a,b; Barnett *et al.*, 1982; Goss *et al.*, 1988). The appearance of the membranes may be affected by ambient light (some fluorescent lights in particular) and it is also necessary for at least 15 g/l of desaturated haemoglobin to be present for cyanosis to be seen. Flushing of the mucous membranes may occur with hypercapnia, but there are other things that will do this, and so it is not pathognomonic. Capillary refill time, if definitely prolonged, is a reasonable indicator of poor circulation, but it too is a relatively insensitive test (Schriger and Baraff, 1991; Baraff, 1993; Gorelick *et al.*, 1993). Capillary refill time depends on ambient temperature, amount of pressure applied to the surface and the body temperature of the patient.

Auscultation of the lungs and trachea should be carried out to try to identify the location and nature of the lesion. Percussion of the lung field may also be helpful in detecting areas of hypo- or hyper-resonance associated with fluid/solid masses or pneumothorax, respectively. If the examination of the patient at this point indicates the need for radiographic or ultrasonographic studies, these should be carried out. These studies may be able to better locate and define a lesion that has been difficult to elucidate on physical examination, and determine the surgical approach that is to be taken.

Preoperative measurement of respiratory volumes can be done relatively simply using a tight fitting mask and a Wright's respirometer or an electronic spirometer. This may help to show whether the patient is hyper- or hypopnoeic (normal minute ventilation for dogs is 210 ± 56 ml/kg/min (Gillespie and Hyatt, 1974) and for cats is 175 ± 158 ml/kg/min (Fordyce and Tenney, 1984)), but it does not define the extent of change as the individual animal's normal minute ventilation is not known. There may also be alterations in the exchange of gas across the alveolar membrane due to the disease process, resulting in hyperpnoea with hypoventilation.

Measurement of blood gases defines the degree of change in the respiratory system. Arterial samples can usually be obtained from a dorsal pedal or femoral artery. The validity of the results from such a sample will depend to some extent on how the animal behaved during the collection of the sample. If the animal is greatly stressed by the procedure it tends to hyperventilate, which may mask the extent of hypoxaemia and decrease the arterial carbon dioxide tension ($PaCO_2$). If a sample is to be taken from a dyspnoeic animal that objects to being restrained, the attempt should be abandoned. Venous samples can be used to obtain information about acid-base status and $PaCO_2$, if the sample can be obtained by free flow without occluding the vessel. A sample from the jugular vein is best used for this as it is the largest accessible vein and is least likely to collapse on to the needle during aspiration.

If a patient has any indication of fluid in the chest, a thoracocentesis should be performed to obtain a sample for further diagnostic investigations. A thoracocentesis is best carried out using a butterfly needle, teat cannula or intravenous catheter. A regular hypodermic needle is very sharp and is more likely to lacerate the lung. It is important to establish that the end of the needle/catheter has entered the thoracic cavity before a negative result is accepted, for example, a short butterfly needle may be too short to reach the pleural space in an obese patient.

Cardiovascular function

Observation of the patient for venous distension and pulsations in the jugular vein should be carried out before handling the animal. Observation of vessels may not be feasible in many breeds because of long hair. After observation of vessels, it is important to feel the pulse and get some sense of its character both centrally (femoral artery) and peripherally (dorsal pedal or ulnar arteries). A weak pulse is usually much more evident at a peripheral vessel than at the central vessel.

Auscultation of the heart must be carried out to characterize any abnormalities. If a murmur or arrhythmia is heard, the clinician needs to decide whether further investigation is required. This must be predicated on the other lesions present in the animal and the resources of the client, but it is generally advised to obtain as much information as possible about cardiac function before anaesthesia. This is particularly the case when a thoracic procedure is contemplated, as the surgery may have significant effects on cardiac function. Radiographs are helpful in delineating the size of the heart and deciding whether left heart failure is present, but much more definitive information can be obtained from ultrasonography. M-mode or 2-dimensional echocardiography can differentiate a pericardial effusion from an enlarged heart and can define the dimensions of cardiac structures and how they relate to normal. Doppler echocardiography can detect abnormal blood flow and can be used to estimate the pressure gradient across stenotic vessels. Ultrasonography can also define the shortening fraction of the heart, which is a measure of contractility. The results from such tests should determine whether the animal is an appropriate candidate for surgical intervention or whether a period of medical therapy is warranted to ensure that myocardial activity is optimized.

An electrocardiogram (ECG) helps to define both changes in the size of the heart (axis deviations) and any arrhythmias encountered during the examination. Again, therapy may be appropriate before the animal is anaesthetized.

An arterial blood sample should be taken if the investigation suggests any right-to-left shunting or low cardiac output. If an animal with a right-to-left shunt has an arterial oxygen tension (PaO_2) of < 60 mmHg (8 kPa) on room air, great care is needed to ensure that a significant increase in right-sided pressures or a decrease in left-sided pressures is not created – both of which could exacerbate the shunt.

Clinical pathology

Before undertaking such a major surgical intervention it is appropriate to obtain a complete blood count and biochemical profile of the patient to rule out further unrecognized intercurrent disease. An increased haematocrit may be evidence of chronic hypoxaemia, while a decreased value may represent chronic illness or blood loss. Anaemia may not be tolerated well in an animal with poor cardiac output, and it is imperative that this be taken into account when making a decision about preoperative or intraoperative transfusion. Dogs and cats tolerate a haematocrit of 0.15–0.2 l/l by increasing cardiac output so that oxygen delivery is maintained. However, an animal with a relatively fixed cardiac output (e.g. aortic stenosis) may barely survive at a haematocrit of 0.3 l/l.

PREPARATION

Pulmonary disease

Any conditions amenable to treatment before an animal is taken to surgery should be dealt with. If the animal has pneumonia that can be treated with antibiotics without risk of developing further infection, this should be done as long as the surgery can be delayed. If the pleural space, pericardium or abdomen are full of air or fluid these should be drained as much as possible before carrying on with the surgery. The animal with ascites has a decreased ability to ventilate and may show significant hypotension if put in dorsal recumbency. The fluid can usually be drained using a catheter (14–16 G) entering the abdomen 3–10 cm from the midline midway between the ribs and the pelvic limb on the right side. If the left side is used, care must be taken to avoid perforating the spleen. Drainage of fluid in this way should be carried out slowly so that there is a slow change of pressure in the abdomen. An animal that has compensated for an increase in intra-abdominal pressure due to ascites may suffer from massive hypotension and cardiovascular collapse if the intra-abdominal pressure is relieved too quickly. This is usually not an issue as it is hard to remove fluid rapidly enough with such a narrow access to the fluid (14 G catheter).

Pleural drainage can be achieved with minimal restraint in most animals, but cats with pleuritis are often extremely fractious and may need an analgesic before carrying out thoracic puncture. Opioids such as oxymorphone and butorphanol provide analgesia while also giving some sedation, which is beneficial in these cases. After administering the opioid, the animal should be placed in an oxygen-rich environment and allowed to rest for 15–20 minutes before attempting to drain the chest. Animals with air or fluid in the pleural space should be evaluated for risk of a rapid return of the fluid after it has been drained. An animal with a pleural effusion could be tapped and drained several hours before thoracic surgery, with minimal chance of the fluid returning within that time. However, an animal that has a haemo- or pneumothorax may have such rapid recrudescence that the only option is to place a chest drain and apply continuous controlled suction. If it is not possible to maintain suction during transport to the operating room, the chest drain should be clamped off or connected to a water trap or Heimlich valve so that air cannot enter the pleural space. The chest drain should be a multifenestrated catheter, which is directed toward the anteroventral quadrant of the thoracic cavity. It should be sutured in place using a technique that will ensure that the fenestrations cannot be pulled out and exposed to the atmosphere. A criss cross (Roman bootlace, Chinese fingercot) pattern is often used for this, but this may still allow for excessive movement in a dog with loose skin. A secure attachment can be achieved by passing the suture through the periosteum on one rib, ensuring that the chest tube will not retract far from that site.

With any surgery involving entry into the thoracic cavity, it is essential to be able to ventilate the patient. This can be achieved by simply having someone squeeze the reservoir bag intermittently, but this is labour intensive so ventilation is usually achieved with the assistance of a mechanical device. Before anaesthetizing the patient, it is important to ensure that the ventilator is functioning and that it will work for that particular animal. This is likely to be a problem with units when they are used on very small or very big patients; some machines are not able to provide small enough volumes of gas for patients weighing <5 kg while others cannot cope with giant breeds weighing 70–100 kg. Although not essential, the authors have found it very helpful to be able to apply positive-end expiratory pressure (PEEP) or continuous positive airway pressure (CPAP) to their patients once the thoracic cavity has been opened. Under normal circumstances the tendency of the lung to collapse is balanced by the tendency of the thoracic wall to spring outwards. Once the chest is opened the 'adhesion' between the chest wall and the lung is broken and the lung collapses to a smaller volume. Once this has happened it is necessary either to increase the tidal volume or to add PEEP/CPAP in order to maintain adequate gas exchange. In the authors' experience, the addition of PEEP/CPAP has been helpful in reducing the atelectasis often associated with intrathoracic procedures. This effect can be achieved by adding a resistance to the expiratory limb of the circuit. The simplest method is to take the expired limb and to pass it through a beaker of water, with the depth of the hose under the water determining the amount of PEEP – if the hose is 7 cm under water, then the PEEP should be 7 cmH$_2$O. The same thing can be achieved by putting the scavenge hose from the ventilator under water, although this should be tested with the individual ventilator as some machines do not work properly when a back pressure is exerted on this side of the circuit. This approach is often inconvenient because it can be hard to scavenge the gas after it has bubbled through the water. Commercial PEEP valves can be purchased that will apply a certain pressure. The valves usually come with preset values of 2.5, 5 and 10 cmH$_2$O, and they can be used in sequence in order to provide 7.5 or 12.5 cmH$_2$O pressure. Some ventilators are equipped with a CPAP setting, and the value required is dialled into the machine. With any of these techniques, a manometer placed in the circuit allows the measurement of the effect produced by the PEEP/CPAP manoeuvre. The authors normally aim for a value of 3-7 cmH$_2$O on the basis of the effects on circulation, gas exchange and surgical access.

When dealing with some tracheal surgeries, it may be necessary to place a tracheostomy tube during the surgery and to be able to continue the delivery of anaesthetic through this new tube, for example, surgeries involving tracheal resection. For these cases it is essential to have a range of sterile tracheostomy or endotracheal tubes (ETTs) and a sterile circuit available so that these can be placed in the surgical field without risk of contamination. Before proceeding with placement of a tracheostomy tube, check that all the connections between tubes are compatible to prevent any delays in switching from one circuit to the other.

If the patient has a pulmonary mass that may be an abscess or a tumour with a necrotic centre, it may be helpful to employ a bronchial blocker to prevent material from the lesion being expelled into the lower ventral lung during surgery (Benumof and Alfrey, 1994). There are some ETTs, designed for humans, which can be used for this purpose in some small dogs (the maximum tube size is 9.5 mm and the catheter used for occluding the bronchus is too short for larger dogs). By using the curves of the tube and catheter, it is possible to direct the catheter into the left or right mainstem bronchus blindly, although it is very difficult to know its exact location in the airway. The catheter also has an end hole, so that it is possible to slowly deflate or reinflate the lung beyond the balloon occlusion. The main disadvantage of these tubes is that the main tube is a 'D' shape, which means that a very small endoscope is needed in order to visualize the placement of the catheter. Another alternative is to use a Fogarty catheter. This can be placed in the airway before the ETT, so that it goes down the side of the ETT. Once the animal is in position, an endoscope can be used to guide the Fogarty catheter into the appropriate bronchus, and then the balloon on the catheter can be inflated to occlude that airway. The two main disadvantages with this technique are that there is no end hole in a Fogarty catheter, and that it is very easy for the catheter to become dislodged and slip back into the trachea. If this happens, an immediate total airway occlusion develops, which requires that the balloon is deflated and the catheter repositioned. The final approach for these cases is to use a double lumen tube, which allows intubation of one mainstem bronchus and functional separation of the other. This has been described a number of times by various authors but has been difficult to apply clinically because of the anatomy of the dog's respiratory tract (see section on thoracoscopy) (Elliott *et al.*, 1991; Garcia *et al.*, 1998; Cantwell *et al.*, 1999). If none of these approaches is possible, the surgeon should clamp the bronchus of the lobe nearest the lesion or, if that is not accessible, clamp the mainstem bronchus until the mass has been removed. Before the transected bronchus is closed, the airway should be suctioned to remove any material from the airway.

Cardiovascular disease

Before carrying out a thoracotomy on a patient with cardiovascular disease, if the procedure can be delayed, it is important to optimize medical therapy that may improve the patient's condition. If vasodilators, inotropes, diuretics or anti-arrhythmic drugs can improve the function of the cardiovascular system, treatment should be instituted for long enough to make a difference. Cats with hyperthyroidism and signs of cardiac changes should be given carbimazole or methimazole for at least 1 week before surgery as the mortality rate is much higher without such treatment.

For patients with bradycardia that is non-responsive to anticholinergic therapy or that have sick sinus syndrome, it is advisable to place a temporary pacemaker until the permanent one can be implanted. This can usually be achieved by placing an introducer (a large thin-walled catheter) into a saphenous vein using local anaesthesia, and then advancing the pacing lead up to the heart from this site. The authors avoid using the jugular vein if possible when placing a permanent transvenous pacemaker, so that both vessels are available for this purpose if needed. If the patient is too small for a saphenous approach, the lead can be introduced via the jugular vein.

An animal with a pericardial effusion of sufficient magnitude to cause a restriction of myocardial function should have the fluid drained before surgery. This is typically carried out using a needle or catheter, and the intent is to drain enough fluid off to release any pressure in the pericardial sac. The animal is usually positioned in left lateral recumbency, and access is gained through the right 4th to 6th intercostal space. An over-the-needle catheter with multiple fenestrations is ideal as the catheter can be left in place during the aspiration of fluid, minimizing the risk of trauma to the heart. Care must be taken not to touch the myocardium to avoid causing accidental puncture of a coronary vessel or promoting cardiac arrhythmias.

The risk of surgical blood loss should be assessed before the procedure and, using the current haematocrit and cardiovascular status of the patient, a decision should be made as to whether blood is going to be needed. If blood is likely to be needed, the necessary arrangements should be made to obtain an adequate supply of cross-matched blood or packed red cells for that patient.

Surgical approach

Both a lateral and ventral approach to the chest involve some risk of damage to the underlying structures as the pleura are incised. The anaesthetist should establish controlled ventilation before the thorax is opened and should be able to stop the ventilation for the brief period required to open the pleura. This reduces the risk of accidental injury to the lung during entry into the chest. A lateral thoracotomy may involve a single intercostal space or may entail the removal of one or more ribs. If surgery involves the heart, mediastinum or oesophagus, it is likely that the surgeon will need to pack off the lung in the surgical field. This should be done carefully so that minimal gas exchange surface area is lost, but it is also appropriate to compress the lung fairly completely since, by reducing the compliance of the upper lung, more gas will be directed to the lower lung field. However, it is expected that this manoeuvre will decrease the available exchange surface resulting in a decrease in the PaO_2.

With a sternal approach it is unlikely that the lung fields need to be compressed, but the alteration in the orientation of the heart can lead to some decrease in venous return, and it may be necessary to increase fluid therapy in order to increase central venous pressure (CVP; preload on the heart). As the surgery proceeds it is often noticed that certain manipulations cause a sudden dramatic decrease in blood pressure. The surgeon and the anaesthetist should work together to define these deleterious events so that their effects can be minimized. It is more common to see cardiac arrhythmias with a ventral approach, and this should be monitored carefully and therapy initiated if the arrhythmias seem to be detrimental to cardiovascular function.

Nitrous oxide (N_2O) is contraindicated during any thoracotomy because of the rapid accumulation of N_2O in gas pockets in the pleura. As the pleural space is well vascularized and is in direct contact with the lung containing N_2O, the N_2O diffuses down the concentration gradient and doubles the volume of a pneumothorax in 10–15 minutes.

Analgesia

Analgesia for thoracotomy can be provided in several ways. A lateral thoracotomy seems to cause less pain than a sternotomy, and many dogs show few signs of pain after a single intercostal incision if other muscle groups have not been transected. An extradural injection with an opioid with or without a local anaesthetic certainly provides some analgesia for a thoracotomy, and it can be given before surgery to provide some preemptive effect (Popilskis *et al.*, 1991, 1993; Pascoe and Dyson, 1993). This also provides bilateral analgesia so it is useful for both a lateral and sternal incision. Intercostal nerve blocks have been used for a lateral approach and provide some analgesia, but when applied before surgery they are unlikely to give analgesia over more than half the thorax. This is because the dorsal branch of the intercostal nerve branches off close to the spinal cord, and it supplies the cutaneous structures to about halfway down the thoracic wall (Kitchell *et al.*, 1980; Bailey *et al.*, 1984). The block can be done more effectively once the chest is opened by injecting the nerves from inside the thorax aiming out towards the

vertebrae where the nerves exit the canal. Interpleural block can be carried out after the chest has been closed (Riegler *et al.*, 1989; VadeBoncouer *et al.*, 1990; Thompson and Johnson, 1991). For a lateral thoracotomy, the animal is placed in dorsolateral recumbency and the local anaesthetic (usually 0.1–0.2% bupivacaine at 1–2 mg/kg) is injected through the chest drain. The anaesthetic tends to go to the most ventral part of the chest and diffuse through the thoracic wall into the intercostal nerves. For a sternotomy, the local anaesthetic is injected through the chest drain with the animal in sternal recumbency. In both instances the animal should be left in that position for at least 10 minutes after the injection, so that the drug has time to get taken up into the relevant tissues.

Monitoring

Monitoring an animal undergoing a thoracotomy must allow the anaesthetist to establish the sufficiency of ventilation, to diagnose arrhythmias and to provide information on changes in cardiac function, especially when the animal has some cardiac disease. The monitoring of ventilation without being able to measure airway pressure, minute volume, end-tidal CO_2 ($ETCO_2$) or $PaCO_2$ is difficult once the chest is open as it does not move in a manner that allows tidal volumes to be estimated. The list of monitoring modalities given above is ordered in increasing desirability. Airway pressure indicates the force being applied to the pulmonary system but does not give any information about gas exchange. It is expected that peak pressures in the 10–15 and 10–20 cmH$_2$O range would be normal for the cat and dog, respectively. If higher pressures are required to achieve adequate inflation, it may be an indication of decreased airway compliance. Minute volume is a more accurate representation of how much gas is being moved in and out of the lungs but still does not indicate whether there is adequate exchange. End-tidal CO_2 should reflect the value for $PaCO_2$, but there is often a discrepancy between the two values and this is not readily predictable. The two values are usually close enough in patients with normal lungs for surgeons not to be greatly under- or over-ventilating the patient, and a capnograph is a non-invasive monitor with continuous sampling that provides rapid feedback on changes in ventilation. Arterial or free flow lingual venous blood gas samples will give the definitive assessment of ventilation. A pulse oximeter is very helpful in cases where desaturation may be expected (e.g. extensive pulmonary disease, right-to-left shunt) or where other techniques for measuring ventilation are not available. A pulse oximeter provides limited information on the early changes associated with ventilation-perfusion mismatching or alterations in shunt fraction, but if desaturation occurs it is likely to be sensed by the monitor and the clinician warned before it is too late. A combination of capnography, arterial blood gas monitoring and pulse oximetry is ideal for these cases as the two non-invasive continuous monitors can be checked intermittently using blood gases, allowing more accurate interpretation of the values displayed. Electrocardiography is essential for these cases to allow diagnosis of arrhythmias. Early diagnosis and management may prevent the heart from going into fibrillation.

Haemodynamic monitoring should include at least some measure of blood pressure – preferably with a transducer attached to an arterial catheter that also allows multiple sampling of blood for blood gas measurement. In some conditions it may also be beneficial to be able to monitor CVP and/or pulmonary arterial pressure.

MISCELLANEOUS CONDITIONS

Trauma

Trauma to the chest wall requiring immediate surgical intervention would include a flail chest, puncture wounds to the thoracic cavity or intrathoracic bleeding. Delayed intervention may occur for fractured ribs, although these are rarely repaired.

An animal with a flail chest may be unable to ventilate normally, and the flail segment is pulled inwards every time the animal inhales. This makes ventilation very inefficient, and the animal may be hypoxaemic and hypercapnic. Some dogs and cats seem to cope quite well with a 3–4 rib flail segment and may not become hypoxaemic. While preparing to anaesthetize such a patient, the inspired gas should be supplemented with oxygen and the anaesthetic technique should be aimed at gaining rapid control of the airway. This is best achieved using drugs with a rapid onset of action, such as thiopentone or etomidate. Propofol has a rapid onset of action, but it should be given slowly to minimize the respiratory depression and hypotension that can occur. Ketamine and tiletamine both take about 60 seconds to take effect, which is not ideal under these circumstances. Opioids, used for induction, also take at least 2 minutes to reach peak effect. Once the animal is intubated, it should be ventilated until the flail segment has been stabilized. Since a fractured rib could damage the lung, it is essential to monitor the patient carefully for signs of pneumothorax during this procedure.

Diaphragmatic hernia

Diaphragmatic hernias may be traumatic or congenital. Traumatic hernias are usually caused by an excessive force being applied to the abdomen causing viscera to rupture through the diaphragm into the chest. Most of these patients present with dyspnoea, although some animals can be totally asymptomatic. The animal may be presented in *extremis* immediately post-trauma, or the hernia may be discovered as an incidental finding from abdominal radiographs or ultrasonograms. The liver is the most common organ to penetrate through a diaphragmatic hernia and so some cases present with ascites and hepatic dysfunction. The severity of the dyspnoea usually relates to the loss of space in the chest

for normal pulmonary function, and it may be helpful, when handling these animals, to stand them on their hind legs and lift them up so their back is perpendicular to the ground. Many of these animals have fractured limbs, pulmonary contusions and myocardial trauma, and these other lesions need to be assessed before proceeding with repair of the diaphragmatic hernia. The timing of the surgical repair is controversial. One author suggests that one should 'never let the sun go down' on a diaphragmatic hernia, even in cases where the diagnosis has been made months after the traumatic incident (Brasmer, 1984). The justification for immediate repair is that it is quite possible for more abdominal content to shift into the thoracic cavity and for animals to become severely dyspnoeic, or even die, overnight, and this author has seen examples of such incidents. The disadvantages of carrying out the repair the same day may relate to scheduling conflicts and wanting to have the animal fully resuscitated and stable before proceeding with the repair. These authors favour the former approach since there is usually time to provide adequate restoration of circulating volume (after trauma), while an animal that decompensates can die in a matter of minutes. Preoperative preparation of the patient is important – cases of acute trauma need to receive adequate fluid therapy and should be preoxygenated before induction.

Premedication with an opioid, at conservative doses, and with an anticholinergic is appropriate. In the recently traumatized patient (< 5 days) these authors would avoid acepromazine as these patients often become more hypotensive with this drug and it can cause splenic enlargement. Preoxygenation should be carried out for 5 minutes using a tight fitting mask in order to increase the inspired oxygen concentration to >95%. The mask should be kept on during induction until the animal is ready to be intubated. Induction with a dissociative agent, propofol or etomidate would be ideal – this allows rapid control of the airway so that the animal can be ventilated immediately. Thiopentone commonly causes splenic enlargement, which could lead to severe respiratory distress if the spleen is wholly or partially in the chest. Once the animal is intubated, positive-pressure ventilation should be initiated. It seems to be important not to re-expand atelectatic lung too rapidly, so the aim should be to use high respiratory frequencies with low peak airway pressures. Oxygenation of the arterial blood should be carefully monitored, as these authors have found it difficult to avoid hypoxaemia if tidal volume is restricted excessively. The concern with rapid re-expansion of the lung is its association with pulmonary oedema (Wilson and Hayes, 1986). It has been suggested that the surfactant-producing type II cells shut down in areas of atelectasis and that when this area of lung is re-expanded the lack of surfactant causes an increase in the forces pulling fluid into the alveoli, leading to alveolar flooding. The aim with these cases is to provide adequate ventilation to prevent hypoxaemia and hypercapnia but not to re-expand the lung. Once the hernia has been repaired and the air evacuated from the chest, the lung will be expanded gradually by the animal – hopefully allowing enough time for reactivation of the type II cells. The usual approach to a diaphragmatic hernia is via a midline laparotomy, with extension of the incision into the sternum if necessary. Some advocate a lateral thoracotomy and repair of the hernia from the anterior surface of the diaphragm (Stokhof, 1986). This approach has been quite successful as long as the location of the hernia has been adequately defined (e.g. right lateral thoracotomy for a right-sided hernia). Before the hernia has been completely repaired, it is helpful to place a chest drain so that air can be drained from the thoracic cavity and the normal negative pleural pressure re-established.

Space-occupying lesions not associated with the cardiopulmonary system: thymoma

The most common tumours to be found in the thoracic cavity, which do not involve the heart or lungs, are thymomas. These can be of considerable size and interfere with pulmonary function by compression of the trachea or affect venous return by compressing the anterior vena cava. Myasthenia gravis is also associated with thymoma and may be recognized by a history of regurgitation or by the presence of a megaoesophagus on thoracic radiographs. This condition may lead to aspiration pneumonia, and so extra care needs to be taken while handling these patients during induction and recovery (see Chapter 16 for details on dealing with megaoesophagus). Patients with myasthenia are normally being treated with an anticholinesterase (physostigmine). This therapy should be given on the morning of surgery if the signs of myasthenia have been relatively severe. The presence of long-acting anticholinesterases may alter the duration of action of some opioids. The response to muscle relaxants is variable, but in general these patients tend to have an increased sensitivity to these drugs. If it is necessary to give a non-depolarizing relaxant (which is rarely the case), the patient should receive small doses while the response is monitored (see Chapter 10 for further details of neuromuscular blocking agents and myasthenia).

The patient should be premedicated according to the severity of compromise caused by the thymoma. Routine premedication would be acceptable in a young active patient with few clinical signs, whereas a patient with prominent signs should be given minimal premedication. Before induction the patient should be preoxygenated and suction apparatus should be immediately available if the animal has a megaoesophagus. The induction drug needs to have a rapid onset in cases of megaoesophagus, but if megaoesophagus is not present, the induction technique is not overly important. Maintenance with an inhalant would be typical. A second intravenous catheter should be placed in case more than one infusion is necessary. Some of these tumours wrap around the major blood vessels, so significant blood loss is possible, and the animal should have blood available for transfusion if needed.

Oesophageal lesions including persistent right aortic arch

Access to the oesophagus in the thorax may require a thoracotomy. Congenital lesions such as persistent right aortic arch (PRAA), or other aortic arch anomalies, may cause a restrictive lesion of the oesophagus. These animals are therefore prone to similar problems to those with megaoesophagus from other causes and should be handled as such. While PRAA is usually an avascular remnant, some of the other anomalies causing oesophageal stricture may be associated with viable blood vessels, and significant blood loss can occur during surgical correction. The patient should have two venous catheters placed, and blood transfusions should be available. For oesophageal tears or foreign bodies, the greatest risks are from infection and pneumothorax. The latter can occur if the foreign object has damaged some lung as well as the oesophagus. If this is likely, due to the nature or position of the foreign body, the animal should have a chest drain placed before intermittent positive-pressure ventilation (IPPV) is initiated.

Pulmonary lesions

Most cases of pulmonary lesions will have some degree of respiratory compromise and will need preoxygenation before induction. Ideally, the mask should be left on for 5 minutes before induction, and it is essential that the mask be left on during induction until the animal is ready to be intubated. If the mask is removed, then the animal will begin to breathe room air and, since there are no oxygen 'stores' in the body, the benefit of preoxygenation will be lost within a few breaths. If the animal will not tolerate a mask, a bag over the head may be tolerated better by some animals – a plastic bag with an oxygen inlet can be placed over the head and closed on to the neck. If this technique is not feasible then it may be necessary to start the induction and place the mask as soon as the animal begins to lose consciousness. Although it may take up to 5 minutes to reach the peak PaO_2, the initial rise is steep and the animal will benefit from even a few breaths of 100% oxygen. Pneumothorax is usually a result of damage to the lung or major airways. If there is any concern that air leakage may continue during the preparation period, a chest drain should be placed and the animal connected to a continuous suction device. If the amount of air in the thorax is minimal and there does not seem to be any ongoing leakage, it may be safe not to place a chest drain provided the time from induction to entrance into the thoracic cavity is short. If it is known that there will be significant ongoing air leakage from pulmonary tissue until the surgeon can oversew or remove the damage, a total intravenous anaesthetic technique should be considered. This is to avoid the leakage of inhalant into the thoracic cavity so that the surgeons and assistants do not have to breathe in the waste anaesthetic gases. For this purpose a propofol/opioid infusion technique is ideal. Propofol is given at 0.1–0.3 mg/kg/min while an opioid such as fentanyl can be given at 0.3–1.0 μg/kg/min. The dose of fentanyl should be limited to no more than 0.4 μg/kg/min in cats. Animals with pulmonary contusions need to be ventilated very carefully because there is some risk that the vessel rupture responsible for the contusion can be opened up again by stretching the lung excessively. Further haemorrhage into the lung may cause a significant loss of gas exchange surface and lead to severe respiratory compromise. Ventilation of these animals should be with low tidal volumes and high frequencies (e.g. 20 breaths per minute, tidal volume = 10 ml/kg).

Preoperatively it is often difficult to differentiate between a pulmonary abscess and a tumour. If it is expected that the lesion may be an abscess or a tumour with a necrotic centre, then the precautions described (see section on preparing patients with pulmonary disease) should be taken. It is also wise to have a suction device available so that the airway can be suctioned if the above measures fail to contain the pus. Any major drainage of pus into the lower lung carries a poor prognosis for the patient.

Another concern with such lesions is that there may be adhesions between the lung and the parietal pleura, such that entry through the pleura results in entry into the lesion. The anaesthetist should be prepared to handle the blood loss or air leakage that can occur under these circumstances.

A lung lobe torsion is usually treated by excision of the lobe, and this is normally a relatively straightforward procedure, especially if it is done using advanced stapling techniques. Apart from the considerations above (preoxygenation, ventilation etc.), there are no major new ones for this surgery.

Chylothorax

Concerns with chylothorax and other pleural effusions relate to the amount of fluid in the chest and with adhesions that may have formed to the parietal pleura, increasing the chance of pulmonary injury when the thoracic cavity is opened. If possible, attempts should be made to drain the fluid off the chest before anaesthesia to improve intraoperative ventilation. Blood loss is minimal if the lymph duct is tied off or a drainage system is implanted into the diaphragm, but it can be substantial if a pleurodesis is performed.

Pericardectomy

Pericardectomy may be undertaken for a pericardial effusion or for a pericardial constriction. Animals with cardiac tamponade, where the intrapericardial pres-

sure approaches the right ventricular diastolic filling pressure, are at immediate risk of circulatory collapse. A pressure of 9 mmHg caused a 60% reduction in cardiac output, while pressures as high as 12–13 mmHg may be tolerated (Koller *et al.*, 1983). Drainage of fluid from the pericardium should be carried out to relieve these symptoms before the animal is anaesthetized. The preferred approach is via sternotomy as this gives the best access to the pericardium, but a lateral approach may be used in some cases. Pericardectomy may also be amenable to endoscopic approaches (see below). If an animal with cardiac tamponade must be anaesthetized, it should be pretreated with fluids to ensure optimum venous return and a technique used which minimizes reductions in myocardial contractility and heart rate (heart rate is usually increased in an attempt to maintain cardiac output in the presence of a reduced stroke volume). Etomidate would be the ideal induction drug for this purpose. Once the animal is intubated, it is recommended that spontaneous ventilation be maintained to minimize any further reduction in venous return. However, it has also been shown that hypercapnia will further decrease cardiac output, so it is better to use IPPV than to allow hypercapnia to develop (Koller *et al.*, 1983). If IPPV is used, it is best to use high breathing frequencies to limit peak airway pressures, and not to use PEEP (Mattilla *et al.*, 1984). Dobutamine is probably the best drug to use to improve cardiac output as it has been shown to delay the onset of tissue hypoxia when compared with norepinephrine (Zhang *et al.*, 1994). However, dopamine also increases cardiac output and improves myocardial perfusion (Martins *et al.*, 1980). Once the tamponade has been reduced, the anaesthetic management of these patients during the pericardectomy is relatively straightforward. Ventricular arrhythmias are common during manipulation of the pericardium, and so lignocaine (lidocaine) should be on hand in case these begin to alter haemodynamic function. Haemorrhage may be marked if a decortication of the epicardium is undertaken, and it is necessary to have adequate supplies of typed and cross-matched blood to cope with any blood loss.

Patent ductus arteriosus

Most animals anaesthetized for correction of a patent ductus arteriosus (PDA) are young and are usually in good health apart from the changes caused by the PDA (see Chapter 14). In the early stages, there are very few myocardial changes associated with a PDA. However, if the ductus is large and/or the lesion has not been recognized early, there can be significant enlargement of the left ventricle with cardiac failure, due to volume overload, occurring terminally. If the animal is operated on before significant changes have occurred, there are few concerns for the anaesthetist. It is expected that the diastolic pressure will be very low in these patients before ligation of the ductus, because of the connection of the systemic circulation to the low resistance pulmonary system. Because of this, phenothiazines and butyrophenones should be avoided for premedication because the α-blockade will tend to decrease systemic vascular resistance (SVR), decreasing diastolic pressure still further. The maintenance of diastolic pressure is important in the effectiveness of coronary perfusion. Systolic pressures are usually normal to high but, because of the low diastolic pressure, the mean pressure is also normal or reduced and is often 50–60 mmHg during the approach to the ductus. Positive inotropes may increase systolic pressure and also increase mean pressure but should only be used if systolic pressures fall below 90 mmHg. Peripheral vasoconstrictors should not be used since an increased SVR will tend to increase the shunt through the ductus and may lead to pulmonary oedema. If there are problems with the dissection of the ductus, it is possible to lose large quantities of blood very quickly. A second intravenous catheter should be placed so that fluids can be given rapidly if needed, although the outcome is rarely favourable if the ductus is ruptured. Before the ductus is ligated it is wise to give an anticholinergic, because the sudden change in blood pressure associated with ligation can elicit a strong baroreceptor reflex which can even cause cardiac arrest. The anticholinergic blocks the vagal part of this reflex. The authors typically use the anticholinergic at the time of premedication, although it could be given closer to the time of ligation. Monitoring of direct arterial blood pressure in these cases is helpful in allowing the assessment of moment to moment changes and is also of use in ensuring that the ductus has been ligated. Typically, there is a sudden increase in diastolic pressure as soon as the ductus is tied off.

Patients with signs of failure or pulmonary oedema should be treated with diuretics and positive inotropes for 1–2 days before surgery. The anaesthetic technique should attempt to maintain myocardial function as much as possible and not cause further decreases in peripheral vascular resistance. Premedication with an opioid-anticholinergic combination is useful, and induction with an opioid-benzodiazepine technique or etomidate ± benzodiazepine is preferred. It could be argued that halothane would be a better anaesthetic than isoflurane for these cases because it has less effect on SVR, but the increased negative inotropic effect and the risk of catecholamine arrhythmias countermand this argument. Maintenance of anaesthesia in these patients should be by a balanced technique combining an opioid and/or a muscle relaxant with the inhalant in order to reduce the negative effects of the inhalant. Patients with a right-to-left shunt are rarely amenable to surgical correction since closure of the duct often results in right heart failure due to the pulmonary hypertension. If such an animal needs to be anaesthetized for part of the diagnostic investigation or for other reasons, the regimen described for the PDA with some degree of heart failure should be used. It is important to maintain or increase SVR while aiming to reduce (or at least not increase) pulmonary vascular resistance.

Non-surgical repair of the PDA is being used more frequently (Grifka *et al.*, 1996; Snaps *et al.*, 1998). For this procedure it is necessary to insert a catheter up the aorta from the femoral artery. The tip of the catheter is positioned at the entrance to the PDA, and a coil is released into the ductus. The coil lodges in the ductus, and blood clots on the coil causing a functional occlusion of the ductus. Anaesthetic techniques for these cases are similar to those described for the surgical approach except that a thoracotomy is not necessary, obviating the requirement for positive-pressure ventilation (although IPPV may be needed for other reasons).

Pulmonic stenosis

Management of dogs with pulmonic stenosis (see Chapter 14) is normally by balloon valvuloplasty, and this does not require a thoracotomy (Brownlie *et al.*, 1991; Martin *et al.*, 1992; Kienle, 1998b). These dogs usually present with right ventricular hypertrophy, and it is rare for them to be in right heart failure. Animals with pressure gradients of <40 mmHg across the stenosis are at low risk of anaesthetic complications and may be handled in a relatively routine fashion. Animals with pressure gradients >40 mmHg may have significant hypertrophy and should be regarded as having an increased anaesthetic risk, although it is uncommon to see problems with these cases until the gradient exceeds 80 mmHg (Kienle, 1998b). The right ventricular hypertrophy makes these animals more prone to reduced myocardial perfusion and ventricular arrhythmias. The anaesthetic technique chosen for these animals should aim to minimize the possibility of bradycardia. Since the right ventricle is thick and non-compliant, cardiac output is more dependent on heart rate than it is in a normal animal. At the same time a tachycardia will tend to increase myocardial oxygen demand while shortening diastole and reducing coronary perfusion. These two changes may lead to myocardial ischaemia and precipitate severe arrhythmias. Premedication should therefore aim to minimize anxiety and prevent tachycardia. Opioids combined with low doses of anticholinergics will usually achieve this aim. Induction of anaesthesia can be carried out using etomidate ± a benzodiazepine as the technique of choice, as there is minimal change in heart rate or contractility. An opioid/benzodiazepine technique can be used as long as an anticholinergic has been given previously, and the heart rate is monitored carefully during induction. Maintenance of anaesthesia can be with an inhalant such as isoflurane, or a balanced technique can be used with the addition of an opioid or N_2O. Lignocaine should be readily available as a first line treatment for ventricular arrhythmias that may occur during therapy. Animals with a dynamic component to their stenosis should receive phenylephrine for hypotension as described below (aortic stenosis).

If a surgical approach is used for this condition, the anaesthetist should prepare as above but add a second venous access and have blood products available for rapid transfusion.

Aortic stenosis

Aortic stenosis (see Chapter 14) is also associated with ventricular hypertrophy as it is also caused by a pressure overload (Kienle, 1998a). Balloon valvuloplasty for this condition has been disappointing (Kienle, 1998a), and the best results with surgical correction have been achieved using cardiopulmonary bypass (Orton and Monnet, 1994) (beyond the scope of this text). Closed aortic valvotomy has also been described. This requires a thoracotomy and there is a significant risk of haemorrhage and cardiac arrhythmias (Linn and Orton, 1992; Dhokarikar *et al.*, 1995). If an animal with aortic stenosis must be anaesthetized for diagnostic procedures or non-cardiac surgery, then most of the comments above (dealing with right ventricular hypertrophy) apply. However, there is more concern with reduction in SVR as coronary perfusion may be reduced if this occurs, and so the phenothiazines and butyrophenones are usually avoided. Management of intraoperative hypotension is also different. Many cases of aortic stenosis have a dynamic component that is exacerbated if a positive inotrope is given. For these animals the authors typically use phenylephrine (2–5 µg/kg slow bolus and infusion of 0.1–1 µg/kg/min) to treat hypotension, as phenylephrine can be titrated to give an α_1-mediated vasoconstriction with minimal positive inotropic effect. For closed aortic valvotomy, the same techniques are used but the animal should be cross matched before surgery and have at least two patent intravenous accesses. Lignocaine infusion may be started before the ventriculotomy (Dhokarikar *et al.*, 1995).

Thoracoscopy

Thoracoscopy may be used for diagnostic purposes (e.g. biopsy of a mass) or for surgical approaches (e.g. pericardectomy, lung lobectomy). The basic procedure involves the introduction of a rigid or flexible fibreoptic endoscope into the thoracic cavity, and the use of air or another gas to create a pneumothorax allowing visualization of intrathoracic structures. One or more other ports are usually placed to allow the introduction of a gas or instruments for surgical manipulation. The approach may be made laterally with the animal in lateral recumbency or ventrally (subxyphoid) with the animal in dorsal recumbency. For the lateral approach it is necessary to collapse the upper lung, and so it is advantageous if selective one lung ventilation (OLV) can be performed (Benumof and Alfrey, 1994). In the dog, the right lung is about 1.5 times the size of the left lung and receives almost 60% of the blood supply (Mure *et al.*, 1998). It is possible to achieve adequate ventilation of the animal

using just the right lung, although some desaturation can occur during the first few minutes (Cantwell *et al.*, 1999). Some of the approaches to OLV are outlined above, but the preferred method is to use a double lumen tube so that if a bilateral thoracoscopic procedure is undertaken each lung can be collapsed down separately. The double lumen tubes that have been used in dogs are the Robertshaw tubes (Figure 15.1), which have a long and short tube with two cuffs (Elliott *et al.*, 1991; Garcia *et al.*, 1998). The longer tube is placed in the bronchus while the shorter tube is supposed to remain in the trachea. Once the cuffs are inflated, the right and left lungs should be functionally isolated from each other. The tubes are supplied as a left and right version, with the right tube having an orifice in the side of the cuff that, in humans, is supposed to be placed at the entrance to the bronchus of the right upper lobe. This does not work well in dogs because of the position of the right apical lobe bronchus, and it is difficult to place an endobronchial tube on the right side without losing ventilation to the right apical and cardiac lobes of the lung (see Figure 15.1). Because of this difference in anatomy, it is usual to use a left-sided Robertshaw tube. The cuffs of these tubes are bright blue so that they are easy to see with the endoscope, and it is

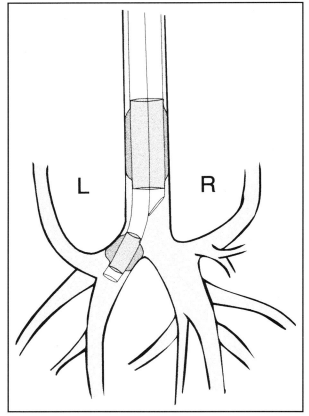

Figure 15.1: *The trachea and bronchi of the dog drawn to show the placement of a Robertshaw tube in the left mainstem bronchus. Note the proximity of the distal end of the tube to the bronchi in the left cranial lobe showing the likelihood of occluding one or more of these bronchi.*

necessary to be able to see the coloured tip to ensure correct placement of the tube. In studies in humans, blind positioning has resulted in high incidences of malpositioning (38–78%) (Benumof, 1993). The endoscope should be passed down both tubes to ensure that the ends of the tubes are in the right place (not impacted against a bronchial wall or that the right tube has not slipped into the left main bronchus), and that the cuff is adequately inflated in the correct position. For the larger sizes of tube (39 and 41 French) a 4.9 mm (outside diameter) bronchoscope will work, but a bronchoscope <4.2 mm will be needed for the smaller tubes (28–37 French).

If a lateral approach is being used, then the dependent lung will be ventilated while the upper non-dependent lung will be collapsed. One lung ventilation seems to be adequate for the removal of CO_2, but there is a significant risk of hypoxaemia because of the loss of exchange area and the shunting of blood through the non-ventilated lung. Strategies to improve oxygen exchange include:

- The application of PEEP to the dependent lung. The combination of gravity, the weight of the heart and surgical manipulation all tend to induce collapse in the dependent lung. The application of PEEP is an attempt to minimize these changes and to hold the airways open. However, the ideal value of the PEEP is not easy to determine since too low a value will not have any effect and too high a value will increase pulmonary intravascular pressure. Pulmonary intravascular pressure may decrease cardiac output and may also shunt blood into the upper unventilated lung. Nevertheless, in humans the application of 10 cmH_2O PEEP to the dependent lung was shown to improve PaO_2 in patients with a PaO_2 <80 mmHg (Cohen et al., 1985)
- The application of CPAP to the non-dependent lung. This is applied to the upper lung before deflation is allowed to occur, or after a large tidal volume, so that the pressure is applied before the lung has collapsed. An adjustable, disposable, CPAP valve can be bought for this application. The CPAP valve is applied to the ETT in the upper lung and oxygen is delivered at 5 l/min. This approach allows some mass diffusion of oxygen into the upper lung and improves oxygenation more than the application of PEEP to the dependent lung alone (Cohen et al., 1988)
- The use of high frequency ventilation to the non-dependent lung. This gives comparable results to the application of CPAP in terms of PaO_2, but interferes less with cardiac output so it provides better oxygen delivery to the tissues (Nakatsuka et al., 1988). In this report on humans, a high frequency jet ventilator (HFJV) was used, set at a rate of 150 breaths per minute.

If it is necessary to turn the dog over and examine the other hemithorax endoscopically, the use of the double lumen tube enables the process to be reversed so that the lung that was collapsed can be re-expanded while the other lung is deflated.

Using the subxyphoid approach for something like a pericardectomy means that it may be unnecessary to use a double lumen tube since both sides may need to be kept at relatively low volumes in order to improve visualization. However, the use of a double lumen tube may allow more flexibility in achieving the best ventilation with the least interference with the surgery. Using PEEP/CPAP for this approach may also be beneficial in improving oxygenation.

Animals undergoing thoracoscopy should be monitored using pulse oximetry so that any desaturation can be recognized and treated promptly. The addition of capnometry, electrocardiography and direct arterial pressure and CVP measurement (CVP will be affected by the amount of air or CO_2 in the chest making it easier to recognize excessive pneumothorax) adds considerably to the ability to recognize problems early and treat them immediately. Once the thoracoscopic procedure has been finished, the air should be removed from the chest and a chest drain placed, so that any remaining air can be removed or any subsequent haemorrhage or air leaks can be recognized.

Bronchoscopy

Most patients undergoing bronchoscopy are likely to have compromised pulmonary function, and so it is important to provide oxygen supplementation. In large animals it is possible to use a standard endoscope and pass it through a diaphragm on an elbow attached to the ETT. A double diaphragm arrangement is less likely to leak and so would be less hazardous to the staff managing the case (Figure 15.2). With this arrangement the animal can be kept anaesthetized with an inhalant delivered in oxygen, thus achieving the best oxygenation possible. It is also feasible to ventilate the animal should this be necessary. In small patients, where it is not possible to pass the endoscope through an appropriately sized ETT, or where the arrangement above is not available, it will be necessary to maintain anaesthesia with an injectable technique. For short procedures this can probably be achieved with most of the injectable anaesthetics, but for longer procedures the authors typically use propofol. This drug will provide a rapidly adjustable depth of anaesthesia with a smooth recovery. For these cases, oxygen can be supplied by three different methods:

- An oxygen source can be attached to one of the channels of the endoscope. This method will deliver oxygen deep into the lung, but that supply may be limited to one lung (if the endoscope is in a bronchus) or it may need to be discontinued if the endoscope's ports are needed for other things (e.g. suction or sampling)

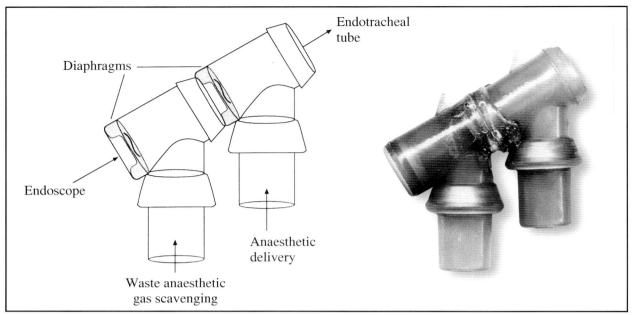

Figure 15.2: *The adapter used for bronchoscopy. The double diaphragm created with this arrangement reduces the amount of anaesthetic spilling into the room while allowing the delivery of inhaled anaesthetics with positive-pressure ventilation if needed.*

- A catheter can be placed in the trachea, and oxygen can be insufflated directly. This method will provide high concentrations of oxygen but does not remove CO_2. Care must be taken that the catheter is securely attached to the tubing so that it does not get dislodged into the trachea
- A catheter can be placed in the trachea and this can be attached to a HFJV. This has the advantage of providing high concentrations of oxygen while also oscillating the gas in the airway and enhancing the removal of CO_2. The authors typically run a HFJV at 180 breaths per minute and adjust the pressure so that they can just see the chest move with each pulse – often giving $PaCO_2$ values in the normal range.

These patients should be monitored carefully and continuously. A pulse oximeter is ideal for these patients since desaturation often occurs, as the bronchoscope blocks off various portions of the lung. The bronchoscope should be moved or completely removed if desaturation occurs. When biopsies are being taken there may be significant haemorrhage into the airway, compromising gas exchange still further. This should be suctioned out using the suction channel on the endoscope if possible. Occasionally a biopsy may rupture an airway or there may be sufficient disease in the lower airway that spontaneous rupture may occur. This will be manifested as a rapid desaturation, an increase in respiratory rate and a change in pulmonary compliance. Evacuation of the air from the pleural space should be undertaken immediately and a chest drain placed to allow further removal of air over the next few hours.

Once the bronchoscopic examination is finished the animal can be intubated and maintained on oxygen. An inhalant can be used to continue anaesthesia if necessary, or the animal can remain on oxygen until it is ready to be extubated.

Postoperative care

Many animals undergoing thoracic procedures are at risk of postoperative hypoxaemia. This can be minimized by taking the following precautions:

- Make every effort to ensure that the animal is normothermic by the time it is recovering. An animal that begins to shiver to warm itself up may increase its oxygen consumption by 300%. If the animal has poor pulmonary function, this extra demand may exacerbate any hypoxaemia
- Ensure that the animal has received analgesics (if necessary), and monitor the recovery carefully so that the animal emerges calmly from the anaesthetic. It may be necessary to give a tranquillizer if the animal becomes agitated during recovery. A rough recovery will be accompanied by huge increases in oxygen consumption, which may contribute to the hypoxaemia
- Place a chest drain and provide timely intermittent drainage or continuous suction if there is any risk of pneumo- or haemothorax. Remove the chest drain as soon as it is deemed safe to do so
- Provide an enriched supply of oxygen. A face mask can be used in the early postoperative period, as long as the animal will tolerate it. A tight fitting mask will allow the delivery of 100%

oxygen but, unless the animal is deeply sedated, this will require someone to be with the animal all the time, and most animals will not tolerate this technique for long. The delivery of 100% oxygen can also be achieved by placing a nasal insufflation catheter during the procedure and beginning oxygen insufflation as soon as the animal is extubated. The efficacy of this approach will diminish with large animals (Fitzpatrick and Crowe, 1986), but it will increase the inspired oxygen fraction (FiO_2) to some extent and it will continue to deliver the oxygen while the animal is being examined or treated. A more certain method of supplying high concentrations of oxygen would be to place the animal in an oxygen cage. The inspired oxygen concentration can be adjusted according to the needs of the patient, but it is hard to handle the animal without losing the benefit of the increased oxygen (Pascoe, 1988)

- If surgery has been carried out on the heart or lungs, the animal must be monitored carefully for signs of respiratory distress, cardiac arrhythmias, congestive failure or shock.

REFERENCES

Bailey CS, Kitchell RL, Haghighi SS and Johnson RD (1984) Cutaneous innervation of the thorax and abdomen of the dog. *American Journal of Veterinary Research* **45**, 1689-1698

Baraff LJ (1993) Capillary refill: is it a useful clinical sign? *Pediatrics* **92**, 723-724

Barnett HB, Holland JG and Josenhans WT (1982) When does central cyanosis become detectable? *Clinical Investigative Medicine* **5**, 39-43

Benumof J (1993) The position of a double-lumen tube should be routinely determined by fiberoptic bronchoscopy. *Journal of Cardiothoracic and Vascular Anesthesia* **7**, 513-514

Benumof JL and Alfrey DD (1994) Anesthesia for thoracic surgery. In: *Anesthesia, 4th edn.* ed. RD Miller, pp. 1663-1755. Churchill Livingstone, New York

Brasmer TH (1984) A is for Airway. In: *The Acutely Traumatized Small Animal Patient*, pp. 55-95. WB Saunders, Philadephia

Brownlie SE, Cobb MA, Chambers J, Jackson G and Thomas S (1991) Percutaneous balloon valvuloplasty in four dogs with pulmonic stenosis. *Journal of Small Animal Practice* **32**, 165-169

Cantwell SL, Duke T, Walsh JP, Remedios AM, Walker D and Ferguson JG (1999) One-lung versus two-lung ventilation in the anesthetized dog: a comparison of cardiopulmonary parameters. *Veterinary Surgery* (In press)

Cohen E, Eisenkraft J, Thys D, Kirschner P and Kaplan J (1988) Oxygenation and hemodynamic changes during one-lung ventilation: effects of CPAP10, PEEP10, and CPAP10/PEEP10. *Journal of Cardiothoracic Anesthesia* **2**, 34-40

Cohen E, Thys DM, Eisenkraft JB and Kaplan JA (1985) PEEP during one lung anesthesia improves oxygenation in patients with low arterial PaO_2. *Anesthesia and Analgesia* **64**, 201

Comroe JH Jr and Botelho S (1947) The unreliability of cyanosis in the recognition of arterial anoxemia. *American Journal of Medical Science* **214**, 1-6

Dhokarikar P, Caywood DD, Ogburn PN, Stobie D and Burtnick NL (1995) Closed aortic valvotomy: a retrospective study in 15 dogs. *Journal of the American Animal Hospital Association* **31**, 402-410

Elliott AR, Steffey EP, Jarvis KA and Marshall BE (1991) Unilateral hypoxic pulmonary vasoconstriction in the dog, pony and miniature swine. *Respiration Physiology* **85**, 355-369

Fitzpatrick RK and Crowe DTJ (1986) Nasal oxygen administration in dogs and cats: experimental and clinical investigations. *Journal of the American Animal Hospital Association* **22**, 293-300

Fordyce WE and Tenney SM (1984) Role of the carotid bodies in ventilatory acclimation to chronic hypoxia by the awake cat. *Respiration Physiology* **58**, 207-221

Garcia F, Prandi D, Pena T, Franch J, Trasserra O and de la Fuente J (1998) Examination of the thoracic cavity and lung lobectomy by means of thoracoscopy in dogs. *Canadian Veterinary Journal* **39**, 285-291

Gillespie DJ and Hyatt RE (1974) Respiratory mechanics in the unanesthetized dog. *Journal of Applied Physiology* **36**, 98-102

Gorelick MH, Shaw KN and Baker MD (1993) Effect of ambient temperature on capillary refill in healthy children. *Pediatrics* **92**, 699-702

Goss GA, Hayes JA and Burdor. JG (1988) Deoxyhaemoglobin concentrations in the detection of central cyanosis. *Thorax* **43**, 212-213

Grifka RG, Miller MW, Frischmeyer KJ and Mullins CE (1996) Transcatheter occlusion of a patent ductus arteriosus in a Newfoundland puppy using the Gianturco-Grifka vascular occlusion device. *Journal of Veterinary Internal Medicine* **10**, 42-44

Kienle RD (1998a) Aortic stenosis. In: *Small Animal Cardiovascular Medicine*, eds. MD Kittleson and RD Kienle, pp. 260-272. Mosby, St Louis

Kienle RD (1998b) Congenital pulmonic stenosis. In: *Small Animal Cardiovascular Medicine*, eds. MD Kittleson and RD Kienle, pp. 248-259. Mosby, St Louis

Kitchell RL, Whalen LR, Bailey CS and Lohse CL (1980) Electrophysiologic studies of cutaneous nerves of the thoracic limb of the dog. *American Journal of Veterinary Research* **41**, 61-76

Koller ME, Smith B, Sjostrand U and Brevik H (1983) Effects of hypo-, normo-, and hypercarbia in dogs with acute cardiac tamponade. *Anesthesia and Analgesia* **62**, 181-185

Linn K and Orton EC (1992) Closed transventricular dilation of discrete subvalvular aortic stenosis in dogs. *Veterinary Surgery* **21**, 441-445

Martin MWS, Godman M, Fuentes VL, Clutton RE, Haigh A and Darke PGG (1992) Assessment of balloon pulmonary valvuloplasty in six dogs. *Journal of Small Animal Practice* **33**, 443-449

Martins JB, Manuel WJ, Marcus ML and Kerber RE (1980) Comparative effects of catecholamines in cardiac tamponade: experimental and clinical studies. *American Journal of Cardiology* **46**, 59-66

Mattilla I, Takkunen O, Mattila P, Harjula A, Mattila S and Merikallio E (1984) Cardiac tamponade and different modes of artificial ventilation. *Acta Anaesthesiologica Scandinavica* **28**, 236-240

Morgan-Hughes JO (1968a) Fluorescent lighting and cyanosis. *Nursing Mirror and Midwives Journal* **126**, 51

Morgan-Hughes JO (1968b) Lighting and cyanosis. *British Journal of Anaesthesia* **40**, 503-507

Mure M, Domino KB, Robertson T, Hlastala MP and Glenny RW (1998) Pulmonary blood flow does not redistribute in dogs with reposition from supine to left lateral position. *Anesthesiology* **89**, 483-492

Nakatsuka M, Wetstein L and Keenan R (1988) Unilateral high-frequency jet ventilation during one-lung ventilation for thoracotomy. *Annals of Thoracic Surgery* **46**, 654-660

Orton EC and Monnet E (1994) Pulmonic stenosis and subvalvular aortic stenosis: surgical options. *Seminars in Veterinary Medicine and Surgery (Small Animal)* **9**, 221-226

Pascoe PJ (1988) Oxygen and ventilatory support for the critical patient. *Seminars in Veterinary Medicine and Surgery (Small Animal)* **3**, 202-209

Pascoe PJ and Dyson DH (1993) Analgesia after lateral thoracotomy in dogs. Epidural morphine vs. intercostal bupivacaine. *Veterinary Surgery* **22**, 141-147

Popilskis S, Kohn D, Sanchez JA and Gorman P (1991) Epidural vs. intramuscular oxymorphone analgesia after thoracotomy in dogs. *Veterinary Surgery* **20**, 462-467

Popilskis S, Kohn DF, Laurent L and Danilo P (1993) Efficacy of epidural morphine versus intravenous morphine for post-thoracotomy pain in dogs. *Journal of Veterinary Anaesthesia* **20**, 21-25

Riegler FX, VadeBoncouer TR and Pelligrino DA (1989) Interpleural anesthetics in the dog: differential somatic neural blockade. *Anesthesiology* **71**, 744-750

Schriger DL and Baraff LJ (1991) Capillary refill – is it a useful predictor of hypovolemic states? *Annals of Emergency Medicine* **20**, 601-605

Snaps FR, McEntee K, Saunders JH, Dondelinger RF, Fellows CG, Lerche P, King G and Tometzki A (1998) Treatment of patent ductus arteriosus by placement of intravascular coils in a pup. *Journal of the American Veterinary Medical Association* **39**, 196-199

Stokhof A (1986) Diagnosis and treatment of acquired diaphragmatic hernia by thoracotomy in 49 dogs and 72 cats. *Veterinary Quarterly* **8**, 177-183

Thompson SE and Johnson JM (1991) Analgesia in dogs after intercostal thoracotomy. A comparison of morphine, selective intercostal nerve block, and interpleural regional analgesia with bupivacaine. *Veterinary Surgery* **20**, 73-77

VadeBoncouer TR, Riegler FX and Pelligrino DA (1990) The effects of two different volumes of 0.5% bupivacaine in a canine model of interpleural analgesia. *Regional Anesthesia* **15**, 67-72

Wilson G and Hayes H (1986) Diaphragmatic hernia in the dog and cat: a 25-year overview. *Seminars in Veterinary Medicine and Surgery (Small Animal)* **1**, 318-326

Zhang H, Spapen H and Vincent JL (1994) Effects of dobutamine and norepinephrine on oxygen availability in tamponade-induced stagnant hypoxia: a prospective, randomized, controlled study. *Critical Care Medicine* **22**, 299-305

CHAPTER SIXTEEN

Gastrointestinal and Hepatic Disease

Rachel C. Bennett and Peter J. Pascoe

INTRODUCTION

Patients with gastrointestinal disease may be suffering from significant metabolic disturbances that may only be recognized with a careful examination of the animal and extensive clinical pathological tests. Deficiencies in blood volume, blood coagulation and electrolytes may make the management of the anaesthetized animal precarious and so it is essential that these things are recognized and managed first.

New technological advances ensure that the management of some cases will change considerably from those described here. The recent introduction of ameroid rings in the management of portosystemic shunts has significantly reduced the risk of post-operative haemorrhage and intestinal ischaemia. Hopefully such innovations will continue to improve the perioperative management of many of these patients.

THE OESOPHAGUS

Clinical conditions of the oesophagus can be divided into three categories: obstructions, disorders of motility and inflammation. Obstructive conditions can result from foreign bodies, strictures and vascular ring anomalies while motility problems refer almost exclusively to megaoesophagus, of which there are a large number of potential aetiologies. Oesophageal inflammation (oesophagitis) is most commonly caused by gastro-oesophageal reflux, which may occur during anaesthesia.

Obstructions

Removal of oesophageal foreign bodies is usually performed under general anaesthesia. The presence of objects within the oesophagus prevents the normal passage of saliva and ingested material into the stomach. Fluid and saliva that have accumulated cranial to the obstruction may move into the oropharynx at the time of anaesthetic induction, increasing the risk of aspiration. Equipment for suctioning the oropharynx and oesophagus should be available.

Anaesthesia of patients with oesophageal foreign bodies requires a 'rapid induction technique' making use of intravenous agents. In this way the anaesthetist is able to gain control of the airway quickly and reduce the risk of aspiration. The need for preoperative sedation will depend on the individual patient, the duration the obstruction has been present and the existence of any other medical conditions. The use of opioids and their potential to cause emesis have not been found to be a problem in these patients. Anaesthesia can be induced with thiopentone, propofol, etomidate or ketamine (see Chapter 8), as all of these agents have a rapid onset of action and can be titrated to effect, reducing the risk of overdose. These induction drugs may be used with diazepam (0.2–0.5 mg/kg i.v.) or midazolam (0.1–0.2 mg/kg i.v.). The animal should be positioned in sternal recumbency with its head elevated during induction. The assistant should keep the head elevated until the endotracheal tube (ETT) has been inserted and the cuff inflated. This precaution is taken to prevent fluid refluxing into the trachea while the airway is unprotected. Once the ETT cuff has been inflated, the oesophagus should be suctioned to reduce the risk of regurgitation. If fluid enters the larynx after the ETT has been placed and the cuff inflated, it is still possible for this fluid to seep past the cuff. Removing material from the oesophagus at this stage will reduce this risk. If the patient does start to vomit or reflux during induction, the head should immediately be lowered below the level of the body – off the end of the table – so that the fluid can drain out. The pharynx should then be swabbed out and cleaned as much as possible before intubation is attempted.

The use of neuromuscular blocking agents has been found to be useful in dogs, where the entire length of the oesophagus is made up of striated muscle. This allows the oesophageal tissue to relax and aids removal of the object either via the mouth or by passage into the stomach. This technique may also be useful in cats, but since the caudal third of the oesophagus is composed of smooth muscle it is less likely to provide full relaxation if the foreign body is in this area. A nondepolarizing drug such as atracurium (0.2–0.3 mg/kg i.v.) should be used for this purpose since a depolarizing drug could cause oesophageal contraction and rupture. The use of neuromuscular blocking agents requires artificial ventilation.

Animals that present for removal of oesophageal foreign bodies or dilation of an oesophageal stricture are at an increased risk of developing an iatrogenic pneumothorax. Signs of pneumothorax may include a change in respiratory pattern (usually an increase in respiratory rate) resistance to manual inflation of the lungs, expansion of the thorax (the diameter of the thorax is increased) and cyanosis. Appropriate measures need to be taken to deal with this problem should it arise (anything from simple drainage with a needle or butterfly in a mild case, to immediately creating a hole in the thoracic wall in the case of tension pneumothorax). Surgery of the oesophagus in the cervical region may be complicated by damage to the laryngeal nerves. Care should be taken during recovery to ensure that laryngeal obstruction does not occur. In cases with mild laryngeal dysfunction the condition is likely to be exacerbated during a rough recovery so it is appropriate to administer tranquillizers/opioids for those animals where this is expected. If the approach to the oesophagus requires a thoracotomy, further details may be found in Chapter 15. If, despite all the precautions taken, it is suspected that the animal has regurgitated, and some fluid has entered the trachea, the cuff should be left inflated during removal of the ETT. The inflated cuff should displace most of the fluid out of the trachea as it is withdrawn.

Megaoesophagus

Motility problems of the oesophagus generally result in megaoesophagus. While surgical correction of the megaoesophagus is rarely attempted, anaesthesia of patients with this condition may be required. In these cases emphasis is again on the need to use a rapid induction technique. Patients should be handled in the manner described above during induction. The oesophagus should be suctioned to remove any liquid or food material that may be present. Thoracic radiography before the procedure may indicate the presence or degree of pneumonia present and may be important in the timing of anaesthesia and surgery if the procedure is elective. Opioids can be used for premedication if required. Propofol is suitable for induction of anaesthesia; not only does it have a rapid onset of action but recovery is also fast. This is particularly advantageous in patients who need to be able to protect their airway as soon as possible after the end of the procedure.

Patients presenting for surgical correction of vascular ring anomalies are generally young. The extent of changes in oesophageal motility will be dependent on the time of diagnosis. Apart from potential alterations in oesophageal tone, the young age of these patients and small size are also important anaesthetic considerations.

In animals that have a megaoesophagus, the pharyngeal region needs to be examined at the end of the procedure to determine whether food material is visible. The pharynx and oesophagus may need to be suctioned out to remove any residual material that could be aspirated during recovery from anaesthesia.

Oesophagitis

Reflux of gastric contents into the oesophagus may result in oesophagitis and stricture formation. Gastro-oesophageal reflux (GOR) during anaesthesia is one of the most common causes of oesophagitis. The lower gastro-oesophageal sphincter is not a true anatomical sphincter but is described as a physiological sphincter. The activity of this so called sphincter is thought to reside in the circular muscle of the oesophageal wall. It is the difference between the lower oesophageal sphincter pressure and the intragastric pressure, termed the barrier pressure (BrP), which determines whether or not reflux occurs. Even if reflux does occur this may not lead to oesophagitis. The likelihood of GOR leading to physical damage increases if the pH of the refluxed fluid is low or excessively high, if the oesophageal mucosa's resistance to injury is reduced (previous oesophagitis, damaged mucus layer) or if the fluid sits in the oesophagus for a long time. The incidence of GOR (as defined by a pH of <4.0 or >7.5 in the oesophagus) was 16.3% and 17.4% in two studies in dogs, yet regurgitation was reported in only three out of 510 dogs studied (0.6%) (Galatos and Raptopoulos, 1995a,b). However, the number of cases of oesophagitis that is reported is far below this incidence of GOR, and it is unclear which predisposing factors are the most important. In humans it has been reported that damage begins to occur if a solution with a pH <2.5 remains in contact with the oesophageal mucosa for more than 20 minutes, yet Galatos and Raptopoulos (1995b) found that the average contact time in dogs was 44 minutes, with no cases of oesophageal stricture being reported postoperatively. In the authors' experience, with many cases being anaesthetized for 5-6 hours, the occurrence of post-operative oesophageal damage is rare. Studies have identified several factors associated with an increased risk of reflux. It is known that many drugs used for anaesthesia decrease the BrP to a greater or lesser extent. They include atropine, glycopyrrolate, xylazine, dopamine, opioids, thiopentone, propofol, halothane and isoflurane. In comparative studies in cats, the BrPs were highest with ketamine or xylazine and ketamine, 54-60% of these values with propofol, 33-38% with thiopentone and 19-21% with alphaxalone/alphadolone (Hashim and Waterman, 1991). In premedicated dogs, the BrP after induction with propofol was 36% of that after thiopentone (while on halothane) (Waterman and Hashim, 1992). In further studies in dogs, the incidence of GOR was reported to be much higher after induction with propofol than after induction with thiopentone (50% versus 18%, respectively) (Raptopoulos and Galatos, 1997).

An increase in intragastric pressure can lead to a greater incidence of GOR. A significantly higher incidence of reflux has been observed in dogs undergoing abdominal procedures compared with those undergoing non-abdominal procedures. In some human hospitals it is routine to place an orogastric tube in all

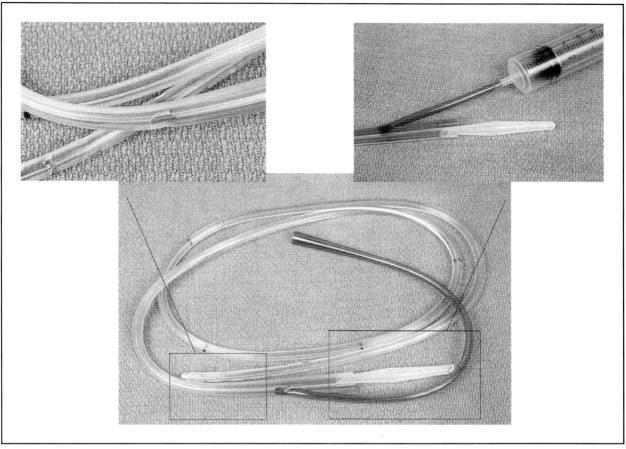

Figure 16.1: *Double lumen suction catheter used to irrigate and suction the oesophagus. Note the placement of a relief hole in the suction lumen, which allows the negative pressure to be released while manipulating the catheter. The irrigation channel has also been cut to allow attachment of the syringe. The piece of tubing that has been cut off can be used as a 'straw' to draw up the saline from a 500 ml bottle.*

patients who are undergoing abdominal procedures. In this way gastric contents can readily be removed during and after surgery.

There is a trend towards a greater incidence of GOR with increasing age. This should be borne in mind when geriatric patients are undergoing surgical procedures that require general anaesthesia. Puppies and kittens are also at an increased risk of experiencing GOR as the lower oesophageal sphincter is incompetent at birth; by 6 weeks of age, lower oesophageal sphincter pressure is still only half that of adults (Strombeck and Guilford, 1996).

Patients with an increased volume of gastric contents are believed to be at a greater risk of developing GOR. It was thought that preoperative fasting reduced the volume of food material in the stomach. However, recent studies in dogs showed that reflux occurred less frequently in animals fed 2–4 hours before the induction of anaesthesia. Prolonged preoperative fasting was associated with decreased gastric pH and an increased incidence of GOR (Galatos and Raptopoulos, 1995a).

Postanaesthetic oesophagitis is seen rarely, despite the fact that GOR is a seemingly frequent occurrence during anaesthesia. The results of studies suggest either that asymptomatic mild oesophagitis occurs,

which is undiagnosed, or that other factors may lead to the production of oesophagitis and stricture formation. At present, these factors await identification. Nevertheless, if gastric or intestinal fluid are regurgitated during anaesthesia, the oesophagus should be flushed out immediately. This can be done efficiently using a double lumen suction catheter (Figure 16.1). The catheter is passed down to the distal oesophagus and connected to the suction pump. A relief hole or clamp should be present in the suction line so that the suction is only applied when the catheter is stationary, as it is very easy to suck oesophageal mucosa into the catheter and damage the mucosa. Once the catheter is positioned, suction is applied and saline infused down the second lumen until the aspirated material is clear and colourless. The suction is stopped, the catheter moved, and the process repeated until the whole of the oesophagus has been lavaged. Even if no more regurgitated material is seen for the rest of the procedure, it is worth repeating this lavage just before awakening the animal.

Oesophagitis should be suspected when animals recovering from general anaesthesia show signs of pain when attempting to swallow, repeatedly attempt to swallow or salivate profusely. Treatment of oesophagitis is aimed at reducing ongoing reflux, resolving inflammation and preventing stricture formation. Decreasing the amount of refluxed acid and pepsin is the mainstay of successful treatment via the use of H_2-receptor antagonists, e.g. cimetidine, ranitidine and famotidine. Prokinetic agents, e.g. metoclopramide and cisapride, increase lower oesophageal sphincter tone and gastric motility thereby decreasing the amount of reflux. Sucralfate is the only mucosal protective drug that has been evaluated for the treatment of oesophagitis. Sucralfate requires an acidic environment for maximal effect, so realistically administration must coincide with the period of reflux, which is difficult to accomplish during general anaesthesia. However, there is support for its use with other forms of therapy such as prokinetic drugs, H_2-antagonists or proton pump inhibitors (Weyrauch and Willard, 1998). In order to allow the oesophagus time to heal, it is important to rest the oesophagus and to provide nutritional support. This can be achieved by placement of a gastrostomy tube. Use of the gastrostomy tube for feeding allows the oesophageal mucosa to rest and reduces the formation of scar tissue, and subsequent development of strictures.

GASTRODUODENOSCOPY

This is a diagnostic procedure that is frequently performed in both cats and dogs and requires general anaesthesia. The anaesthetic protocol used in these cases depends on the health status of the patient. Some veterinary anaesthetists use opioids routinely for premedication (e.g. oxymorphone 0.02–0.05 mg/kg, morphine 0.1–0.5 mg/kg, butorphanol 0.1–0.4 mg/kg). However, others prefer to avoid the use of opioids since morphine with atropine, in particular, increases the tone of the antral portion of the stomach and duodenum making it harder for the endoscope to pass through the pyloric sphincter (Donaldson *et al.*, 1993). To avoid the changes associated with opioids, it is preferable to use no premedication where appropriate or to use acepromazine or a dissociative drug for premedication.

These animals often have a history of chronic vomiting with some degree of pre-existing dehydration. Administration of intravenous fluids before the procedure helps to replace some of this deficit. At the very least, intravenous fluids should be administered throughout the procedure. Anaesthesia can be induced with any of the commonly used induction drugs – thiopentone, propofol, etomidate, alphaxalone/alphadolone, ketamine and diazepam, or tiletamine and zolazepam. Anaesthesia is maintained with an inhalant such as halothane or isoflurane in oxygen. The use of nitrous oxide (N_2O) is controversial in these patients due to its ability to diffuse into gas-filled spaces – that is, it further increases gastric or duodenal volume during the procedure. This can, however, be managed as long as the volume of gas in the gastrointestinal (GI) tract is monitored and removed when it becomes excessive.

Careful monitoring of anaesthetic depth in these patients is essential as the fibreoptic endoscopes are expensive and fragile. The damage caused by an animal that begins to chew while the endoscope is in place can rapidly be expensive. Routine anaesthetic monitoring of these patients includes electrocardiography, indirect blood pressure, temperature probe and pulse oximetry. The use of the pulse oximeter allows arterial haemoglobin saturation to be monitored. Inflation of the stomach during the procedure may cause cranial displacement of the diaphragm leading to a reduction in functional residual capacity and hypoxia, identified by rapid desaturation. If this occurs, the stomach should be deflated until saturation improves, before continuing.

PERCUTANEOUS PLACEMENT OF GASTROSTOMY TUBES

The concerns for carrying out percutaneous placement of gastrostomy tubes are similar to the above, except that it is unnecessary to go through the pylorus, so opioids may be used for premedication. Animals requiring the placement of a gastrostomy tube are often debilitated, and so it is important to ensure that they are well prepared preoperatively. This may include restoring circulating volume, increasing colloid oncotic pressure and dealing with anaemia and coagulation defects. If an endoscope is used for the procedure, it is imperative that the animal does not awaken while the endoscope is in place (see above).

THE STOMACH AND INTESTINES

Surgery of the stomach and GI tract can involve a wide range of conditions that may be acute in onset or more longstanding. Alterations in volume status are common and may be severe in patients with GI disease. Acute volume depletion can result from GI bleeding, hypersecretion accompanied by inadequate fluid replacement, or third space losses. In addition to hypovolaemia, GI and metabolic diseases may lead to electrolyte and acid-base disturbances. Malnutrition is a common feature of many GI disorders because these patients have digestive impairment or malabsorption with increased metabolic demands due to illness. In human medicine it has been shown that nutritional support greatly improves patient outcome as well as reducing mortality. Apart from the metabolic disturbances, these patients may also be experiencing severe discomfort and/or pain.

It is important to assess electrolytes, packed cell volume (PCV), total protein (TP) and acid-base status before anaesthesia. This enables more informed decisions to be made regarding fluid therapy preoperatively. Ideally, circulating blood volume should be restored before anaesthesia, thereby improving cardiovascular stability. 'High' gastrointestinal obstruction tends to lead to metabolic alkalosis due to the loss of acidic gastric contents, whereas loss of duodenal contents results more commonly in metabolic acidosis. Animals that are considered to be alkalotic benefit from an acidifying solution such as 0.9% saline. Those that are acidotic are generally treated with lactated Ringer's solution or acetated polyionic solutions. Weight loss leads to a decrease in the volume of distribution of many drugs. This means that a given dose of an agent will have an enhanced effect when compared with the same dose administered to a normal healthy individual. Injectable anaesthetic drugs are present as bound and unbound fractions within the bloodstream. It is the free or unbound portion of the drug that is pharmacologically active, while the fraction that is principally bound to albumin is inactive. Animals that are hypoproteinaemic show an enhanced response to an injectable drug. For this reason it is important to administer drugs slowly and to effect, thereby avoiding the tendency to overdose these patients.

Gastric dilatation and volvulus

Gastric dilatation initiates hypovolaemic shock due to a reduction in venous return. The dilated stomach obstructs blood flow through the caudal vena cava, while the increased gastric pressure also decreases blood flow through the portal vein. The obstruction to flow in both the vena cava and portal vein leads to a decrease in venous return and a corresponding reduction in cardiac output and a failure to maintain normal tissue perfusion. Therefore it is essential to try to stabilize these patients before anaesthesia and surgery by deflating the stomach and administering intravenous fluids in an attempt to restore circulating blood volume.

Pretreatment blood samples provide an initial reference point and allow the efficacy of treatment to be assessed later. Laboratory information that is pertinent to these cases includes blood gases, plasma electrolytes, PCV, TP, urea and blood glucose. If indicated, measurement of activated clotting time, colloid oncotic pressure and plasma lactate will give further useful information. Volume resuscitation is usually performed with a balanced electrolyte solution at 40–90 ml/kg. Hypertonic saline may provide a more rapid initial resuscitation, but it should be followed by routine crystalloid therapy (see Chapter 11). Colloids may also provide a more sustained restoration of circulating volume. Polygelatins have been widely used for this purpose, with few adverse side effects. Hetastarch may interfere with coagulation, but its propensity for this seems to be less than that of the dextrans; dextrans may significantly prolong bleeding times in some patients.

It is useful to have at least two intravenous catheters in place in order to allow rapid volume resuscitation and easy intravenous access during surgery. Several different solutions and drugs may need to be adminis-

tered during the course of the anaesthetic, some of which are incompatible. For example, sodium bicarbonate should not be given with dopamine or solutions containing calcium; blood products, where citrate has been used for anticoagulation, should not be given with solutions containing calcium such as lactated Ringer's solution.

Premedication may be achieved with the use of an opioid at a reduced dose if the animal is very depressed. In cases where the animal is extremely debilitated, no premedication may be deemed necessary. Animals should be preoxygenated via a face mask. If possible, monitoring equipment should be placed before the induction of anaesthesia. Electrocardiographic pads on the feet allow the heart rate and rhythm to be assessed throughout the induction process. A Doppler probe over a peripheral artery allows non-invasive measurement of blood pressure and is also an indicator of peripheral perfusion. The Doppler technique has been shown to be the most reliable non-invasive indicator of hypotension in small animals (Dyson, 1997; Caulkett *et al.*,1998). If an arterial catheter has been placed, then direct blood pressure monitoring can be used. Anaesthesia may be induced with a combination of opioid and benzodiazepine (e.g. fentanyl 0.01–0.02 mg/kg i.v. and diazepam 0.2–0.5 mg/kg i.v., sufentanil 0.005 mg/kg i.v. and midazolam 0.1–0.6 mg/kg i.v., oxymorphone 0.1–0.2 mg/kg i.v. and diazepam 0.2–0.5 mg/kg i.v., or methadone 0.1–0.6 mg/kg i.v. and diazepam 0.2–0.5 mg/kg i.v.). Alternatively an agent such as etomidate in combination with diazepam would be suitable. These drug combinations have minimal impact on the cardiovascular system, and for this reason they are commonly used in hypovolaemic animals undergoing surgery. Whichever induction technique is employed, it is important to administer drugs slowly and to effect; in this way the risk of overdose is greatly reduced. In theory ketamine and diazepam would be acceptable. Ketamine increases sympathetic tone via release of noradrenaline from postganglionic nerve terminals. Blood pressure is maintained, there is little effect on myocardial contractility and respiration is not greatly impaired. However, there is concern about the use of ketamine in patients who already have increased sympathetic tone. In these individuals the authors have seen a dramatic decrease in blood pressure after the induction of anaesthesia. Ketamine should therefore be used judiciously in patients with gastric dilatation. Thiopentone and propofol are known to cause hypotension and respiratory depression after intravenous administration. Thiopentone has also been shown to induce ventricular arrhythmias (ventricular bigeminy or trigemy), and propofol may sensitize the myocardium to catecholamines, so for these reasons thiopentone and propofol would not be the agents of choice in patients with increased sympathetic tone. If it has not been possible to decompress the stomach before anaesthesia it is important to begin intermittent positive-pressure ventilation (IPPV) as soon as possible after intubation. In order to achieve adequate ventilation it may be necessary to use very high inspiratory pressures (30–40 cmH$_2$O), and the negative effect this has on the circulation may necessitate further fluid therapy to increase blood volume. The agent (or agents) used to maintain anaesthesia depends on the response of the patient. Anaesthesia can be maintained with isoflurane in oxygen. Isoflurane is relatively insoluble, so changes in anaesthetic depth can be implemented quite rapidly, and recovery tends to be fast. Isoflurane is preferable to halothane as it does not sensitize the heart to the effects of high concentrations of circulating catecholamines. It has a dose-dependent depressant effect on cardiovascular and respiratory function causing hypotension and hypoventilation. In these patients it may be more appropriate to employ a balanced technique using a potent opioid and in addition to this a neuromuscular blocking agent. Opioids have been shown to cause a significant reduction in the minimum alveolar concentration (MAC) of inhalants, but do not result in hypotension; in this way the unwanted side effects of the volatile anaesthetic may be minimized. Use of potent opioids such as fentanyl and sufentanil cause profound respiratory depression. These patients usually need to be mechanically ventilated to prevent hypoventilation and respiratory acidosis. It is important to remember that positive pressure ventilation will cause a drop in systemic blood pressure through a reduction in venous return. In those individuals that are already hypovolaemic, the effect of IPPV is often more severe.

Anaesthetic monitoring should include electrocardiography, measurement of blood pressure (ideally measured directly), temperature probe, arterial blood gases and monitoring of acid–base status. There are several portable blood gas monitors now available, and these may be convenient to use in practice where there are no clinical laboratory facilities. If neuromuscular blocking agents are to be administered, then a peripheral nerve stimulator should be used to monitor the blockade.

Measurement of pH, arterial blood gases, bicarbonate and base excess allows the anaesthetist to determine the cause of an acidosis or alkalosis. Severe metabolic acidosis is commonly treated with sodium bicarbonate (NaHCO$_3$). The quantity of bicarbonate (HCO$_3^-$) can be calculated using the following formula:

$$\text{NaHCO}_3 \text{ (mmol)} =$$
$$\text{Base excess (mmol/l)} \times \text{bodyweight (kg)} \times 0.3$$

It is common practice to calculate the deficit and then aim to replace one-third to one-half of this over a 20–30 minute period, as rapid administration of

NaHCO$_3$ is associated with hypotension and acidosis of the central nervous system (CNS). The magnitude of the systemic acidosis can then be reassessed and further HCO$_3^-$ given if required. It is important to realize that administration of NaHCO$_3$ will lead to an increase in partial pressure of arterial carbon dioxide ($PaCO_2$). Ventilation may need to be augmented in order to prevent a further respiratory acidosis if the animal is not already being ventilated.

Cardiac arrhythmias are associated with gastric distension-volvulus in the dog (Muir and Lipowitz, 1978). If these arrhythmias are present before surgical intervention the prognosis is worse, but it is not clear what the influence of early anti-arrhythmic therapy may have on this. Monitoring by electrocardiography allows the anaesthetist to detect arrhythmias and instigate treatment if required. Lignocaine (lidocaine) is used to treat ventricular premature contractions either as a bolus or by infusion (1–2 mg/kg boluses followed by an infusion of 50–120 µg/kg/min). If an infusion is used, the animal should be monitored carefully for signs of lignocaine toxicity as the rate of elimination of lignocaine may be decreased in these animals. Other anti-arrhythmic drugs that may be of benefit alone or in addition to lignocaine include procainamide and quinidine (Muir and Bonagura, 1984).

It is useful to monitor PCV and TP during surgery as torsion of the stomach and spleen on occasions can cause rupture of major blood vessels. The extent of blood loss is not apparent until intravenous fluid administration restores blood volume and highlights an earlier period of blood loss. Packed cell volumes in the range of 10–12% have been measured in individuals who have bled preoperatively. Major haemorrhage requires administration of either packed red blood cells or fresh whole blood. When there is a significant drop in PCV, then loss of both clotting factors and platelets also becomes a problem. Loss of clotting factors can be treated with fresh frozen plasma or fresh plasma. Frozen plasma (frozen at least 24 hours after collection) is deficient in the labile factors V and VIII. Low platelet numbers require treatment with platelet-rich plasma or fresh whole blood. Platelets do not survive the freezing process.

THE LARGE INTESTINE, RECTUM AND PERINEUM

Surgery for perineal hernia should include an examination to determine whether the urinary bladder is involved, and tests to rule out azotaemia. These patients may be geriatric and therefore consideration must be given to the potential for other medical conditions, e.g. cardiac disease or renal disease. Conversely, those individuals presented for surgery to correct atresia ani are usually only a few days old. In this instance consideration must be given to their small size and the

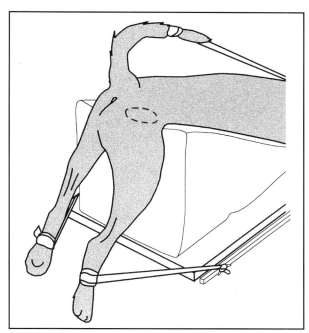

Figure 16.2: Positioning of a dog on a perineal stand for perineal surgery. Note the sandbag under the pubis (dotted circle). This raises the abdomen a little, decreases intra-abdominal pressure and permits the diaphragm to move more easily. Care must be taken to avoid too much tension on the leg ties, to prevent nerve/muscle damage.

potential for hypothermia and hypoglycaemia (if the surgical time is prolonged), with the additional risk of significant blood loss.

Patients requiring surgery for perineal hernia are usually positioned with their head down on a sloping table or perineal stand (Figure 16.2). This results in diaphragmatic compression, and impairs the ability of the animal to ventilate. Intermittent positive-pressure ventilation may be required to prevent hypoventilation. Ventilation can be monitored by the use of respirometers to determine tidal and minute volume, capnography to measure end-tidal CO_2 (ETCO$_2$), and also blood gas analysis if it is available. Placing a pad or sandbag underneath the animal's pubis partially suspends its abdomen and improves the ability of the animal to breathe. Nerve damage to the hind limbs is also a potential complication. This can occur if the legs are extended caudally for long periods or if the legs are tied forward with pressure against the quadriceps.

In cats undergoing colectomy, it has been noted that they can become profoundly hypotensive with a poor response to positive inotropes and vasoconstrictors. The incidence of this complication has been significantly reduced by decreasing the amount of colonic manipulation performed under anaesthesia. This means that if an enema is needed it is used before surgery, and the colon is resected with its contents *in situ* rather than trying to empty it out. This colonic manipulation may cause release of bacteria or endo-toxin into the circulation causing the hypotension and lack of response to therapy.

LAPAROSCOPY AND LAPAROSCOPIC SURGERY

Laparoscopy and laparoscopic surgery usually involve the insufflation of gas into the abdominal cavity to improve visibility. This pneumoperitoneum can lead to a number of concerns for the anaesthetist. The gases that have been used to create a pneumoperi-toneum include air, N_2O, helium and CO_2. Carbon dioxide seems to be the preferred gas, as it is rapidly absorbed after the procedure, leaving little gas trapped in the abdomen. The gas is insufflated into the abdo-men through a needle (usually a Verres needle), and the intra-abdominal pressure should be monitored. This increased intra-abdominal pressure will affect ventilation and circulation, and it is important to understand the changes that are likely to occur. The increased forward pressure on the diaphragm will tend to reduce the functional residual capacity of the lungs and make it harder for the patient to ventilate. This may be exacerbated if the patient is placed in a head down position to facilitate visualization of ab-dominal structures. Consequently, it is best if these animals are intubated and ventilated throughout the period when the intra-abdominal pressure is increased. Application of 5 cmH$_2$O positive end expiratory pres-sure (PEEP) may help to reduce atelectasis. The use of CO_2 to inflate the abdomen can also lead to an increase in arterial CO_2, and it is best if PaCO$_2$ and/or ETCO$_2$ is monitored during anaesthesia. The effect of the increased abdominal pressure on the circulation is dependent on the magnitude of the increase. In a recent study it was shown that 12 mmHg was a relatively safe pressure while at a pressure of 16 mmHg there was a significant decrease in cardiac output with increased systemic vascular resistance (SVR) – central venous pressure (CVP) and mean arterial pressure did not change very much (Ishizaki *et al.*, 1993). In humans intra-abdominal pressures of 20–40 mmHg are commonly used for gynaecological procedures, resulting in even more dramatic changes in cardiac output and SVR.

Although it is a rare complication, a gas embolus can occur, with fatal results if it is not recognized and treated immediately. This is most common during the initial insertion of the Verres needle and insufflation – penetration into a vessel or organ may lead to rapid massive embolization (Gilroy and Anson, 1987). It can also occur during the procedure, when manipula-tion of the abdominal viscera can lead to vascular damage and uptake of gas. The best way to diagnose this (transoesophageal Doppler) is not readily avai-lable and is not generally recommended as a routine monitor even in humans. A capnograph will show an initial sudden rise in ETCO$_2$ (if CO_2 is being used as the insufflation gas) followed by a decrease as the delivery of CO_2 to the lung is impaired by the decrease in cardiac output. An oesophageal stethoscope may allow a new-onset 'washing machine' or 'mill wheel' murmur to be heard. The patient may become cyanotic and show a sudden decrease in blood pressure. If any of these signs are seen, the abdomen should be deflated immediately, the animal placed in left lateral recumbency and a central venous line inserted to try to remove the gas by aspirating from the right side of the heart. Blood pressure and cardiac function should be monitored carefully during this time and cardiopulmonary resuscitation started if necessary. Carbon dioxide is rapidly cleared from the circulation and resuscitation is more likely to be successful after a CO_2 embolus compared with one of air or N_2O.

Gas may also leak into the thorax and create a pneumothorax. The anaesthetist should pay careful attention to changes in pulmonary compliance, and relate such changes to any alterations in intra-abdominal pressure during the procedure. If the abdominal pressure suddenly decreases with no obvious leakage from one of the instruments, it may mean that gas has escaped into the thorax.

The actual choice of anaesthetic technique will largely depend on the condition of the patient. Due to an increase in catecholamine release during pneumoperitoneum, it is wise to avoid the use of halothane unless acepromazine has been used for premedication. There is also some slight risk of an increase in vagal tone, so an anticholinergic is warranted for this procedure. Other inhalants (e.g. isoflurane, sevoflurane, desflurane) or injectable drugs (e.g. propofol) can be used for maintenance but, as indicated above, the animal should be intubated and ventilated. The use of N_2O is controversial – if N_2O has been used for insufflation, then N_2O in the breathing circuit will not diffuse into the pneumoperitoneum, but if other gases are used, diffusion occurs with an increase in intra-abdominal pressure over time. If an embolus occurs then the volume of the embolus will be increased by the N_2O and may make the animal more refractory to treatment. Muscle relaxants may be used to improve relaxation of the abdominal wall and thereby decrease the intra-abdominal pressure required to maintain adequate visualization of abdominal structures.

THE LIVER

Hepatic circulation and volatile anaesthetics

Volatile anaesthetics affect the liver principally through changes in the circulation. All currently available volatile agents decrease cardiac output and reduce liver blood flow in proportion to systemic arterial pressure. All volatile anaesthetics undergo some metabolism in the liver, and metabolites have been shown in urine for many weeks after general anaesthesia. In humans, the detrimental effects on circulation and the presence of metabolites that are potentially hepatotoxic have been

claimed as the basis of postanaesthetic hepatitis. Also in humans, there have been case reports of postanaesthetic hepatitis after exposure to enflurane, isoflurane (Sinha et al., 1996) and sevoflurane. It is unclear, however, how these drugs cause hepatitis. Halothane hepatitis in humans is thought to result from an immune-mediated response to halothane metabolites, and perhaps some genetic factor (Elliott and Strunin, 1993). At present there are no means of predicting susceptible individuals. Comparative studies of halothane, enflurane, sevoflurane, desflurane and isoflurane suggest that isoflurane, sevoflurane and desflurane may be the agents of choice in patients with liver disease, since they have the least effect on hepatic circulation (Merin et al., 1991; Frink et al., 1992). There are case reports of hepatic damage in dogs after the use of both halothane and methoxyflurane (Ndiritu and Weigel, 1977; Gaunt et al., 1984), although the case reports associated with halothane provide weak evidence for the involvement of this drug. It would be prudent to use isoflurane, desflurane or sevoflurane in animals with a history of liver disease. The effects of these agents on the circulation through the liver may be less pronounced than the other agents, the amount metabolized is small and there are no case reports of hepatitis after isoflurane administration in small animals. Sevoflurane has the potential to be hepatotoxic via the production of Compound A (a breakdown product of sevoflurane when it comes into contact with soda lime or baralyme). However, the concentrations of Compound A reached in circle systems while running at least 2 l/min of oxygen are unlikely to reach toxic values.

Anaesthesia for surgical correction of portosystemic shunt

The liver plays an important role in many functions within the body, e.g. protein, lipid and carbohydrate metabolism, production of plasma proteins, clotting factors and also the metabolism and excretion of drugs. Animals with portosystemic shunts (PSSs) tend to have increased total bilirubin, bile acids and fasting ammonia concentrations, white blood cell count and hepatic enzymes (alkaline phosphatase (AP), aspartate transaminase (AST), alanine aminotransferase (ALT)). In some cases such animals may have prolonged bleeding times, although this is not common. They tend to have decreased urea, blood glucose and TP concentrations and PCV, often with especially low albumin values. Dogs and cats with PSS are also prone to hepatic encephalopathy, which may manifest as anything from mild depression to coma. When dealing with these cases, it is important to prepare them for surgery so that medical management minimizes the signs of hepatic encephalopathy if possible. The postoperative progression of neurological signs (especially seizures) may contribute to a negative outcome. Medical management may include a low protein diet (with an increased ratio of branched chain to aromatic amino acids), lactulose and antibiotics. This therapy may be able to control the hepatic encephalopathy by reducing the production of ammonia and other putative toxins such as mercaptans. Therapy with branched chain amino acids may help to restore normal neurotransmitter function in the brain.

Central depressant drugs may have an exaggerated response in patients with hepatic disease. Increased cerebral sensitivity results from an increase in the number of central γ-aminobutyric acid (GABA) receptors during chronic liver failure. Hepatic dysfunction results in a decrease in the ability of the liver to metabolize and inactivate drugs. A reduction in plasma proteins means that the volume of distribution of drugs that bind to albumin is reduced. A decrease in the volume of distribution can lead to a relative drug overdose. The clearance of drugs with a high hepatic extraction ratio is affected by reductions in hepatic blood flow, which occurs in PSS and cirrhosis.

Preoperatively, the analysis of the biochemical profile and haematology should indicate whether it is likely that intraoperative colloids and/or blood products will be needed. Animals with intrahepatic shunts are more likely to lose blood during the surgery, and a cross match should be done for whole blood or packed red cells. It is important that the available blood should be relatively fresh (<1 week old) since ammonia concentrations increase with storage time, and the administration of more ammonia to these patients may compromise the neurological outcome. Similarly, plasma products that are used should be fresh or fresh frozen to reduce the ammonia burden given to the patient. Brain ammonia concentrations may be increased with an alkalosis, so it is important not to hyperventilate these patients.

As these animals have a poorly developed liver with abnormal circulation, it is preferable to avoid using drugs that require extensive metabolism or, alternatively, to use agents that may be reversed. Studies looking at several opioid analgesics indicate that these agents have little or no adverse effects on the liver. The actions of these agents may be enhanced in patients with hepatic dysfunction due to increased cerebral sensitivity and an increase in the unbound fraction of the drug. Opioids generally provide good cardiovascular stability, but intravenous morphine administration in dogs is known to cause histamine release. In this species, histamine leads to spasm of the hepatic vein, which results in hepatic congestion. Opioids are metabolized in the liver, and their effects may be prolonged in animals with PSS. However, in the only pharmacokinetic study of an opioid (pethidine (meperidine)) in these patients, there was no ability to predict which patients would have an altered pharmacokinetic profile (Waterman and Kalthum, 1990). Opioids can also cause a significant reduction in urine output as a result of release of antidiuretic hormone, although this may be balanced by their attenuation of the stress response.

Premedication with an opioid and atropine is appropriate. Young animals seem to be sedated well with low doses of opioids. The use of phenothiazine tranquillizers is not recommended, in part due to their relatively long duration of action, their effect on systemic blood pressure and their tendency to lower the seizure threshold. In humans, chronic doses of phenothiazines have been shown to produce hepatic injury. In rare cases, jaundice has developed after a single dose of a phenothiazine tranquillizer. The mechanism is thought to be a result of sensitivity to the drug, and the jaundice produced is attributed to cholestasis. Butyrophenones are less likely to induce hepatic injury in humans than phenothiazines, but these drugs often have a longer duration of action than the phenothiazines and also need to be metabolized in the liver. The use of α_2-agonists is not recommended due to the profound cardiovascular effects of these drugs.

Anaesthesia can be induced with either propofol or isoflurane in oxygen, delivered via a face mask, the animal intubated and anaesthesia maintained with isoflurane. Thiopentone may result in prolonged recoveries, and while ketamine has been used in these cases, it is not ideal because of the CNS side effects produced and because it is generally given with a benzodiazepine. Benzodiazepines should probably be avoided since endogenous benzodiazepine-like substances have been implicated in the pathogenesis of hepatic encephalopathy. Isoflurane is the inhalant of choice in patients with hepatic disease, as there is minimal hepatic metabolism and it causes minimal change in hepatic blood flow. Sevoflurane and desflurane also cause minimal change in hepatic blood flow and may be useful for these cases. The use of a mask induction obviates the need for parenteral anaesthetic agents with the necessity of hepatic metabolism. Isoflurane is relatively insoluble, and therefore induction of anaesthesia is rapid. These patients are often hypotensive even at light levels of anaesthesia, and therefore it is helpful to use a balanced technique. The use of neuromuscular blocking agents provides good muscle relaxation without the need for high vaporizer settings. Atracurium is the neuromuscular blocking agent of choice as it undergoes Hofmann elimination – that is, the molecule breaks down spontaneously at normal pH and body temperature and therefore does not rely on hepatic metabolism.

A peripheral intravenous catheter is placed before induction of anaesthesia to allow the administration of intravenous fluids. If the animal has a TP value <50 g/l, a colloid (hetastarch or polygelatins) or fresh frozen plasma at 5 ml/kg/h can be administered throughout anaesthesia. This provides volume support, helps to maintain plasma oncotic pressure and also allows administration of clotting factors if fresh frozen plasma is used. It is not routine to run clotting profiles on these patients before anaesthesia, although they may be deficient in these factors due to impaired liver function. If necessary, a second intravenous catheter may be placed either peripherally or centrally. A central venous catheter allows measurement of CVP, which may be of use in deciding on whether to partially or totally occlude the shunt. If the CVP decreases rapidly by 2-4 cmH$_2$O when the shunt is temporarily occluded it may suggest a failure of venous return because of underdeveloped hepatic vasculature (Swalec and Smeak, 1990). A partial occlusion or use of an ameroid ring may be preferable in these cases. In order to be able to measure CVP and use the line for venous access, a multilumen catheter is preferable. A CVP catheter can also be used postoperatively when small peripheral catheters might have clots or be pulled out.

Blood pressure should be monitored in these patients because they often become hypotensive – 59% in one series of cases (Forsyth and Ilkiw, personal communication). This can be done using an indirect technique such as a Doppler probe, or preferably using a direct technique with an arterial catheter. The dorsal pedal artery is used most commonly but radial, auricular and lingual arteries can also be catheterized percutaneously. Monitoring direct arterial blood pressure allows rapid changes in pressure to be observed, and this is particularly useful when the shunt is being ligated. Arterial lines also provide a means of obtaining samples for blood gas analysis. Packed cell volume and TP can be monitored during the procedure. Although blood loss is not common with extrahepatic PSS, it is more likely with intrahepatic shunts. Blood glucose is measured after the induction of anaesthesia, and hypoglycaemia is treated by administration of 5% dextrose in the intravenous fluids. A peripheral nerve stimulator can be placed before draping if neuromuscular blocking agents are to be administered.

Monitoring body temperature is important in small patients, as they have a large surface area to volume ratio and readily lose body heat both as a result of the surgical preparation and the open abdominal cavity. In one study a decreased body temperature at the time of recovery was associated with a poor prognosis (Bostwick and Twedt, 1995). The authors maintain temperature using warm water blankets underneath, and hot air blankets over, the patient. The hot air blankets can be trimmed to fit the patient or even draped over the patient with a hole cut over the surgical site. These blankets are extremely effective at maintaining and/or increasing body temperature. It is important to ensure that the warm air is flowing into the blanket. Application of the heated air directly on to the skin for prolonged periods can result in injury.

Postoperative analgesia can be provided by the use of parenterally administered opioids and also via administration of extradural morphine. Lumbosacral extradural morphine injection is ususaly performed after the induction of anaesthesia. Preservative-free morphine is given at 0.1 mg/kg, diluted to a volume of 0.3 ml/kg, with a maximum volume of 6 ml. Despite the fact that surgery is generally via a cranial abdominal approach, the use of lumbosacral extradural morphine seems to provide appreciable postoperative pain relief. Some clinicians have expressed concern that the provision of good postoperative analgesia masks the signs associated with portal hypertension or intra-abdominal haemorrhage, but in the authors' experience this has not been the case.

These individuals require careful postoperative monitoring for 24–48 hours due to the risk of portal hypertension after ligation of the shunt vessel; with the advent of the ameroid ring, the likelihood of this serious complication is somewhat reduced since the shunt vessel is gradually occluded over a number of days to weeks. Seizures may also occur postoperatively; these are generally refractory to the normal methods of treatment. The aetiology of these seizures is presently unclear. It has been proposed that the signs of hepatic encephalopathy are due to the presence of endogenous benzodiazepine ligands which act within the CNS. Seizures may result from a reversal of the anticonvulsant effects of the benzodiazepines or from a severe benzodiazepine withdrawal syndrome. If the presence of a shunt leads to stimulation of brain receptors for benzodiazepines, post-shunt ligation seizures may result from a withdrawal of the endogenous benzodiazepine after the shunt is ligated (Aronson *et al.*, 1997).

Liver biopsy

Liver biopsy can be performed using a Trucut needle rather than via laparotomy. This procedure is facilitated by the use of ultrasound imaging to identify the hepatic tissue. The use of pethidine has been advocated in these patients because it reduces the tendency of animals to pant. If the patient cannot be adequately restrained using intramuscular pethidine it may be necessary to use a drug such as propofol. This is mainly metabolized in the liver, although other sites may be involved (e.g. kidney), and even in severe hepatic disease recovery seems to be rapid. Another advantage of this drug is that it can be given in small doses to induce chemical restraint without having to anaesthetize the animal. Typically, it can be titrated to calm the animal without complete loss of consciousness – doses in the range of 1–2 mg/kg often work for this purpose. If this is not feasible, for example, with a cat that is difficult to restrain to obtain an intravenous access, it may be necessary to use a mask or box induction with isoflurane, sevoflurane or desflurane. Once the animal is restrained (and not panting) it is easier for the ultrasonographer to view the biopsy needle as it enters the liver lobe.

Haemorrhage is a major risk of biopsy, and it is important to image the liver after the biopsy procedure to assess whether significant haemorrhage has occurred. Liver biopsy should only be performed if the clotting times and platelet numbers are normal.

Anaesthesia for conditions of the gallbladder and biliary tract

Morphine has been shown to cause constriction of the sphincter of Oddi with an associated increase in pressure within the common bile duct. The pressure may increase 10-fold with a duration of effect of 2 or more hours. For this reason morphine is contraindicated in patients with conditions of the gallbladder and biliary tract. Pethidine and fentanyl, which have both been recommended for use in these patients, may also increase constriction at the sphincter of Oddi and so may not be desirable, although pressures in the bile duct do not increase as much as with morphine. Pentazocine also increases sphincter constriction, but nalbuphine and buprenorphine seem to have minimal effect (Isenhower and Mueller, 1998). Butorphanol increases the pressure more than nalbuphine but less than fentanyl (McCammon et al., 1984).

Biliary tract disease resulting in cholestasis can impair absorption of fat-soluble vitamins such as vitamin K. If the disease has been present for some time this may result in a prolonged prothrombin time. For this reason it may be advisable to measure clotting times before surgery, or simply to supplement with parenteral vitamin K to restore the prothrombin time to normal. Treatment can require 24–48 hours of repeated intramuscular injections to be effective. If surgery needs to be performed sooner, the use of fresh frozen plasma should be considered in order to replace factors II, VII, IX and X.

PANCREATIC DISEASE

Animals presented for removal of an insulinoma have few major considerations, but care needs to be taken in the regulation of glucose concentrations (see Chapter 19). These animals are used to having low blood sugars, and so no attempt should be made to restore the value to normal until the tumour has been removed. If a large bolus of glucose is given, it may stimulate further release of insulin with a resultant hypoglycaemia. Patients with insulinoma are often put on 2.5% dextrose overnight once they have been taken off food. It is important to monitor blood glucose concentrations frequently in the perioperative period since hypoglycaemia or hyperglycaemia may develop. Hypogylcaemia is more dangerous because of its effects on the CNS. Intravenous infusion of 2.5–5% dextrose can be administered to treat hypoglycaemia. Hyperglycaemia is deleterious because hyperosmolar coma and ketoacidosis may occur. A hyperglycaemic response may be seen after successful tumour resection. Hyperglycaemia is treated with insulin until euglycaemic levels are restored.

Premedication of these patients may include an opioid and an anticholinergic drug. The opioids do not affect blood glucose concentrations. Increases in plasma amylase and lipase have been recorded in humans after the administration of morphine. This is believed to result from the spasm of the sphincter of Oddi. However, in dogs the bile duct is separate from the pancreatic ducts so this is not a concern, although it may affect cats, where 80% have a single pancreatic duct joined to the bile duct and the sphincter of Oddi. Nalbuphine, buprenorphine or butorphanol would be the best choices for cats.

Any of the commonly used induction agents would be satisfactory, with the possible exception of propofol. There is concern regarding the use of propofol and the development of pancreatitis postoperatively. Acute pancreatitis has been reported to occur after anaesthesia in a few human patients where propofol had been used for induction (Wingfield, 1996). It is unclear whether or not these patients had pre-existing subclinical pancreatitis or if their pancreatitis was related to propofol. The lipid component of the emulsion may predispose to hyperlipidaemia. Triglyceride concentrations were increased in patients on prolonged propofol infusions. Propofol also inhibits nitric oxide synthase, which is hypothesized to contribute to the association between propofol and acute pancreatitis. There is one report of a human patient developing pancreatitis after prolonged propofol infusion (9 weeks) resulting in severe hypertriglyceridaemia (Metkus et al., 1996). At the present time it is unclear exactly what the relationship is between the use of propofol and the occurrence of pancreatitis, although it is unlikely that an induction dose of propofol will contribute significantly to the risk of pancreatitis.

In these individuals it may be beneficial to place a single or multi-lumen central catheter during anaesthesia. This allows blood samples to be collected for measurement of blood glucose concentrations, and also provides access to a central vein for the administration of total parenteral nutrition (TPN) should the need arise.

In cases of acute pancreatitis the indications for immediate surgical intervention are limited. However, some of these cases undergo laparotomy as part of the diagnosis, and it may not be realized until the time of laparotomy that the prime cause of the condition is pancreatitis. The anaesthetic regimen described above would be appropriate for such cases. While hypocalcaemia is a rare complication associated with pancreatitis, it is necessary to measure calcium concentrations before anaesthesia. Hypoglycaemia is relatively common with severe pancreatitis, so this should be checked and treated if present (Hess et al., 1998). Postoperatively the animal must be kept off food to allow the pancreas to 'rest', and fluid therapy must be managed with care to ensure that the animal does not become hypokalaemic. Some of these patients have been placed on TPN while they are unable to eat normally. This will reduce the effects of a negative nitrogen balance, but recent investigations suggest that certain well defined diets given through feeding tubes may preclude the use of this approach. Animals with pancreatitis are often in pain and they may not respond well to standard opioid therapy. To further improve analgesia an extradural catheter can be placed at the time of surgery. Analgesia can then be provided using morphine (15 μg/kg/h) and/or a dilute solution of bupivacaine (0.1–0.2% at 35 μg/kg/h). If the latter is titrated carefully, it is possible to get a sensory block with minimal effect on motor function in some animals.

THE ACUTE ABDOMEN

These patients are often haemodynamically unstable and in pain. It is useful to the anaesthetist to obtain as much information about the metabolic status of the patient before surgery, and also to try and stabilize these individuals before surgery. Depending on the time of day that an animal arrives, laboratory facilities may be limited. However, it should be possible to obtain a PCV and TP concentration at the very least. Blood glucose and urea concentrations should be measured, and also electrolytes and blood gases if feasible.

An abdominal tap can give information regarding the nature of fluid within the abdomen, e.g. haemo-abdomen or septic abdomen. This may be important in deciding what form of fluid therapy to use or whether the animal's blood needs to be cross matched. An activated clotting time (ACT) gives some information about the intrinsic and common pathways of the clotting cascade. A prolonged ACT may indicate that plasma is required to treat a coagulation defect. This may be useful in the case of a septic abdomen where there is a risk of disseminated intravascular coagulation. Assay of the buccal mucosal bleeding time may be indicated to assess platelet function before surgery. Extensive blood loss can lead to a decrease in platelet numbers and clotting factors and may be an indication for the use of fresh whole blood as a means of volume support.

Preoperative stabilization requires the administration of fluids to restore circulating blood volume. This is often performed with crystalloids initially. Low TP concentrations and/or a low colloid oncotic pressure can indicate the need for colloid administration.

An animal with a septic abdomen requires rapid attention in order to repair and remove the source of the sepsis or endotoxaemia. However, there is usually time to stabilize the patient before going to surgery. In some cases of haemoabdomen there may be little time to do anything if the patient is to survive. There has been considerable debate as to when a haemoabdomen should be explored – some clinicians believe that it is never appropriate, while others think that most of them should be explored surgically. The clinical signs that determine when it is necessary to do a laparotomy are not easy to define. This has been made harder with

recent evidence from humans suggesting that fluid resuscitation should be limited in patients with major vessel trauma since it tends to increase the egress of blood, making abdominal tamponade more likely and making it more difficult to find the lesion. Even if it is decided to take the animal directly to surgery with minimal resuscitation, it is essential to obtain adequate venous access so that fluids can be given rapidly once the bleeding has been controlled. In cats, and dogs weighing <5 kg, it is usually feasible to place an 18 G catheter into a jugular vein. In most dogs weighing between 5 and 15 kg it is feasible to place a 16 G catheter in a cephalic vein, while in dogs weighing >15 kg access with a 14 G catheter is normally attainable.

Anaesthesia for these patients should take into account the physical status of the patient at the time of preanaesthetic evaluation. Many of these animals do not require premedication because of the depression associated with the condition. If premedication is deemed to be helpful (some sedation is required or a pre-emptive analgesic effect is needed), then the opioids have proved to be most useful under these conditions. The dose should be tailored to the condition of the animal. Induction is carried out using either an opioid technique (dog) or etomidate (dog or cat), with careful titration of the dose. With opioid induction, it is sometimes helpful to spray the larynx with lignocaine to facilitate intubation. Maintenance involves the use of the minimum amount of inhalant, together with other drugs. Nitrous oxide can be used as long as there is no significant risk of hypoxaemia associated with the condition. Small doses of opioids may be used to supplement the inhalant. These can be given by intermittent injection or by a continuous infusion. If intermittent injection is used, the subsequent doses should be tailored to the pharmacokinetics of the drug and the response of the patient. Ketamine may also be used to supplement anaesthesia in these cases, but care must be taken since it is possible that significant depression of cardiac function may occur in animals with minimal sympathetic reserve – these animals already have high sympathetic activity, so they are likely to have little reserve. The authors do not have enough experience with this technique to recommend appropriate doses.

Since these animals are haemodynamically unstable, the monitoring of blood pressure is critical. The use of direct arterial monitoring is preferable to indirect monitoring because it can be carried out continuously and can provide moment-to-moment feedback on therapy. Monitoring of CVP and/or pulmonary vascular pressures will add useful information in the management of these cases, but care must be taken not to spend too long on attaching monitors to an animal that can only be saved by rapid surgical intervention. The maintenance of body temperature is also important in these patients. Hypothermia can be associated with coagulopathies, cardiac arrhythmias, delayed recovery and shivering during recovery, which may use up much needed metabolic resources. Keeping these animals warm is not easy because they often have abdominal viscera exposed and are receiving fluids that are usually at room temperature or lower, if blood products are being used. The anaesthetist should be aggressive in trying to get the fluids warmed to body temperature to avoid this effect. This can be as simple as passing the fluid line through a beaker of warm (41–42°C) water or using purpose-built equipment for warming fluids. Methods that warm the fluid as near to the patient as possible, and which can cope with rapid rates of infusion, are preferred. In humans, the concern with hypothermia is so great that, in surgery for damage control, one of the main aims of delaying the definitive surgery is to ensure that the patient is normothermic at the time of reoperation.

REFERENCES

Aronson L, Gacad R, Kaminsky-Russ K, Gregory C and Mullen K (1997) Endogenous benzodiazepine activity in the peripheral and portal blood of dogs with congenital portosystemic shunts. *Veterinary Surgery* **26**, 189–194

Bostwick DR and Twedt DC (1995) Intrahepatic and extrahepatic portal venous anomalies in dogs: 52 cases (1982–1992). *Journal of the American Veterinary Medical Association* **206**, 1181–1185

Caulkett NA, Cantwell SA and Houston DM (1998) A comparison of indirect blood pressure techniques in the anesthetized cat. *Veterinary Surgery* **27**, 370–377

Donaldson LL, Leib MS, Boyd C, Burkholder W and Sheridan M (1993) Effect of preanesthetic medication on ease of endoscopic intubation of the duodenum in anesthetized dogs. *American Journal of Veterinary Research* **54**, 1489–1495

Dyson D (1997) Assessment of 3 audible monitors during hypotension in anesthetized dogs. *Canadian Veterinary Journal* **38**, 564–566

Elliott R and Strunin L (1993) Hepatotoxicity of volatile anaesthetics. *British Journal of Anaesthesia* **70**, 339–348

Frink EJJ, Morgan SE, Coetzee A, Conzen PF and Brown BRJ (1992) The effects of sevoflurane, halothane, enflurane, and isoflurane on hepatic blood flow and oxygenation in chronically instrumented Greyhound dogs. *Anesthesiology* **76**, 85–90

Galatos AD and Raptopoulos D (1995a) Gastro-oesophageal reflux during anaesthesia in the dog: the effect of preoperative fasting and premedication. *Veterinary Record* **137**, 479–483

Galatos AD and Raptopoulos D (1995b) Gastro-oesophageal reflux during anaesthesia in the dog: the effect of age, positioning and type of surgical procedure. *Veterinary Record* **137**, 513–516

Gaunt PS, Meuten DJ and Pecquet-Goad ME (1984) Hepatic necrosis associated with use of halothane in a dog. *Journal of the American Veterinary Medical Association* **184**, 478–480

Gilroy BA and Anson LW (1987) Fatal air embolism during anesthesia for laparoscopy in a dog. *Journal of the American Veterinary Medical Association* **190**, 552–554

Hashim MA and Waterman AE (1991) Effects of thiopentone, propofol, alphaxolone-alphadolone, ketamine and xylazine-ketamine on lower oesophageal sphincter pressure and barrier pressure in cats. *Veterinary Record* **129**, 137–139

Hess RS, Saunders HM, Van Winkle TJ, Schofer FS and Washabau RJ (1998) Clinical, clinicopathologic, radiographic, and ultrasonographic abnormalities in dogs with fatal acute pancreatitis: 70 cases (1986–1995). *Journal of the American Veterinary Medical Association* **213**, 665–670

Isenhower H and Mueller B (1998) Selection of narcotic analgesics for pain associated with pancreatitis. *American Journal of Health-System Pharmacy* **55**, 480–486

Ishizaki Y, Bandai Y, Shimomura K, Abe H, Ohtomo Y and Idezuki Y (1993) Safe intraabdominal pressure of carbon dioxide pneumoperitoneum during laparoscopic surgery. *Surgery* **114**, 549–554

McCammon RL, Stoelting RK and Madura JA (1984) Effects of butorphanol, nalbuphine, and fentanyl on intrabiliary tract dynamics. *Anesthesia and Analgesia* **63**, 139–142

Merin RG, Bernard JM, Doursout MF, Cohen M and Chelly JE (1991) Comparison of the effects of isoflurane and desflurane on cardiovascular dynamics and regional blood flow in the chronically instrumented dog. *Anesthesiology* **74**, 568–574

Metkus AP, Trabulsy PP, Schlobohm RS and Hickey MS (1996) A firefighter with pancreatitis. *Lancet* **348**, 1702

Muir W and Bonagura J (1984) Treatment of cardiac arrhythmias in dogs with gastric distention-volvulus. *Journal of the American Veterinary Medical Association* **184**, 1366–1371

Muir W and Lipowitz A (1978) Cardiac dysrhythmias associated with gastric dilatation-volvulus in the dog. *Journal of the American Veterinary Medical Association* **172**, 683–689

Ndiritu CG and Weigel J (1977) Hepatorenal injury in a dog associated with methoxyflurane (a case report). *Veterinary Medicine: Small Animal Clinician* 545–550

Raptopoulos D and Galatos AD (1997) Gastro-oesophageal reflux during anaesthesia induced either with thiopentone or propofol in the dog. *Journal of Veterinary Anaesthesia* **24**, 20–22

Sinha A, Clatch R, Stuck G, Blumenthal S and Patel S (1996) Isoflurane hepatotoxicity: a case report and review of the literature. *American Journal of Gastroenterology* **91**, 2406–2409

Strombeck DR and Guilford WG (1996) Pharynx and esophagus: normal structure and function. In: *Strombeck's Small Animal Gastroenterology, 3rd edn*, pp. 202–210. WB Saunders, Philadelphia

Swalec KM and Smeak DD (1990) Partial versus complete attenuation of single portosystemic shunts. *Veterinary Surgery* **19**, 406–411

Waterman AE and Hashim MA (1992) Effects of thiopentone and propofol on lower oesophageal sphincter and barrier pressure in the dog. *Journal of Small Animal Practice* **33**, 530–533

Waterman AE and Kalthum W (1990) The effect of clinical hepatic disease on the distribution and elimination of pethidine adminstered post-operatively to dogs. *Journal of Veterinary Pharmacology and Therapeutics* **13**, 137–147

Weyrauch E and Willard M (1998) Esophagitis and benign esophageal strictures. *Compendium on Continuing Education for the Practicing Veterinarian* **20**, 203

Wingfield TW (1996) Pancreatitis after propofol administration: Is there a relationship? *Anesthesiology* **84**, 236

CHAPTER SEVENTEEN

Urogenital Disease

Avril E. Waterman-Pearson

INTRODUCTION

Three main factors need to be considered when anaesthetizing patients with urinary tract disease. These are:

· The effect of drugs on renal function
· The effect of renal disease on drug metabolism
· Fluid and electrolyte balance.

The kidneys normally receive about 25% of cardiac output. The glomerular filtration rate (GFR) is usually about 20% of the renal plasma flow (RPF). For each 100 ml of glomerular filtrate, approximately 1 ml appears as urine. The kidneys regulate water and electrolyte balance and excrete hydrogen ions and nitrogenous waste products (urea and creatinine). The excretion of nitrogenous waste products is the least important function with regard to anaesthesia.

ANAESTHESIA AND RENAL FUNCTION

In the conscious animal, autoregulation of renal blood flow (RBF) occurs between mean arterial blood pressures of 80–180 mmHg, i.e. RBF is independent of blood pressure in this range. In hypovolaemic states, however, RBF may decrease more than blood pressure as a result of renal vasoconstriction. If hypovolaemia is corrected quickly (<4 hours), renal vasoconstriction wears off rapidly. If correction is delayed, the vasoconstriction can persist for several days. During general anaesthesia, however, this mechanism is obtunded and once circulating volume is restored, vasoconstriction abates rapidly.

Agents used for general anaesthesia cause functional disturbances rather than direct nephrotoxic effects. The exception to this is methoxyflurane. This does have specific nephrotoxic effects in humans as a result of its metabolism, which yields free fluoride ions. There are, however, few well documented cases of methoxyflurane-related renal failure in dogs.

Anaesthetic agents reduce RBF and therefore GFR by causing arterial hypotension. Pre-existing hypovolaemia will clearly exacerbate these effects. The effect is proportional to the depth of anaesthesia, and at surgical planes of anaesthesia RBF may be decreased by 45%. Nitrous oxide (N_2O), however, has a minimal effect on RBF.

Increased sympathetic tone also predisposes to renal vasoconstriction and reduced RBF, despite causing moderate rises in arterial blood pressure. This was particularly evident with old drugs such as ether and cyclopropane, although thiopentone also tends to cause some afferent arteriolar constriction, but the effect is less marked. Inadequate depth of anaesthesia, hypoxia and hypercapnia can also increase sympathetic tone and produce a vasoconstrictive response. Renal vasoconstriction redirects blood flow away from cortical nephrons, and this may be associated with sodium retention.

The stress of surgery and anaesthetic drugs such as barbiturates and opioids (e.g. morphine) also induce the release of antidiuretic hormone (ADH), which promotes sodium and water retention postoperatively. Conversely, phenothiazines may reduce ADH secretion, which together with their vasodilating effect tend to induce the production of dilute urine.

The aims of the anaesthetist must therefore be to:

· Maintain normovolaemia
· Maintain an adequate depth of anaesthesia
· Avoid drugs that affect marginal renal function
· Avoid hypoxia and hypercapnia.

DRUGS AND RENAL DISEASE

Renal disease affects the pharmacological actions of drugs both directly and indirectly.

Uraemic animals have impaired levels of consciousness and require a smaller dose of anaesthetic than normal animals to achieve a given effect.

Metabolic acidosis frequently accompanies renal failure and affects renal excretion of drugs, especially weak acids (e.g. barbiturates). More importantly, by decreasing the degree of ionization of a weakly acidic drug, metabolic acidosis increases the active fraction of an injected dose.

Renal disease causes a decrease in plasma protein concentrations, which together with uraemia reduces protein binding of drugs. In uraemia, the percentage of barbiturate that is unbound often doubles (from around 28% to 56%).

Drugs that have active metabolites can also have unexpectedly prolonged effects in renal disease. This can affect drugs such as morphine (its metabolite being morphine-6-glucuronide), ketamine (norketamine) and diazepam (oxazepam).

Potassium (K^+) excretion may be impaired. If hyperkalaemia becomes severe, the deleterious effect on myocardial function reduces cardiac output, which has a marked indirect action on pharmacodynamics by altering the volume of distribution of any drugs administered.

Only non-lipid soluble drugs, which are active in an ionized form and are water soluble at physiological pH, are excreted unchanged in the urine. Examples include digoxin, gallamine, neostigmine, atropine and certain antibiotics (neomycin, tetracyclines). Most anaesthetic drugs undergo biotransformation and, as long as their metabolites are inactive, there is no significant prolongation of their action in renal disease. There are some drugs that are primarily excreted and they are probably best avoided in renal disease, e.g. pancuronium and phenobarbitone.

CASE MANAGEMENT

Two types of scenario are commonly encountered in small animal practice:

- Animals with an acute problem where anaesthesia is specifically required for correction of that problem
- Animals with chronic renal disease where anaesthesia is required for an unrelated problem. These animals may be coping with varying degrees of compensation.

It is absolutely vital to assess the degree of dysfunction. This is achieved by reference to the patient's history, clinical examination and laboratory tests, which not only provide information on the present state of the patient but also help to guide future treatment and provide assistance in assessing risk. Essential laboratory information includes:

- Blood urea, creatinine, [K^+] and pH
- Haematocrit and haemoglobin concentration
- Urinary specific gravity and an estimate of the volume of urine being produced.

The reason for anaesthesia is also a major consideration. Unless the surgery is life saving, an animal with renal problems should always be stabilized first.

Chronic renal failure

Either dehydration or overhydration may be present in chronic renal failure. Glomerular failure will cause a reduction in GFR, so that water is not delivered to the tubules and overhydration may result. In contrast, with pyelonephritis or obstructive disorders, GFR is normal but reabsorption fails and animals become dehydrated. Chronic renal failure may also cause:

- Hypertension and secondary cardiac failure, which can greatly reduce the animal's ability to tolerate general anaesthesia
- Increased capillary permeability, resulting in an increased urinary loss of protein, hypoproteinaemia and an increased risk of pulmonary oedema
- Chronic anaemia, which reduces the animal's tolerance to a reduction in tissue perfusion induced by anaesthetic drugs.

Elderly dogs and cats frequently suffer from some degree of renal impairment. They may require surgery for a variety of unrelated conditions, and the 'golden rule' is not to impair renal function further as a consequence of anaesthesia.

During anaesthesia the key is to maintain normal fluid balance, avoid any water deprivation, maintain normotension and ensure that there are no episodes of intense renal vasoconstriction. It is essential to perform a thorough preanaesthetic examination, paying particular attention to the cardiovascular and respiratory systems for signs of, for example, oedema, dyspnoea or hypertension. Preoperative assessment of urea, creatinine, K^+, haemoglobin and haematocrit are advisable in all elderly animals admitted, even for routine procedures. The placement of an intravenous catheter and fluid therapy during anaesthesia are mandatory (0.18% saline with 4% dextrose is suitable). Ideally, arterial blood pressure should be monitored. Fluid administration may need to be rapid (10–15 ml/kg/h) to support blood pressure.

It is important to maintain adequate levels of anaesthesia and to avoid drugs that cause sympathetic stimulation and renal vasoconstriction. Therefore, drugs such as ketamine and α_2- adrenoceptor agonists should be avoided.

Non-steroidal anti-inflammatory drugs (NSAIDs) that block the normal renal protective response to hypotension are also best avoided preoperatively. Carprofen, which has only very weak cyclo-oxygenase inhibitory activity, seems to be the safest drug in this respect.

Renal failure also produces a tendency to glucose intolerance, and fructose or sorbitol are preferable sources of calories in these patients.

Anaesthetic technique

Good oxygenation is essential. Premedication may be best avoided if the degree of renal function is severe;

otherwise an opioid such as pethidine will provide both sedation and analgesia. If possible, preoxygenation is beneficial. Induction should be carried out slowly; some dogs tolerate a mask induction with isoflurane in a 1:2 mixture of O_2/N_2O. However, most patients are best managed by the slow intravenous administration of propofol, which may be preceded by a low dose of midazolam (0.2 mg/kg) intravenously. The dose of propofol required may be considerably less than that needed in normal patients and this is a situation where it is essential to dose to effect. An initial dose of 1–2 mg/kg is often all that is required to allow application of a mask. If there is any evidence of anaemia, it is vital to give at least 50% oxygen during the procedure. Adequate ventilation is necessary to maintain normocapnia and intermittent positive-pressure ventilation (IPPV; facilitated by non-depolarizing neuromuscular blockade) may be required to achieve this.

Acute renal failure

If acute renal failure is prerenal (due to hypovolaemia), the animal's condition can usually be rectified by judicious use of fluid therapy. Primary drug- or toxin-induced renal tubular damage is less common and these animals are rarely presented for anaesthesia.

Postrenal failure

These cases are acute emergencies and require sedation or anaesthesia in order to treat the primary cause. Postrenal failure occurs when urinary excretion is prevented, either as a result of traumatic injury to the urinary tract (ruptured ureter, bladder or urethra) or obstruction to outflow (usually due to urethral calculi, but occasionally as a result of nerve damage).

These patients will be suffering from potentially life-threatening metabolic derangements, including:

- Dehydration (as a result of impaired intake), vomiting and fluid shifts into the peritoneal cavity
- Hyperkalaemia, as renal excretion of K^+ is impaired
- Acidosis, as renal excretion of H^+ is impaired
- Uraemia.

Very occasionally, if vomiting is very severe, animals may become hypochloraemic, which can mask the metabolic acidosis and in some cases cause a metabolic alkalosis with a paradoxical hyperkalaemia. However, this is rare.

These metabolic derangements must be treated before anaesthesia and surgery are contemplated. Precipitous action may be fatal.

In addition to the metabolic changes, these animals will have reduced respiratory function because of physical restriction to diaphragmatic excursion by the distended abdomen. If drainage of urine is too rapid (as may occur at laparotomy), the sudden loss of pressure can lead to a dangerous reduction of peripheral vascular resistance, resulting in severe hypotension. It is therefore important to drain off accumulated urine slowly.

In cases where there is obstruction to outflow, secondary renal tubular damage may occur and these patients may suffer from postrelease polyuria. This can lead to continued dehydration unless treated.

Preanaesthetic treatment

Initial examination and assessment must include evaluation of the animal's metabolic status, by checking:

- Haematocrit
- Plasma electrolytes
- pH and bicarbonate ($[HCO_3^-]$), if possible.

If the acidosis is mild to moderate (base deficit 5–7 mmol/l), the lactate in Hartmann's solution is usually sufficient to correct the disorder when combined with other measures. More often, the base deficit is more severe (10–15 mmol/l) and additional HCO_3^- is required.

Hyperkalaemia is life threatening because serious cardiac dysrhythmias (atrioventricular blocks and cardiac arrest) frequently develop, exacerbated by the acidosis (plasma $[K^+]$ increases by 0.6 mmol/l for every 0.1 decrease in pH). It is unwise to anaesthetize a patient with a plasma $[K^+]$ >5.5 mmol/l for an elective procedure: concentrations >6.0 mmol/l are likely to be accompanied by dysrhythmias, and at >7 mmol/l there are profound electrocardiographic changes. Once plasma $[K^+]$ is >8 mmol/l, severe dysrhythmias and sudden cardiac arrest are serious possibilities, especially if arrhythmogenic drugs (e.g. halothane) are also used. At plasma $[K^+]$ >9 mmol/l, cardiac arrest can occur without warning, even without the complicating factor of anaesthesia.

The classic electrocardiographic changes seen with hyperkalaemia are helpful prognostic indicators of the efficacy of treatment (in the absence of real-time laboratory data). 'Peaking' of the T-wave occurs when $[K^+]$ reaches 7–8 mmol/l, the QRS complex widens at $[K^+]$ >8 mmol/l and at about the same time the P-wave is lost, leading to a biphasic pattern on the electrocardiogram (ECG).

Treatment of hyperkalaemia is essential before anaesthesia is contemplated. Fortunately most cases respond dramatically to the following measures:

- Intravenous administration of Hartmann's or dextrose saline with added bicarbonate (at a rate of 2.5 mmol/l)
- Slow drainage of accumulated urine from the abdomen
- Peritoneal dialysis/lavage with potassium-free fluid
- Urethral catheterization to reduce further leakage of urine into the peritoneum, if appropriate.

Severe cases may additionally require intravenous calcium to antagonize cardiac effects of K^+ (0.5 ml/kg of 10% calcium gluconate), and the administration of glucose and insulin to promote cellular uptake of K^+.

Anaesthetic technique

Premedication: Uraemia greatly increases sensitivity to anaesthetic drugs, and doses must be adjusted accordingly. Sedatives are helpful in smoothing induction and recovery and in reducing stress and therefore sympathetic tone. This decreases catecholamine release and exacerbation of myocardial irritability. Although phenothiazines have been used at very low doses in mild cases, it is probably safer to avoid them. Opioids provide good sedation and produce minimal cardiovascular depression. They may be used alone or in combination with low doses of benzodiazepines, which have the advantage of anticonvulsant activity – many very uraemic patients have a tendency to convulse. While the routine use of atropine has declined, many of these patients have a bradycardia, and addition of an anticholinergic to the premedication can be helpful.

Induction: Placement of an intravenous catheter is essential. The choice of induction agent is not critical, but the dose should be given slowly and to effect because the patient is likely to display an increased sensitivity to all agents, including barbiturates and propofol. In addition, circulation time is likely to be slow, so that rapid injection may lead to overdose. The situation is made worse by dehydration, metabolic acidosis and hypoproteinaemia. There is some merit in using a drug combination for induction. Propofol with an opioid (e.g. alfentanil) or a benzodiazepine (e.g. midazolam) works particularly well.

Inhalation induction of anaesthesia must be dealt with cautiously, although in extremes, isoflurane by mask at low concentrations can be sufficient to allow intubation.

Maintenance: It is vital to maximize the delivery of oxygen to the tissues, so a minimum inspired oxygen concentration of 50% is essential. The addition of N_2O allows the delivery of volatile agents to be reduced. Isoflurane, with its small arrhythmogenic effect, is the volatile agent of choice, although halothane is a relatively safe alternative. The inspired concentration of isoflurane can be minimized by the judicious use of short-acting intravenous opioids to provide analgesia (e.g. fentanyl or alfentanil).

Respiratory inadequacy leads to respiratory acidosis, increasing the risk of severe dysrhythmias and cardiovascular compromise. Respiratory minute volume must therefore be maintained by IPPV, if necessary. This may be facilitated by the use of non-depolarizing muscle relaxants, the most suitable of which are vecuronium and atracurium. With IPPV, careful attention must be paid to the respiratory pattern, so that venous return and cardiac output are not compromised.

Fluid therapy
A polyionic solution such as Hartmann's is the most appropriate choice (with added HCO_3^- if needed), at a rate of 10 ml/kg/h. If there is evidence of severe hypovolaemia (especially if the problem is traumatic in origin), a colloid will be the most effective way of restoring circulating blood volume and blood pressure.

Monitoring
In addition to vital functions such as pulse rate, mucous membrane colour and respiratory rate and pattern, these patients should ideally have arterial blood pressure monitored. Mean arterial blood pressure should be maintained above 70 mmHg to protect RBF and GFR. Also, because serious disturbances in cardiac rhythm are likely, an ECG is invaluable. It will provide prompt warning of severe dysrhythmias so that appropriate drug treatment can be given.

Real-time monitoring of plasma $[K^+]$ and acid–base status is also desirable in these cases if a stat analyser is available. This allows HCO_3^- administration to be titrated carefully, thus obviating any risk of over correction and the development of an iatrogenic alkalosis.

Recovery period
Careful and close monitoring is required well into the postoperative period. It is essential that urine output is maintained at least at a rate of 1 ml/kg/h. Fluid therapy should be continued for a minimum of 6–12 hours. Diuretics may need to be considered if urine production is inadequate, even when rehydration is complete. Plasma $[K^+]$, urea and $[HCO_3^-]$ require serial checks – hypokalaemia may develop after relief of an obstruction and may need attention.

In addition to these specific measures, the more general aspects of postoperative care – warmth, comfort and analgesia – should not be neglected.

THE GENITAL SYSTEM

Neutering procedures
Neutering procedures are the most frequent indications for anaesthesia in dogs and cats. Fortunately, these procedures are generally carried out on healthy young animals, and no special considerations apply beyond those that are applicable to any major surgical intervention.

Technically, ovariohysterectomy can be difficult in obese bitches. There is some merit in considering the use of drugs that provide some degree of muscle relaxation, either specific neuromuscular blocking agents or the intraoperative administration of low doses of a benzodiazepine, which certainly helps to provide muscle relaxation.

Pyometritis

This is a condition of mature bitches, most commonly over 6 years of age, although it is occasionally seen in younger animals. It is hormonally mediated, and animals vary in the severity of their clinical disease. It is much less common in cats and has a less distinct relation with oestrus. Ovariohysterectomy is the treatment of choice, and is routine provided the animal's cardiovascular status is normal.

Patients are usually dehydrated as a consequence of polyuria, vaginal discharge, vomiting and occasionally diarrhoea. Intravenous fluid therapy before anaesthesia is therefore essential, to at least correct the deficit in circulating blood volume that may be present. Occasionally such patients may be very sick, often associated with *Escherichia coli* infection and endotoxaemia. In this situation, colloids are often required in large volumes as well as other supportive measures before, during and after surgery.

Other conditions

Dogs may present with testicular tumours that have undergone torsion. These constitute surgical emergencies, and the major anaesthetic considerations relate to the presence of shock and also the intense pain that this condition causes. Careful attention should be paid to supporting the circulation and to using a combination of a potent opioid and an NSAID to provide analgesia.

Anaesthetic technique

The anaesthetic technique for animals with pyometritis or testicular torsion should avoid the use of sedative premedicants. The marked cardiovascular depression caused by α_2-adrenoceptor agonists is potentially life threatening. Phenothiazines are also best avoided because of their long duration and hypotensive effects. These patients are depressed, and a suitable dose of opioid is generally all that is required to calm the patient and provide pre-emptive analgesia.

During surgery, care should be taken to maintain adequate perfusion of vital organs and effective alveolar ventilation. If facilities are available, oxygen saturation (pulse oximetry), arterial blood pressure, and concentrations of expired carbon dioxide and inspired oxygen should be monitored. Anaesthesia should be maintained with a volatile agent (halothane or isoflurane) vaporized in at least 50% oxygen. Incremental analgesia may be provided by the administration of additional doses of a short-acting opioid during surgery and an NSAID such as carprofen (at the start of surgery) or ketoprofen (at the end of surgery).

FURTHER READING

Doyle PT and Briscoe CE (1976) The effect of drugs and anaesthetic agents on the urinary bladder and sphincters. *Journal of Urology* **48**, 329–335

Gibaldi M (1977) Drug distribution in renal failure. *American Journal of Medicine* **62**, 471–474

Kaufmann G Mc (1984) Renal function in the geriatric dog. *Compendium of Continuing Education* **6**, 1087–1095

Prescott LF (1972) Mechanisms of renal excretion of drugs (with special reference to drugs used by anaesthetists). *British Journal of Anaesthesia* **44**, 246–251

Reidensburg MM (1977) The biotransformation of drugs in renal failure. *American Journal of Medicine* **62**, 482–485

CHAPTER EIGHTEEN

Caesarian Section

Chris Seymour

INTRODUCTION

Caesarian section may be performed either electively or, more usually, as an emergency procedure for dystocia that is not amenable to medical treatment or fetal manipulation. Although most parturient animals are young and healthy, those requiring emergency surgery may present in an exhausted and debilitated condition. These patients are often brought to the clinic outside normal working hours, when veterinary and nursing resources may be stretched. These factors will affect the risks to the patient and will influence the type of anaesthetic technique selected.

The fundamental requirements of any anaesthetic technique for Caesarian section are the provision of adequate anaesthesia for the mother and minimal fetal depression. Anaesthetic drugs must cross the blood–brain barrier to exert an effect, but because they also cross the placental barrier to fetuses with equal ease, selective maternal depression is not possible. It is therefore important to maintain placental oxygen flux during anaesthesia so that maximum fetal viability is ensured.

APPLIED PHYSIOLOGY OF PREGNANCY

A number of physiological changes occur during pregnancy and parturition that are relevant to the anaesthetic management of the patient during Caesarian section.

- Both cardiac output and blood volume increase. Plasma volume may increase more than the increase in red cell mass, which causes a dilutional anaemia. The effect of the dilutional anaemia is reduced by the increase in cardiac output and also by a right shift in the haemoglobin dissociation curve, thereby increasing oxygen delivery to the tissues. The increase in blood volume enables the animal to tolerate better the blood losses at parturition. Blood is also returned to the circulation when the uterus involutes after delivery

- It is often stated that hypotension may occur when the animal is restrained in the supine position for surgery, as a result of compression of the aorta and vena cava by the enlarged uterus. This has, however, been questioned by Probst and Webb (1983), who showed that supine hypotension did not seem to occur in anaesthetized bitches at term. However, the animals studied were relatively small (between 9 kg and 16 kg)

- Cardiac reserve decreases, and heart failure can occur in animals with cardiac disease that were well compensated before pregnancy

- Both the minute volume of ventilation and oxygen consumption increase. Functional residual capacity (FRC), defined as the lung volume at the end of a normal expiration, is also reduced owing to cranial displacement of the diaphragm by the enlarged uterus. The reduced FRC, combined with the increase in oxygen consumption, means that periods of apnoea can cause rapid arterial haemoglobin desaturation. Preoxygenation by mask before induction of anaesthesia is therefore advisable. The decrease in FRC and the increased minute volume also speed equilibration between inspired and alveolar anaesthetic concentrations, making gaseous induction of anaesthesia faster

- The risk of vomiting and aspiration increases owing to pressure placed on the stomach by the gravid uterus. Increases in serum progesterone concentration slow gastric emptying and also reduce tone in the gastro-oesophageal sphincter. All patients should therefore be regarded as having a full stomach, regardless of when they last ate

- Renal blood flow and glomerular filtration rate increase, reducing serum urea and creatinine concentrations. A mild decrease in serum albumin concentration occurs because of the increased blood volume

- Potency of inhalational anaesthetics increases, possibly as a result of the increase in serum progesterone concentrations

- Placental blood flow decreases in response to three main factors – hypotension, uterine contractions and vasoconstriction (which can occur as a result of sympathetic activation during light planes of general anaesthesia)
- Well oxygenated umbilical venous blood from the placenta normally has a low PO_2 of about 40 mmHg (5.3 kPa). To compensate for this, fetal haemoglobin has a greater affinity for oxygen (its dissociation curve is shifted to the left) than maternal haemoglobin. This results in greater haemoglobin oxygen saturation for any given PO_2, and increases fetal oxygen flux.

ANAESTHETIC TECHNIQUES

The technique selected depends on experience, facilities within the practice and the amount of assistance available.

Most drugs given to the mother diffuse across the placenta into the umbilical vein. From here, drugs pass to the fetal liver (where they may be metabolized) and the fetal vena cava via the ductus venosus, where they are diluted by blood returning from caudal parts of the body. To some extent, the fetal heart and brain are protected from perfusion with blood containing high concentrations of anaesthetic by these natural buffering mechanisms. In addition, drugs given as a single bolus and that are cleared rapidly from maternal blood, such as propofol, are only presented to the fetus in high concentrations for short periods. Other drugs given throughout the course of anaesthesia, such as the volatile agents, continuously cross the placenta along their concentration gradient. Care in the choice and administration of anaesthetic drugs is therefore vital if lively neonates are required. The techniques described below are summarized in Figure 18.1.

Extradural (epidural) anaesthesia

This technique is described in detail in Chapter 6. The advantages are that fetuses are not exposed to depressant general anaesthetic drugs and, because the mother stays conscious, the risks of vomiting and aspiration

Technique	Drugs used	Dose	Comments
Extradural (epidural) anaesthesia	Lignocaine 2% Bupivacaine 0.5% (Both drugs with or without 1:200,000 adrenaline)	1 ml/4.5 kg 1 ml/4.5 kg	Usual need for sedation limits the usefulness of the technique. More assistance required at a time when this may be limited. Lactated Ringer's solution given at a loading dose of 20 ml/kg to prevent hypotension
Neuroleptanalgesia	Etorphine hydrochloride/ methomeprazine (Immobilon SA) Diprenorphine hydrochloride (Revivon)	0.5 ml/5 kg i.m. 0.25 ml/kg i.v. Given at same doses as Immobilon SA. Pups given 0.1 ml Revivon at delivery	**Severe** respiratory and cardiovascular depression. Supplemental oxygen therapy during surgery strongly recommended. Only consider if no alternative available. **Do not use in cats**
General anaesthesia: Dogs	Pethidine Midazolam Propofol Halothane or isoflurane	1–2 mg/kg i.m. 0.1–0.2 mg/kg i.v. 4–6 mg/kg i.v. 1–2% either in 100% oxygen or in a 50:50 mixture of oxygen/ nitrous oxide	Method of choice in most cases. Intubation essential to protect airway from aspiration of vomitus. Lactated Ringer's solution throughout surgery at basal rate of 10 ml/kg/h
Cats	Pethidine *Either* propofol or alphaxolone/alphadolone Halothane or isoflurane	1–2 mg/kg i.m. 4–6 mg/kg i.v. 4–6 mg/kg i.v. 1–2% either in 100% oxygen or in a 50:50 mixture of oxygen/ nitrous oxide	Midazolam (0.2 mg/kg i.m.) and ketamine (5 mg/kg i.m.) given as premedication to cats will reduce doses of intravenous induction agents by at least 50%

Figure 18.1: Suggested protocols for anaesthesia in patients presenting for Caesarian section.

are reduced. Earlier introduction of neonates to the mother is also possible than when depressant anaesthesia is used. Relaxation of abdominal muscle is excellent. The disadvantages are that the technique is technically challenging, and the heavy sedation usually required in dogs and cats causes fetal depression. For this latter reason the advantages over general anaesthesia are greatly reduced. Local anaesthetics in the extradural space not only block pain fibres but also block fibres of the sympathetic nervous system as they emerge from the spinal cord, causing vasodilation. This results in hypotension and an increased tendency for surgical bleeding. Both these factors reduce placental blood flow and may cause fetal hypoxaemia.

Hypotension may be minimized by the infusion of lactated Ringer's solution at a loading dose of 20 ml/kg, given over a 20 minute period, preferably while performing the block. Fluids can then be continuously infused throughout the procedure at a basal rate of 10 ml/kg/hour. If facilities are available for measurement of arterial blood pressure, vasopressors may also be used to counteract hypotension. Ephedrine (0.025–0.05 mg/kg i.v.) is preferred because it does not cause uterine vasoconstriction.

Either lignocaine (lidocaine) 2% or bupivacaine 0.5% may be used. The use of preparations containing adrenaline (at a dilution of 1:200,000) will hasten the onset of block. Bupivacaine is theoretically preferable because its slower absorption into the circulation reduces fetal exposure. Lignocaine, however, has a faster onset of action (between 5 and 10 minutes), and the duration of block (about 2 hours), although shorter than that produced by bupivacaine, should be more than adequate for the procedure. Ropivacaine is a new amide local anaesthetic with a similar duration of action to bupivacaine, but with lower toxicity. Its use in animals is yet to be properly evaluated.

Occasionally local anaesthetic spreads more cranially than expected. This has been attributed to engorgement of epidural plexuses, pressure waves in the epidural plexuses associated with abdominal contractions, stenosis of intervertebral foramina or excessive epidural fat.

Cranial spread of local anaesthetic causes a loss of vascular tone in cranial segments and hence tends to cause hypotension. If such spread extends to the cranial thoracic spine, the sympathetic nerves responsible for maintaining heart rate may be blocked, causing bradycardia and exacerbating hypotension. The possibility of such side effects predicates careful monitoring of the cardiovascular system and easy availability of treatment for hypotension (e.g. plasma volume expanders and ephedrine).

Generally, a dose of local anaesthetic of 1 ml/4.5 kg injected into the extradural space at the lumbosacral junction produces analgesia sufficient for Caesarian section.

Neuroleptanalgesia

This technique refers to the administration of a tranquillizer in combination with a potent opioid. Although this method is rarely used as the primary anaesthetic technique, opioids in combination with acepromazine or benzodiazepines are often used in low doses to make handling easier and to reduce the dose of induction and maintenance anaesthetics.

The use of neuroleptanalgesics as primary anaesthetic agents may be a useful technique if there are no facilities for giving inhalational anaesthetics. The method is not, however, suitable for cats. Their use as a primary anaesthetic causes hypotension in the bitch, as well as severe respiratory depression in both the bitch and the puppies, which may not be fully reversed after giving opioid antagonists. Another disadvantage is that the bitch may move in response to loud noises.

The only commercially available neuroleptanalgesic mixture now licensed for use in dogs in the UK is one that contains 0.074 mg/ml etorphine hydrochloride and 18 mg/ml methotrimeprazine. The effects of etorphine may be antagonized by the administration of diprenorphine hydrochloride. The manufacturers recommend that when these drugs are used in parturient bitches, each puppy should be given 0.1 ml diprenorphine hydrochloride intramuscularly after delivery to counteract the depressant effects of etorphine.

Neuroleptanalgesia should be considered only if there is absolutely no alternative.

General anaesthesia

This is the method chosen for most patients, providing that facilities for giving inhalational agents are available. General anaesthesia is reliable and familiar and provides the best possible operating conditions.

Premedication

The degree of premedication required is determined by the condition of the animal on presentation.

Anticholinergic agents: The routine use of these drugs remains controversial. Advantages include reduction of salivation and prevention of excessive vagal tone when traction is applied to the uterus. They may, however, produce unwanted tachyarrhythmias and increase the possibility of reflux of gastric contents. Their use is probably best restricted to those cats receiving ketamine (as this drug can induce profuse salivation) and to the treatment of bradycardia. Glycopyrrolate (0.01 mg/kg i.m. or i.v.) is the preferred drug because its highly ionized molecule does not cross the placental barrier. It is also said to increase the pH of gastric contents, so that if aspiration of vomitus occurs, pulmonary damage is less severe.

Phenothiazines: These drugs (e.g. acepromazine) cause hypotension as a result of α_1-adrenergic blockade, thus reducing placental blood flow. They will also cross the placental barrier, inducing fetal depression. Their effects cannot be specifically antagonized, and their duration of action may be as long as 8 hours. Their use before Caesarian section is not advised, except perhaps in very nervous or aggressive dogs. In these circumstances the dose should not exceed 0.02–0.03 mg/kg.

Benzodiazepines: In dogs, midazolam may be given intravenously in small doses (0.1–0.2 mg/kg) just before the administration of an intravenous induction agent, which seems to smooth both induction and recovery from anaesthesia. If necessary, unwanted depression can be reversed with flumazenil, a specific benzodiazepine receptor antagonist. In fractious cats, midazolam may be given by intramuscular injection at a dose of 0.2 mg/kg in combination with ketamine at 5 mg/kg. Both drugs can be combined in the same syringe. Use of the combination reduces subsequent doses of intravenous induction agents by at least 50%.

α₂-Adrenergic agonists: These drugs (e.g. medetomidine) are powerful sedatives with desirable analgesic properties (particularly visceral analgesia). They often induce vomiting, which may be needed in the obstetric patient. They cause profound respiratory depression and bradycardia and their use is best avoided in parturient animals, even though specific receptor antagonists are available.

Analgesics: Provision of adequate analgesia for the mother is often a neglected area because of worries about respiratory depression in the neonates. All opioids readily cross the placenta but are safe to use in small doses before induction of anaesthesia. The author prefers the use of pethidine (meperidine) at a dose of 1–2 mg/kg in both dogs and cats. In dogs, morphine at a dose of 0.1–0.2 mg/kg has also been advocated because it induces vomiting in many cases and may ensure an empty stomach before induction of anaesthesia. In women, morphine is not used because neonates seem more sensitive to its respiratory depressant effects than they do to other opioids. Of the nonsteroidal anti-inflammatory drugs, carprofen is the only one licensed for preoperative use. It is not, however, recommended for use in pregnant animals and is best avoided in the obstetric situation.

Metoclopramide: This drug can be included in premedication at a dose of 0.2–0.4 mg/kg intramuscularly or intravenously. It acts as an anti-emetic and increases gastric motility. Cimetidine (5–10 mg/kg i.m. or i.v.) is an H₂-receptor antagonist and may also be given to increase gastric pH.

Induction
The decision whether to induce anaesthesia by volatile agents or by intravenous drugs will be determined partly by personal preference and also by the size, condition and temperament of the patient. Regardless of the method chosen, it is preferable to give oxygen via a face mask for 3–5 minutes before induction to prevent arterial desaturation should periods of apnoea occur, although in a large fractious dog this may not be possible. It is also advisable to insert an intravenous cannula, not only for immediate venous access, but also to enable fluids to be given as soon as the animal is asleep.

Inhalational induction: This is achieved by gradually introducing a volatile agent into the inspired gas mixture. Generally the carrier gas used is either 100% oxygen or a 50:50 mixture of oxygen/nitrous oxide. The gas is delivered through a face mask attached to an appropriate circuit such as an Ayre's T-piece (for cats and small dogs weighing up to 8 kg), Bain or circle system. It is vital that the correct flow rate for the selected circuit is used.

Either halothane or isoflurane can be used, although the latter is preferable because its lower solubility in blood results in faster induction and recovery. Hypovolaemic patients, however, may not tolerate its potent vasodilatory properties particularly well. It must be remembered that because of reduced FRC and increased minute volume of ventilation during pregnancy, gaseous induction is usually faster than normal, especially with the less soluble agents. Also, the increased potency of volatile agents at term means that lower inspired concentrations are usually needed to induce anaesthesia. With both halothane and isoflurane, concentrations greater than 2% only should be used and then with great care.

The main disadvantage of this method is that because loss of consciousness is slow, vomiting and aspiration may occur before endotracheal intubation can be achieved.

Intravenous induction: This has the advantage that loss of consciousness is rapid, and the airway may be secured immediately.

- Propofol, at a dose of 4–6 mg/kg, is the drug of choice because of rapid recovery. Experience suggests that slower administration (>20 seconds) reduces both the dose required and the incidence of apnoea. Propofol crosses the placenta readily, but because plasma clearance is rapid, the fetus is exposed to high concentrations for only a relatively short period
- Alphaxolone/alphadolone may also be used safely in cats because it too undergoes rapid clearance from the circulation. Doses of 4–6 mg/kg produce minimal respiratory depression. The disadvantage is the possibility of hypersensitivity reactions developing in the mother

- Midazolam (0.2 mg/kg) and ketamine (2 mg/kg), combined in the same syringe, may also be used for intravenous induction of anaesthesia in cats, providing these drugs have not been used for premedication. Extravascular injection results in a violent reaction because the solution has a low pH. Recovery to normal behaviour can be prolonged, which may delay the time at which kittens can be safely introduced to the mother. Such drug combinations are also used in dogs in the USA
- Thiopentone (thiopental) and methohexitone (methohexital) may be used at doses just sufficient to permit endotracheal intubation. When these drugs are used at half their normal induction doses, fetal depression is minimal.

When an intravenous induction agent is used, it is generally recommended that about 10–15 minutes is allowed to elapse before the fetuses are delivered, to allow plasma concentrations of the drug to decline, thus reducing neonatal depression. This would normally be about the time taken for surgical exposure of the uterus after preparation and positioning of the patient. Clipping the surgical site before induction is worthwhile.

Guinea pigs are also occasionally presented for Caesarian section. In these patients induction and maintenance of anaesthesia with isoflurane in oxygen, delivered via a face mask and an Ayre's T-piece, is the preferred method.

Maintenance
A cuffed endotracheal tube must be inserted as soon as possible after induction of anaesthesia and the cuff inflated to protect the airway from aspiration of gastric contents.

An infusion of lactated Ringer's solution is started at a basal rate of 10 ml/kg/h. If blood losses during surgery are great, Ringer's solution can be substituted with a synthetic plasma expander such as gelatinized calf protein or dextran. If there are facilities for blood pressure measurement, periods of hypotension can be monitored and treated with ephedrine (0.025–0.05 mg/kg i.v.).

The most satisfactory method of maintenance of general anaesthesia is by the use of inhalational agents. Either 100% oxygen or a 50:50 mixture of oxygen/nitrous oxide is used as the carrier gas. Giving inspired oxygen at a concentration of at least 50% will result in livelier neonates. It is uncertain whether puppies have diffusion hypoxia associated with the use of nitrous oxide. This potential danger can be eliminated by discontinuing the nitrous oxide just before delivery. Either halothane or isoflurane are added at the lowest possible concentration to maintain maternal unconsciousness (usually between 1% and 2%). Isoflurane is preferable because recovery is faster than with halothane. In dogs, it has also been shown that use of propofol

or isoflurane for induction, with isoflurane maintenance, is associated with reduced neonatal mortality at 7 days after surgery (P.F. Moon, personal communication). The increased cost of isoflurane needs to be balanced against the potential value of improved outcome. The newer, even less soluble volatile agents, desflurane and sevoflurane, could offer greater advantages and deserve further evaluation. In women, halothane and isoflurane at concentrations greater than 0.5 MAC (minimum alveolar concentration) have been associated with increased postpartum haemorrhage as a result of delayed uterine involution, but this does not seem to be a serious problem in animals. This contrast may be related to anatomical differences in placentation between humans and animals.

The fresh gas mixture should be delivered via an appropriate circuit. An accurate vaporizer is essential.

Neuromuscular blocking drugs may be used to reduce anaesthetic maintenance requirements. These drugs are highly ionized at physiological pH and do not cross the placenta, hence they do not cause fetal or neonatal paralysis. Because these drugs paralyse skeletal muscles, including the diaphragm, their use requires the availability of a means of controlling breathing by positive pressure ventilation. This may be an individual assigned to compress the rebreathing bag, or a suitable automatic ventilator. If the use of neuromuscular blocking agents is anticipated, newer drugs such as atracurium are preferable because they are rapidly eliminated from the body and have few cardiovascular side effects. For further details see Chapter 10.

Although a light plane of anaesthesia is highly desirable, care must be taken not to keep the animal too lightly anaesthetized, otherwise stress-induced vasoconstriction can adversely affect placental blood flow. Reynolds (1998) states that anaesthesia is normally too short to have significant fetal effects, whereas maternal stress caused by inadequate anaesthesia is a potential cause of fetal hypoxia, a far more damaging situation.

As soon as the neonates have been delivered, further doses of an opioid analgesic can be given to the mother as required so that adequate pain relief is continued into the postoperative period. Ecbolics such as oxytocin may also be given once the uterine incision has been closed, to promote uterine involution. The use of oxytocin before delivery can cause transient hypotension and reduce placental blood flow.

Monitoring of anaesthesia may not always be ideal when assistance is limited, because attention is mainly directed at resuscitation of neonates. In this respect the use of monitoring equipment, such as a reliable pulse oximeter, can be useful. An oesophageal stethoscope may be used by either the surgeon or nurse, enabling both hands to remain free. Facilities for the non-invasive measurement of blood pressure (e.g. Doppler, Dinamap) are invaluable.

Maternal recovery from anaesthesia

Once the endotracheal tube has been removed, attendants should be particularly vigilant for vomiting. Vomitus may include not only the last meal but also ingested placentae from neonates delivered before surgery. Patients should be kept on a recovery trolley until in sternal recumbency, so that if vomiting does occur a head-down position can be achieved quickly. The availability of suction equipment can also be a lifesaver at this stage.

Neonates should be introduced to the mother as soon as possible and encouraged to suckle at the earliest opportunity. Constant supervision is necessary until the bitch has recovered to full consciousness and proper coordination, so that the young are not inadvertently harmed.

Postoperative problems are rare but include haemorrhage, hypovolaemia and hypothermia, and peritonitis from exposure to uterine fluids.

CARE OF THE NEONATE

Before induction of anaesthesia, a suitable receptacle for the neonates should be prepared. This should contain plenty of absorbent bedding material, and an infrared lamp may be suspended at a suitable distance above the receptacle. Hypothermia is a great risk in neonates because of their higher surface area:bodyweight ratio and immature thermoregulatory mechanisms. Immediately after delivery, the neonate should be placed in a clean dry and warm towel, and membranes and fluid quickly cleared from the face and mouth. Suction facilities are invaluable. Quite vigorous rubbing may be used, both to dry the neonate and to stimulate breathing. Swinging the neonate to clear fluids probably does not help much and may even be harmful. Mouth to mouth resuscitation can also be used if there is difficulty in taking the first breath, or the trachea may be intubated to enable positive pressure ventilation with oxygen. Once respiration is established, oxygen should be given if a neonate seems weak or cyanosed. A slow heart rate is a sign of neonatal hypoxia. The onset of vigorous vocalization denotes good lung expansion. Once respiration is well established, the umbilical stump should be treated with povidone-iodine solution and then tied about 2.5–5.0 cm from the body wall with sterile suture material.

The use of naloxone and respiratory stimulants such as doxapram may be considered, but their use is no substitute for good resuscitation technique.

In humans, the Apgar score has been developed as a guide to viability of the neonate, and is performed at 1 and 5 minutes after delivery. Up to 2 points for each of five variables are awarded, thus giving a maximum score of 10. The variables scored are heart rate, respiratory effort, muscle tone, colour and reflex irritability. Extremely vigorous neonates have scores between 8 and 10. The score taken at 1 minute in human neonates positively correlates with survival. This system deserves further evaluation in animals.

REFERENCES AND FURTHER READING

Hall LW and Clarke KW (1991) Anaesthesia for obstetrics. In: *Veterinary Anaesthesia, 9th edn*, pp. 355-362. WB Saunders, London

Hellyer PW (1991) Anesthesia for Cesarian section. In: *Textbook of Small Animal Surgery, 2nd edn*, pp. 2300-2304. WB Saunders, Philadelphia

Morgan GE and Mikhail MS (1996) Maternal and fetal physiology and anesthesia. In: *Clinical Anesthesiology, 2nd edn*, pp. 692-704. Appleton and Lange, Stamford, Connecticut

Paddleford RR (1992) Anesthesia for Cesarian section in the dog. In: *Veterinary Clinics of North America:Small Animal Practice*, ed. SC Haskins and AM Klide, pp. 481-484. WB Saunders, Philadelphia

Probst CW and Webb AI (1983) Postural influence on systemic blood pressure, gas exchange and acid/base status in the term-pregnant bitch during general anesthesia. *American Journal of Veterinary Research* **44**, 1963-1965

Reynolds F (1998) Commentary. *British Journal of Anaesthesia* **80**, 688-689

Tranquilli WJ (1992) Anesthesia for Cesarian section in the cat. In: *Veterinary Clinics of North America: Small Animal Practice*, ed. SC Haskins and AM Klide, pp. 484-486. WB Saunders, Philadelphia

Tranquilli WJ, Lemke KA, Williams LL, *et al.* (1992) Flumazenil efficacy in reversing diazepam or midazolam overdose in dogs. *Journal of Veterinary Anaesthesia* **19**, 65-67

CHAPTER NINETEEN

Endocrine Disease

Craig Johnson

INTRODUCTION

The endocrine system plays a major role in the maintenance of the body's internal environment and the regulation of growth and development. Many important physiological systems, such as glucose and calcium homeostasis, are controlled by the endocrine system, which utilizes complex negative feedback loops based on the release of hormones into the blood. The target organs of different hormones can vary from small groups of cells in specific tissues, for example, the prostaglandins of the female reproductive cycle, to all the cells of the body, for example, insulin. This means that the effects of various hormones can be widespread and dramatic and also that disorders of the endocrine system can have far-reaching effects upon the body.

The endocrine system is important in anaesthesia in two ways. First, its function is affected by physiological insults such as surgical procedures. An endocrine response to surgery, which is usually called the stress response, is seen to a greater or lesser extent in healthy patients. Second, the alterations in function caused by disorders of the endocrine system can alter the response of the patient to anaesthesia and cause additional perioperative management problems for the anaesthetist.

THE STRESS RESPONSE

The stress response is the term used to cover the response of a normal endocrine system to a noxious stimulus. In general terms, the stress responses elicited by different noxious stimuli are qualitatively similar and only vary in their magnitude and duration. Stress responses can be caused by a variety of noxious stimuli in various combinations. The stimuli (or stressors) are detected by the body in various ways, and the response is orchestrated by the hypothalamo-pituitary axis, which acts as a common pathway in the generation of the response. The sensory and effector arms of the stress response are illustrated in Figures 19.1 and 19.2, respectively.

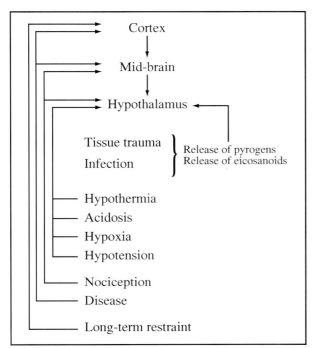

Figure 19.1: Sensory arm of the stress response.

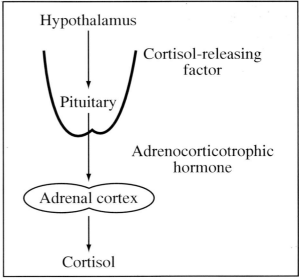

Figure 19.2: Effector arm of the stress response. Cortisol is used as an example of a hormone produced by the stress response.

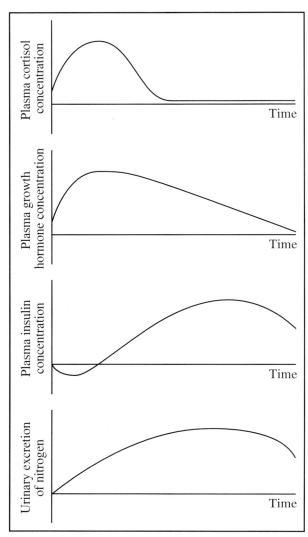

Figure 19.3: Metabolic and hormonal changes associated with the stress response.

The stress response initiates a number of alterations in metabolic activity that can persist for several days after the stress of surgery. The changes are aimed at preserving homeostasis in the face of stimuli that are a serious threat to life. In the initial phase of the stress response, the body conserves sodium and water and enters a catabolic state with negative nitrogen balance. Later in the course of the response an anabolic phase is entered. The first phase aims to preserve blood volume (and thus tissue perfusion) and ensures that there are adequate metabolic substrates in the blood for the continuation of function of the vital organs. Increased plasma catecholamine concentrations form an integral part of this phase of the stress response diverting blood flow to the essential organs of the body. There are also increases in other catabolic hormone concentrations, such as glucagon and cortisol, and concomitant decreases in anabolic hormone concentrations, such as insulin and testosterone. The second phase of the stress response begins the process of healing damaged tissues. Metabolism becomes largely anabolic, with the increased cellular uptake of substrates and the manufacture of proteins. The changes in plasma hormone concentrations and metabolic nitrogen balance that occur in both phases of the stress response are summarized in Figure 19.3. The two phases are sometimes referred to as the ebb and flow of the stress response.

The alterations in endocrine function which comprise the stress response are appropriate to the preservation of life after 'natural' insults such as severe trauma. Unfortunately many of the stimuli that initiate a stress response (Figure 19.1) occur in the surgical patient. In this situation the stress response may be less appropriate. For example, where careful attention is paid to perioperative fluid balance, the sodium conservation seen in the stress response is not required. It may actually be detrimental to the patient and can exacerbate such conditions as congestive heart failure and acute renal failure.

The stress response can be decreased by reducing the number and magnitude of noxious stimuli to which a patient is subjected during anaesthesia. Good anaesthetic practice should ensure that stressors such as hypoxaemia, hypothermia, hypotension, acidosis etc. are minimized throughout the course of the anaesthetic. In addition, the perception of nociceptive stimuli can be minimized by the use of carefully planned multimodal analgesia.

Some anaesthetic agents, such as the α_2-agonists and etomidate, seem to block the stress response in the effector arm rather than reduce sensory input. This direct blocking of the response itself, rather than reduction by the removal of stressors, can be detrimental to the patient. It seems that the inability to mount a stress response in situations where the body perceives that one is required can be very dangerous and even result in the death of the patient. It may be advisable to stimulate a stress response artificially by the administration of glucocorticoids in patients where the endogenous stress response may be inhibited by, for example, hypoadrenocorticism, hyperadrenocorticism or chronic steroid therapy. In these cases, production of endogenous corticosteroid is not regulated by the normal mechanisms and so the endocrine changes that characterize the stress response may only be triggered in response to an increase in steroid hormone concentrations greater than that which the body is able to produce. Exogenous steroids can be used to initiate the stress response, allowing the patient to respond to the stressful situation in a relatively normal way.

ANAESTHESIA FOR ENDOCRINOPATHIES

The adrenal gland
The adrenal glands are composed of two parts: the inner medulla and the outer cortex. The medulla secretes the catecholamines adrenaline and noradrena-

line, while the cortex secretes cortisol, aldosterone and over 30 other steroidal hormones. The cortical hormones are involved in many regulatory processes such as sodium homeostasis and the stress response. Diseases of the adrenal glands usually involve release of too much or too little of one or more of the above hormones. The wide range of target organs of the adrenal hormones mean that these diseases can have dramatic effects upon the patient.

Cushing's disease (hyperadrenocorticism)

Cushing's disease is due to the secretion of excessive amounts of glucocorticoids by the adrenal cortex. This may be due to adrenal neoplasia or to the overstimulation of a normal adrenal gland by excessive amounts of adrenocorticotrophic hormone produced by a pituitary tumour. Patients with Cushing's disease often have polyuria/polydipsia and are prone to sodium retention. Alterations in the structure of connective tissue result in the classic pendulous abdomen seen in these animals and can have implications for the ability of the tissues to heal after surgery. This abdominal conformation together with muscle wasting, which is commonly seen, can result in poor ventilatory function during anaesthesia in extreme cases. Treatment of Cushing's disease is usually achieved by medical therapy, but animals with this condition often require anaesthesia and present particular problems for the anaesthetist. The main clinical signs relevant to the anaesthetist are listed in Figure 19.4.

Skin thinning and reduced elasticity can make placement of intravenous cannulae difficult. Care should be taken with cannulae or other intravenous injections, as alterations in collagen formation can make patients prone to bruising. Animals with hyperadrenocorticism may be hypercoagulable and can be at increased risk of pulmonary thromboembolism. This may be apparent radiographically (although they usually have a normal chest radiograph) or may be seen as dyspnoea, cyanosis, trembling and/or apprehension. Treatment is symptomatic and should be aimed at increasing inspired oxygen fraction and supporting the cardiac output. Heparinization will prevent the formation of new clots, but will not dissolve those that have already formed. An initial dose of 50 IU/kg heparin intravenously should be followed by an infusion of 5–50 IU/kg/h with the aim of prolonging activated clotting time by two or three times the reference value.

Addison's disease (hypoadrenocorticism)

The main clinical signs relevant to the anaesthetist are listed in Figure 19.4. Most patients with Addison's disease are stabilized with medical therapy at the time of surgery. The main problem is their inability to mount an appropriate stress response to surgery similar to that seen in healthy animals. Healthy patients undergoing major surgery develop a five- to 10-fold

Condition	Clinical change
Cushing's disease	Slow tissue healing Polydipsia/polyuria Hypercoagulability Muscle wasting Skin changes Lethargy
Addison's disease	Bradycardia Dehydration Syncope Polydipsia/polyuria Weight loss Weakness Lethargy
Diabetes mellitus	Loss of glucose homeostasis Ketoacidosis Reduced liver function Polydipsia/polyuria Weight loss

Hyperthyroidism	Hypertrophic
	    cardiomyopathy
	Hypertension
	Altered temperament
	    (usually for the worse)
	Compromised hepatic
	    function
	Compromised renal
	    function
	Weight loss
	Usually aged

Hypothyroidism	Bradycardia Hypotension Megaoesophagus Obesity Lethargy
Oestrogen-secreting neoplasia	Non-regenerative anaemia Thrombocytopenia Pyrexia Immunosuppression

Figure 19.4: Major clinical signs for the common endocrinopathies relevant to the anaesthetist.

increase in cortisol production. If the patient is unable to produce this increase in endogenous glucocorticoid, it is important that exogenous therapy is provided to prevent adrenal crisis and circulatory collapse in the perioperative or postoperative periods.

Minor elective surgery can usually be carried out safely if intravenous hydrocortisone is administered at 4–5 mg/kg at induction of anaesthesia. For major elective surgery this should be followed by oral administration of 0.5 mg/kg prednisolone twice daily for 3 days. If complications such as fever or ongoing blood or protein loss continue, then prednisolone should be continued until these have resolved. After resolution, prednisolone therapy can be removed by using a weaning dose regimen. Despite the importance of perioperative glucocorticoid administration, the drug should be withdrawn as soon as possible after surgery as side effects may include delayed healing and immunosuppression leading to an increased risk of postoperative infection.

Phaeochromocytoma

This is a rare tumour of the cells of the adrenal medulla, which secrete catecholamines. The resultant over-response to stressful stimuli makes the patient with phaeochromocytoma subject to sudden episodes of tachycardia and hypertension, which are often accompanied by tachydysrhythmias. Surgical manipulation of these masses can precipitate the secretion of large amounts of catecholamines, and the anaesthetist should be ready to deal with sudden changes in heart rate and blood pressure. Arrhythmias such as premature ventricular contractions and ventricular tachycardia may also occur without warning. It is useful to have appropriate doses of drugs used in the treatment of these complications drawn up into syringes before the induction of anaesthesia. As a minimum, a β-blocker such as esmolol (0.1–0.5 mg/kg) combined with an increased isoflurane concentration should be able to control moderate increases in blood pressure. In extreme circumstances, an α-blocker such as phentolamine or a venodilator such as nitroprusside may also be required. In addition to these, a selection of anti-arrhythmics such as lignocaine (lidocaine) and bretylium may be useful. It should be remembered that the concentration of circulating catecholamines decreases after clamping of the venous drainage from the mass. Sudden hypotension may follow and thus it is desirable to use short-acting agents to control intraoperative hypertension.

Disorders of glucose homeostasis

The two most common conditions in this group are diabetes mellitus and insulinoma. These conditions result in either a functional lack of (diabetes mellitus), or abundance of (insulinoma), circulating insulin. In both cases the normal homeostatic mechanisms are breached, and the animal loses its ability to regulate blood glucose concentration adequately. Long-term effects upon the body's metabolic processes can be dramatic, resulting in various conditions such as chronic intermittent hypoglycaemia, ketoacidosis and dehydration. During the perioperative period, there can be sudden alterations in plasma glucose concentration, which are masked by anaesthesia and so can go unnoticed. In the worst instance, severe brain damage can occur which does not become apparent until the end of the period of anaesthesia.

The metabolic and endocrine changes brought about by anaesthesia and surgery will alter the balance of glucose homeostasis in these patients, and so the maintenance of perfect balance is not a realistic goal even in patients that are well controlled by medical therapy. The aims of the anaesthetist should be first to prevent hypoglycaemia at any time during management of the case, to prevent prolonged or severe hyperglycaemia (and the development of ketoacidosis) and to maintain normal fluid and electrolyte balance.

Diabetes mellitus

Diabetic patients present for surgery for a variety of procedures. Some procedures are an essential part of the management of the condition (e.g. bitch in season requiring ovariohysterectomy), some will be indirectly related to the condition (e.g. cataract removal) and some will be unrelated to the diabetes. Except in emergency situations, anaesthesia should only be undertaken once the diabetes is adequately controlled by medical management. Animals that are not properly controlled may be ketoacidotic and/or have unpredictable changes in blood glucose concentrations during anaesthesia. Ketoacidotic patients often have severe metabolic dysfunction, including altered protein binding and hepatic function. This can make them unusually sensitive to anaesthetic agents and can greatly increase the duration of action of these drugs. The main clinical signs relevant to the anaesthetist are listed in Figure 19.4.

Diabetic patients are controlled by many different regimens, which are tailored to suit their condition and their owner's lifestyle. During the perioperative period, the normal insulin and feeding routine should be adhered to as closely as possible, and the details of drug administration and feeding should form part of the history taking when the patient is admitted. It is useful if the patient can be admitted one or two days before surgery to allow the nursing team to become familiar with the animal's routine and to allow preoperative tests to establish the health status of the patient. This is particularly important if the clinicians are not those who usually deal with the patient (e.g. at a referral centre).

Anaesthesia and surgery should be carried out so as to minimize interference with the animal's routine. It is usually possible to limit alterations to this routine to the day of surgery. This requires a degree of flexibility in the timing of anaesthesia and the details of the anaesthetic protocol used. The suggested management plan set out below and in Figure 19.5 is appropriate for a patient ordinarily receiving a single dose of insulin in the morning.

The anaesthetic should be scheduled first on the operating list and should include short-acting agents wherever possible so that the patient can return to its normal routine as early as possible. The insulin dose should be divided into two halves, the first given at the time of premedication and the second held back for later. Blood glucose should be measured at induction of anaesthesia and at least every 15 minutes until the patient regains consciousness. The timing of surgery should mean that the procedure is over long before the animal approaches its glucose nadir, but hypoglycaemia can occur during surgery without obvious signs, resulting in cerebral damage that is only apparent upon recovery from anaesthesia. Throughout anaesthesia, efforts should be made to keep blood glucose concentrations towards the top end of, or just above, the normal range. A moderate hyperglycaemia for the duration of anaesthesia does not have any lasting consequences and provides a buffer against the patient becoming hypoglycaemic between blood glucose measurements. A low normal blood glucose concentration can usually be adequately increased by the use of 4% dextrose saline at a routine maintenance rate of 5–10 ml/kg/h. If this does not prove adequate, then an infusion of hypertonic glucose should be started to further increase blood glucose concentrations. The administration of dextrose saline at increased rates should be avoided as it can result in serious water loading, leading to pulmonary oedema. Infusions containing glucose should always be given through a different cannula to that used for taking samples for blood glucose analysis.

After surgery the patient should be offered food as soon as it seems able to eat. Half an hour after it has eaten a test amount of food without regurgitating or vomiting, it should be given the remainder of its morning feed and insulin. The second feed of the day

should be given at the normal time, unless surgery was prolonged, in which case it should be delayed to coincide with peak insulin effect. On the days after surgery, the normal feeding regimen and insulin doses should be adhered to. The metabolic response to surgery alters metabolic rate and energy balance on the days after surgery, and glycosuria is often seen. As long as the patient remains bright and does not become hypoglycaemic, any attempts to re-stabilize the diabetes should be delayed until about the fourth day after surgery.

The above approach to the perioperative management of a diabetic patient is intended as an example. Many stable diabetic patients are managed using regimens that are different from the above, and anaesthesia should be altered to fit in with their requirements, rather than attempting to alter their routine in the days before surgery.

Unstable ketoacidotic diabetic patients can be very poor candidates for anaesthesia. They should be treated and their insulin requirements stabilized before surgery whenever possible. When these patients present for emergency procedures they are often best managed using a triple infusion of insulin, glucose and potassium, which can be continued into the recovery period until stabilization of the diabetes can be attempted. Infusion rates should be adjusted according to the response of the patient, and blood glucose, potassium and ketone body concentrations should be monitored closely. Recommended initial infusion rates are: insulin 0.5–1 IU/kg/h, potassium 0.5 mmol/kg/h, dextrose saline 5–10 ml/kg/h. These patients often have greatly impaired hepatic function, and any drugs that rely upon hepatic metabolism should be used cautiously.

Insulinoma

Insulinomas are adenocarcinomas of the β cells of the islets of Langerhans. They secrete insulin, resulting in intermittent bouts of hypoglycaemia, which may be accompanied by neurological signs, ataxia, exercise intolerance and syncope. Insulinomas often metastasize to the liver, but removal of the pancreatic tumour can result in remission for 12 months or more. Partial pancreatectomy is the most common reason that patients with insulinomas require anaesthesia.

Surgical resection of an insulinoma presents several challenges for the anaesthetist. Patients with chronic hypoglycaemia are at risk of developing cerebral damage after sudden decreases in blood glucose concentration. In addition, a tumour can secrete large amounts of insulin into the blood when it is handled by the surgeon. This can result in particularly severe hypoglycaemia and the need for rapid infusion of glucose. Blood glucose concentrations must be monitored closely throughout the perioperative period and especially during manipulation of the pancreas. The normal mechanisms of glucose homeostasis are often suppressed by the high circulating insulin concentra-

| **Premedication** |
| Give one-half normal insulin dose |
| **Anaesthetic induction (do first in morning list)** |
| Measure blood glucose on induction of anaesthesia |
| • If low give glucose infusion
    If normal use dextrose saline as
    maintenance fluid
    If high use polyionic maintenance fluid
    (without dextrose) |
| **Perioperative period** |
| Measure blood glucose every 15 minutes throughout anaesthesia |
| • Adjust fluids as above |
| **Postoperative period** |
| Give small amount of food as soon as patient able to eat
Give morning feed and remaining insulin 30 minutes after first eating
Give evening meal as usual |

Figure 19.5: Suggested plan for management of a patient with controlled diabetes mellitus.

tion, and so patients often have symptoms of diabetes mellitus in the postoperative period. This can result in the development of hyperglycaemia and the need for a reduced rate of glucose administration after resection of the mass. The administration of exogenous insulin is often required for some time after surgery.

Surgery of the pancreas also risks the development of acute pancreatitis. This can lead to serious and even fatal complications. The anaesthetic management of pancreatic surgery and patients with pancreatitis is described in Chapter 16.

The thyroid and parathyroid glands

Hyperthyroidism

Hyperthyroidism is commonly seen in cats with tumours of one or both thyroid glands, but only very rarely in dogs. There are several treatment options for this condition, one of which is surgical excision of the affected thyroid gland. This is the usual reason for anaesthesia of these patients.

Cats with hyperthyroidism present with a variety of clinical signs, many of which have important implications for the management of anaesthesia. The main clinical signs relevant to the anaesthetist are listed in Figure 19.4. Animals presenting for surgical removal of the thyroid mass are often poorly controlled by medical management and therefore often difficult to anaesthetize safely. In these cases, there can be a degree of tension between conflicting perioperative goals. For example, the temperament of the patient would suggest the use of a deeply sedative premedicant, but the cardiovascular and metabolic compromise favour minimal sedation. The cardiovascular disease would also suggest maintaining anaesthesia with minimal doses of anaesthetic agents, but the effects of catecholamine release due to inadequate anaesthesia can be catastrophic.

The details of the final anaesthetic plan vary from case to case, depending upon the relative severity of the various signs. In cats with a relatively healthy cardiovascular system, opioid-based premedication can be followed by propofol or alphaxalone/alphadolone as induction agents. Where the cat's temperament or degree of cardiomyopathy would make restraint for intravenous cannulation dangerously stressful, an induction chamber can be used with isoflurane to produce a slow and relatively stress-free induction. When induction of anaesthesia proceeds before intravenous access is secured, a cannula should be placed as soon as possible, as sudden changes in cardiovascular function may require the urgent administration of intravenous drugs.

Anaesthesia should be monitored very closely to ensure that adequate anaesthesia is achieved without a dangerous degree of cardiovascular depression. Even so, sudden changes can occur and it is advisable to have a number of drugs drawn into syringes at hand. Atropine (0.1 mg/kg), a β-adrenergic antago-

nist such as esmolol (0.1–0.5 mg/kg) and an intravenous anaesthetic agent such as propofol will cope with bradycardia, tachycardia and inadequate anaesthesia. It is advisable to have an emergency resuscitation box to hand in case of more severe complications. Further details of emergency boxes can be found in Chapter 24.

Patients should be monitored closely in the postoperative period for signs of hypocalcaemia. It is possible to inadvertently remove the parathyroid glands with the thyroid gland, leading to the development of hypocalcaemia. This complication can be treated by the administration of calcium (5–15 mg/kg to effect).

Hypothyroidism

Hypothyroidism is a common chronic endocrinopathy of the elderly dog. Animals affected with this condition usually require anaesthesia for unrelated conditions. The main clinical signs relevant to the anaesthetist are listed in Figure 19.4. In addition to these, the presence of concurrent diseases such as hypoadrenocorticism and diabetes mellitus should be ruled out before undertaking anaesthesia for elective procedures.

Anaesthesia of patients with hypothyroidism should be carried out with care. Particular attention should be paid to cardiovascular function, as alterations in myocardial function can result in reduced contractility and hypotension. Negative inotropic drugs should be avoided. This is particularly true of halothane, which can cause a pronounced reduction in contractility since sarcoplasmic calcium uptake can already be reduced. Care should be taken to ensure that these patients are adequately fasted as megaoesophagus and reduced gastrointestinal motility can occur in this disease. The placement of a cuffed endotracheal tube should always be a priority in these cases.

Recovery from anaesthesia can be slow due to a slow metabolic rate and tendency to develop hypothermia during anaesthesia. Care should be taken to keep these patients warm throughout anaesthesia and recovery, and the airway should be protected for as long as possible into the recovery period.

Hyperparathyroidism

Primary hyperparathyroidism is rare in dogs and very rare in cats and is usually due to an adenoma of the parathyroid gland. Removal of these masses results in sudden changes in plasma calcium concentration and should not be attempted unless facilities for monitoring plasma ionized calcium are available. Where this surgery is undertaken, calcium should be given by infusion with the aim of keeping calcium concentrations stable over the course of the perioperative period.

Oestrogen-secreting tumours (Sertoli cell tumours)

Many neoplasms that secrete endocrinologically active substances have been described. The majority of cases can be treated in a similar manner to animals with excessive amounts of the particular hormone for other reasons. For example, hyperadrenocorticism may have various aetiologies, but the anaesthetic implications for each are similar. Oestrogen-secreting testicular tumours are unusual in that they secrete hormones not usually present in the male animal. They are principally found in the dog, but have been reported in the cat. The main clinical signs relevant to the anaesthetist are listed in Figure 19.4.

Of principal concern are the anaemia and thrombocytopenia that are due to bone marrow depression and which may persist even after removal of the mass. If the animal is only moderately affected, the choice of an anaesthetic technique that does not depress cardiac output, together with close attention to haemostasis during surgery may be sufficient. In more severe cases a transfusion of fresh whole blood may be indicated at the time of surgery to support oxygen delivery and improve clotting function. This should support the patient through the perioperative period and give the bone marrow time to regenerate.

SUMMARY

The above discussion has dealt with anaesthesia for patients with common endocrine disorders. There are many more unusual disorders of this system. When planning management strategies for these cases the best starting point is a thorough understanding of the underlying pathophysiology of the condition. In most cases, the major concern is how best to monitor and compensate for a specific failure of the patient's homeostatic mechanisms. It should, however, be remembered that these animals may be unable to compensate for major stressors, and so the anaesthetic protocol should be chosen to minimize the metabolic insult of the surgical procedure.

CHAPTER TWENTY

Neurological Disease

Jacqueline C. Brearley and Karen Walsh

INTRODUCTION

Animals with neurological disorders may present for anaesthesia for a variety of reasons: as part of the diagnostic process, for treatment of the disorder or for entirely unrelated reasons (Figure 20.1). Some breeds of dog have an increased propensity for certain conditions. For example, chondrodystrophic breeds, such as Basset Hounds and Dachshunds, have a high incidence of intervertebral disc protrusion, Dobermann Pinscher dogs have an increased incidence of spinal canal stenosis and elderly Boxers may have an increased incidence of brain tumours.

Some understanding of normal neuroanatomy, physiology and pathology is essential if the anaesthetist is to understand the reaction of the patient to anaesthesia and to optimize the patient's condition pre-, intra- and postoperatively.

CENTRAL NERVOUS SYSTEM

Neuroanatomy relevant to anaesthesia

The central nervous system (CNS) consists of the spinal cord and the brain and is protected by the bony surrounds of the vertebral column and the skull. However, due to the inflexible nature of bone, the CNS is not only protected by these structures but also trapped by them. The intracranial cavity volume is filled by the brain (80%), cerebrospinal fluid (CSF, 10%) and blood (10%). As the total volume is fixed, if there is an increase in the volume of one component the volume of the other components decreases or the intracranial pressure rises (the Monroe-Kellie doctrine) which may temporarily or permanently damage the nervous tissue (see section on Neurophysiology and Anaesthesia below).

The brain can be subdivided anatomically into the cerebrum, brainstem and cerebellum. Conscious function and higher information processing takes place in the cerebrum. Fundamental functions (e.g. respiration, homeostasis, cardiac regulation) are controlled from the brainstem, and the cerebellum controls proprioception and muscular coordination. All of the central nervous tissue is covered with three protective fibrous membranes — the meninges (Figure 20.2). Between the arachnoid and pia mater is the subarachnoid space, which is filled with CSF. This space extends down the spine to the lumbosacral region. In the dog the subarachnoid space extends to between L7 and S1; in cats it extends rather more caudally to S1.

For diagnostic procedures
Imaging - radiography, computed tomography, magnetic resonance imaging
Cerebrospinal fluid sampling
Biopsies - muscle/nerve/tumours
Electrodiagnostic procedures

For treatment
Decompressive spinal surgery:
dorsal laminectomy
ventral slot
fenestration of disc spaces
Stabilization techniques
Removal of tumours
Shunt surgery
Sedation for status epilepticus

For treatment unrelated to neurological condition
Intracranial:
Neural dysfunction (e.g. epilepsy)
Increased intracranial pressure:
Space-occupying lesion e.g. blood, tumour
Decreased CSF drainage
Spinal:
Neuronal disease
- degenerative
- storage
- transmitter imbalance
Spinal compression
- intervertebral disc protrusion
- dynamic instability - congenital (e.g. Dobermanns)
- acquired (trauma/fractures)
- congenital vertebral abnormalities (e.g. atlanto-occipital subluxation, cervical stenosis)

Figure 20.1: *Types of neurological patient presenting for anaesthesia.*

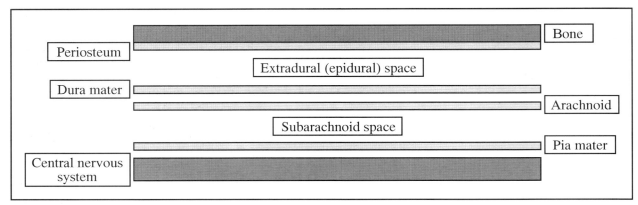

Figure 20.2: Schematic of the meninges.

CNS blood supply and blood–brain barrier

Blood supply to the brain in the dog is via the internal carotid and basilar arteries. In the cat a third source, the anastomotic artery, also contributes blood to the brain. The spinal cord is supplied by the ventral artery, which anastomoses with the segmental spinal arteries.

The blood–brain barrier (BBB) is formed by the cerebral capillary endothelium, the basement membrane and astrocyte foot processes. Unlike other capillary beds, the endothelial junctions between the cells are very narrow (1 nm). This renders the BBB impermeable to large or polar molecules but permeable to lipid-soluble agents e.g. anaesthetic drugs. These tight endothelial junctions are disrupted in inflammation, trauma and acute hypertension.

NEUROPHYSIOLOGY AND ANAESTHESIA

The function of the CNS is information processing and control of effector organs. This is achieved by cells communicating with each other by release of neurotransmitters that alter the ion permeability of neighbouring cells via receptors. Many of the drugs used in anaesthesia exert their effects by interaction at these receptors. Thus, sedation by α_2-agonists is thought to be mediated via presynaptic adrenoceptors in the locus coeruleus region of the brain, and their muscle relaxant properties mediated via adrenoceptor projections on to GABAminergic (γ-aminobutyric acid) inhibitory neurones.

As mentioned above, increases in intracranial volume must be met either by changes in volume of one of the intracranial components or by increased intracranial pressure (ICP). When an intracranial structure increases in volume, an increase in ICP is minimized initially by displacement of cranial CSF into the spinal subarachnoid space and by compression of veins that shifts blood into the jugular veins. If a sample of CSF is taken by cisternal puncture in these circumstances, the sudden release of pressure by the puncture may result in herniation of the cerebellum under the tentor-

ium with subsequent brainstem barotrauma. This is manifest by respiratory arrest, bradycardia or cardiac arrest. Thus, if increased ICP is suspected, CSF sampling should be done with great caution and should be accompanied by close monitoring. Once the compensatory mechanisms of displacement of CSF and venous compression have reached their limits, further small increases in intracranial volume cause large increases in ICP, decrease cerebral perfusion and compromise in turn delivery of nutrients to, and removal of waste products from, the brain. Because of its high metabolic rate (around 20% total oxygen consumption) the brain is very susceptible to such ischaemic damage. The brain receives approximately 15% of the cardiac output, and the majority of the brain blood volume is contained within venous capacitance vessels. Ordinarily, increasing cerebral blood flow (CBF) increases the volume of blood contained in the intracranial blood vessels at any instant and this increases ICP. In patients with intracranial trauma, malformations or masses, the anaesthetist may influence outcome by controlling ICP via alterations in CBF.

The major physiological factors that influence ICP are cerebral perfusion pressure, arterial carbon dioxide tension ($PaCO_2$), arterial oxygen tension (PaO_2) and cerebral metabolic activity. Cerebral blood flow is closely coupled with metabolic activity or neuronal activity.

Cerebral perfusion pressure

This is the pressure gradient between mean arterial blood pressure (MAP) and ICP (or cerebral venous pressure, whichever is greater). Ordinarily, increasing this pressure gradient tends to increase CBF. However, in the normal animal, CBF stays fairly constant as long as MAP is between 50 and 150 mmHg. This autoregulatory response is thought to be mediated either through action of a vasodilatory metabolite or a direct arterial myogenic response. Arterial pressures of <50 mmHg result in decreased CBF, and pressures >150 mmHg cause increased CBF and, hence, increased ICP. While autoregulation is less efficient under anaesthesia, CBF is best maintained at normotension. In anaesthetized patients with intracranial lesions, it is crucial to monitor systemic blood pressure and maintain it within normal limits by judicious use of vasodilator drugs or positive inotropic agents.

Coughing, vomiting, positioning that compromises the jugular veins and badly applied intermittent positive-pressure ventilation (IPPV) with high and/or prolonged airway pressures, tend to increase the pressure in the venous outflow from the brain and cause distension of intracranial veins. Therefore these processes tend to increase ICP and must be avoided by careful attention to technique when anaesthetizing patients with intracranial lesions.

Arterial carbon dioxide and oxygen tensions

Cerebral blood flow is very sensitive to changes in $PaCO_2$; there is a 4% increase in CBF (or 0.04 ml/100 g increase in cerebral blood volume) for every 1 mmHg increase in $PaCO_2$ in the range of 30–60 mmHg. Thus, hypoventilation and its accompanying hypercapnia increase ICP and are, therefore, life threatening in the patient with an intracranial space-occupying lesion. However, hyperventilation leads to hypocapnia that can result in vasoconstriction, which is sufficient to limit oxygen delivery to the brain.

The arteries and veins in damaged regions of the brain often lose their capacity to autoregulate flow. Under these circumstances, when undamaged areas of the brain respond to vasodilatory stimuli (e.g. hypercapnia), blood may be shunted away from these vasoparalysed areas, producing 'intracerebral steal'; this may cause ischaemia and exacerbate the damage. Conversely, if intact areas vasoconstrict in response to appropriate stimuli (e.g. hypocapnia), the vasoparalysed areas may have blood shunted towards them ('inverse steal').

The sensitivity of the cerebral circulation to changes in $PaCO_2$ dictates that any patient that may have increased ICP should be mildly hyperventilated to slight hypocapnia ($PaCO_2$ ~30 mmHg). This is sufficient to produce modest vasoconstriction but maintain normal CBF distribution.

The response to oxygen is much less dramatic than the response to carbon dioxide. If the PaO_2 decreases to <50 mmHg, vasodilation is stimulated. With high oxygen tensions mild vasoconstriction takes place but this is generally insignificant in all but extreme cases.

In practice, hypoxia should be avoided by allowing the patient to breathe a gas mixture that is oxygen enriched.

Influence of anaesthetic agents on ICP

Opioids have been said to be contraindicated in patients with head injury. In spontaneously breathing animals, the degree of respiratory depression caused by high dose opioids may be sufficient to cause a degree of hypercapnia that results in significant vaso-dilation and increases ICP. In animals with controlled ventilation the effects of opioids are less clear. Opioid-induced relative hypotension may decrease perfusion pressure and so could either increase or decrease ICP depending on the animal's circumstances. In general, opioids are best avoided in spontaneously breathing animals, but may be used as adjuncts to anaesthesia in animals with controlled ventilation.

Barbiturates and propofol have been found to be equally cerebroprotective. In one study, human patients anaesthetized with propofol were found to have improved oxygen delivery to the brain compared with patients anaesthetized with thiopentone. Propofol has the advantage of being suitable for continuous infusion, and so total intravenous anaesthetic techniques can be used to avoid inhalational agents.

Both halothane and isoflurane seem to cause cerebral vasodilation and may increase ICP. At a given $PaCO_2$ and depth of anaesthesia, ICP is less with isoflurane than with halothane. Given this and considering the other properties of the drugs, low doses of isoflurane are probably preferable to halothane if inhalational agents are to be used. The influence of desflurane and sevoflurane are yet to be fully established, although there is some evidence that sevoflurane may have some proconvulsant properties similar to enflurane. Nitrous oxide (N_2O) is a potent cerebrocortical vasodilator, causing more vasodilation than either halothane or isoflurane. This, in conjunction with the risks of expansion of air emboli and pneumocephalus in craniotomies, indicates that N_2O should be avoided during intracranial surgery or in patients that may have increased ICP.

Cerebral protection during and after CNS injury

CNS injury is often divided into primary and secondary injury. Primary injury is characterized by direct trauma, concussion and haemorrhage. It is generally traumatic in origin and almost immediate in onset. Secondary injury develops minutes to hours later and may be independent of primary trauma. It is characterized by neural ischaemia. Factors contributing to secondary injury include hypoxia, hypercapnia, hypoglycaemia, decreased cerebral perfusion, systemic hypotension, cerebral arterial spasm and transtentorial and cerebellar herniation.

The onset of ischaemia is associated with loss of intracellular adenosine triphosphate (ATP). ATP is fundamental to maintaining a normal stable transmembrane electrical potential difference. Hence, ischaemia destabilizes neural cells, allows the release of excitatory neurotransmitters (e.g. glutamate) and disrupts intracellular calcium homeostasis.

Until recently, neuronal protection was based on hypothermia, corticosteroids, judicious use of intravenous fluids and the use of neuroprotective drugs (e.g. barbiturates).

Moderate hypothermia (2–3°C below normal body temperature) has been shown to be effective in reducing neural damage. The mechanism for neuroprotection with hypothermia may involve an overall decrease in metabolic rate and reduced release of excitatory neurotransmitters (e.g. glutamate) during neural injury. Although more severe hypothermia is also protective, the cardiac effects of extreme hypothermia make elective hypothermia technically difficult to manage without cardiopulmonary bypass.

Corticosteroids (e.g. methylprednisolone 30 mg/kg i.v.) are associated with improved outcome after acute spinal trauma if they are given within 8 hours of injury and followed by an infusion of methylprednisolone (5.4 mg/kg) for the subsequent 23 hours. If they are given more than 8 hours after the acute injury, no beneficial effects are seen.

In the case of oedema and inflammation associated with neural tumours, corticosteroids (e.g. dexamethasone 0.5 mg/kg) will improve the condition of the animal.

Because the intact BBB is not permeable to ions, iso-osmotic crystalloid solutions should be used. Hypo-osmotic solutions exacerbate brain oedema by permitting movement of water into the brain from the vasculature. Lactated Ringer's solution is slightly hypo-osmotic compared with plasma and should probably be avoided in patients with increased ICP. If crystalloids are required, then 0.9% (w/v) sodium chloride, or other iso-osmotic solutions, should be used. Hypertonic saline may be beneficial in resuscitation of the circulation, because it should draw oedema fluid out of the brain. Colloid solutions have some advantages in patients with CNS injury because they do not contribute to brain oedema; unfortunately, they may also inhibit coagulation and exacerbate any bleeding tendency. Mannitol is often used to reduce brain swelling acutely in circumstances where ICP may be sufficient to cause cerebellar herniation. A dose of 0.5 g/kg i.v., given over 20 minutes, is generally effective. This may be repeated up to three times in 24 hours. A continuous infusion of 0.05 g/kg/h may also be used. Mannitol is a simple sugar in hypertonic solution and principally acts as an osmotic diuretic, although it also decreases blood viscosity and, thereby, improves tissue perfusion. It requires an intact BBB to maintain an osmotic gradient that facilitates water flux from the cerebral interstitium. The major disadvantage of this therapy is the risk of hyperosmolarity and hypernatraemia. If mannitol is being given by infusion, or in repeated doses, serum osmolarity should be monitored to ensure that it does not exceed 320 mOsm, otherwise rebound oedema and/or renal failure may ensue.

Barbiturates are cerebroprotective by decreasing the cerebral metabolic rate. This effect is modest compared with the protective effects of mild hypothermia.

The theoretical benefits of L-NAME (a nitric oxide inhibitor), NMDA (N-methyl-D-aspartate) antagonists, calcium channel blockers and other therapies aimed at limiting neuronal disruption have yet to be verified in clinical trials.

ANAESTHESIA AND EPILEPTIC ACTIVITY

Conditions that disrupt intrinsic neural function, for example, epilepsy, are often affected by anaesthetic agents. Idiopathic epilepsy is common in dogs but quite rare in cats. Drugs that are reported to promote the onset of seizures are the phenothiazines, enflurane and ketamine, and so these drugs should be avoided in known epileptics. Anaesthetic regimens for procedures that may cause seizures (e.g. myelography) should also avoid the above mentioned drugs.

Seizure activity after myelography is probably due to the irritant nature of the contrast material, and the increase in pressure in the subarachnoid space caused by the volume of contrast agent injected. The incidence of seizures after myelography can be minimized by:

- Using the contrast agent iohexol, rather than metrizamide
- Using lumbar injections of contrast agent, rather than cisternal injections, whenever possible
- Minimizing the total volume of contrast agent injected and the rate of its injection
- Ensuring that the patient is kept anaesthetized long enough to permit redistribution and elimination of the contrast agent from the meninges. This usually takes around 45 minutes after injection
- Taking special care in patients with obstructive lesions in the cervical spinal canal. Injection of contrast medium into the cisterna magna in such patients may cause the medium to spread into the cranial vault, rather than caudally into the spinal canal. The time for dispersal of the agent may be prolonged in these patients
- Maintaining the patient in a head-up position. The specific gravity of contrast agents is greater than CSF and so they flow away from the brain with gravity when the head is higher than the spinal canal
- Intravenous crystalloid fluids may be used to promote diuresis and increase elimination of contrast agent.

Medetomidine has been shown to promote epileptiform activity but is also thought to be cerebroprotective by altering cerebral metabolic rate. Propofol, while associated with excitatory activity (muscle tremors, hiccups), has been used to treat status epilepticus, and there are reports of an anticonvulsant effect of this drug.

Anaesthesia may be the symptomatic treatment of choice for status epilepticus if the seizures cannot be controlled by intermittent intravenous or rectal benzodiazepines. Total intravenous sedation or light general anaesthesia is generally used with a variety of drugs being employed. Traditionally, pentobarbitone, either intermittently or by infusion, is used as the first-line agent while the animal is stabilized on phenobarbitone. The initial loading dose of pentobarbitone is in the order of 13 mg/kg, with an infusion rate of 1–2 mg/kg/h to effect. The aim is to have sedation as light as possible without seizures. Propofol and midazolam have been used in the same way.

Nevertheless, it must be borne in mind that chronic administration of phenobarbitone to control epileptic seizures induces the hepatic P450 enzyme system and alters the pharmacokinetics of other drugs, including some anaesthetic agents, that are metabolized by this system.

SPINAL CORD TRAUMA AND ANAESTHESIA

Surgery on the vertebral column is most commonly performed for one of the following reasons:

- Decompressive surgery to relieve pressure on the spinal cord (e.g. dorsal laminectomy, ventral slot technique or fenestration of disc spaces to remove intervertebral disc material)
- Stabilization of vertebral column instability (e.g. atlanto-occipital subluxations, fractures or subluxations, dynamic instability in Dobermanns and Great Danes).

Anaesthesia is also performed on animals with spinal cord conditions for diagnostic purposes (e.g. myelography and other imaging modalities, electrophysiology and CSF sampling).

In general, the more cranial the lesion, the more likely the anaesthetist is to encounter problems in maintaining cardiovascular and respiratory stability. Positioning for surgery can also compromise ventilation by thoracic compression or restriction of diaphragmatic movement. It is often preferable to ventilate these patients soon after induction of anaesthesia, although this may introduce complications for the surgeon: IPPV increases venous pressure by increasing intrathoracic pressure, which results in dilation of the paravertebral venous sinuses. If these sinuses are punctured during surgery, haemorrhage is often difficult to control because of their anatomical location. Close cooperation between the surgeon and anaesthetist is required in these circumstances.

Other important considerations during anaesthesia include adequate pain control and vagal reflexes.

Animals with intervertebral disc disease often present with severe pain, which may be relatively recent in onset or may have been present for some days. In each case, 'upregulation' of nociceptive pathways may occur, resulting in pain that may be difficult to control and that may cause difficulty in achieving a stable plane of surgical anaesthesia. Multimodal analgesia is advisable in these situations. If corticosteroids are indicated for spinal trauma, non-steroidal anti-inflammatory drugs (NSAIDs) should be avoided. However, if the time since trauma is >6 hours, there is no indication for corticosteroids and NSAIDs can be used for pain control. Prostaglandin-sparing NSAIDs (e.g. carprofen) are the only ones recommended for preoperative use unless blood pressure is to be closely monitored and controlled. In addition, opioids provide good analgesia and reduce the dosages of agents used for induction and maintenance of anaesthesia. Morphine, methadone, oxymorphone or papaveretum can all be given preoperatively. Partial agonists (buprenorphine, butorphanol and pentazocine) may be used but have the disadvantage of antagonizing any subsequent short-acting analgesics (e.g. fentanyl) given intraoperatively to provide analgesia during periods of intense surgical stimulation.

Bradycardia is not uncommon during spinal surgery and may be due to either direct vagal stimulation or a vagal response to pain. It usually responds to anticholinergics, but their routine use for premedication is not generally recommended. Symptomatic treatment with anticholinergics is recommended if the heart rate falls rapidly as severe bradycardia may compromise cardiac output and hence tissue perfusion. Prevention is aided by ensuring adequate analgesia and depth of anaesthesia. Note should be made that potent μ-opioid receptor agonists may cause bradycardia in their own right, especially if given intravenously.

Surgical trauma of the spinal cord may manifest as bradycardia, apnoea, tachypnoea or tachycardia.

PERIPHERAL NEUROLOGICAL DISEASE

Distal to the spinal cord, dysfunction may occur in the afferent or efferent nerves or at the level of the muscle itself (Figure 20.3). In general, anaesthesia has little effect on afferent function. Efferent nerve dysfunction can lead to secondary muscle weakness. Locomotor dysfunction is not life threatening, but weakness of the respiratory and laryngeal muscles may lead to respiratory insufficiency and lack of airway protective mechanisms. Although there is little that can be done about these conditions, they should be recognized before anaesthesia. The use of neuromuscular blocking agents should probably be avoided in such patients to prevent exacerbation of the condition and

Afferent peripheral nerve pathology Lack of sensation leading to dysfunction Increased activity e.g. neuralgias

Efferent peripheral nerve pathology
Secondary muscle weakness (locomotor,
    respiratory, airway protection, oesophageal
    function)

Muscle pathology Interaction with neuromuscular blocking agents   (respiratory function)

Figure 20.3: *Effects of peripheral nervous system disease.*

prolongation of blockade. One example of such a condition is myasthenia gravis, in which an autoimmune reaction occurs to acetylcholine receptors. It is characterized by profound muscle weakness. It is often associated with tumours of the thymus, the excision of which requires a thoracotomy (see Chapter 15). If neuromuscular blocking agents are required, extreme prolongation of their effect should be anticipated, and a test dose of approximately 1/10th of the normal dose should be used initially. Weakness of the oesophageal musculature often results in megaoesophagus, predisposing the animal to regurgitation and inhalation pneumonia (see Chapter 16). Thus thoracic auscultation and chest radiography are important parts of the preoperative assessment in these patients. Evidence of pulmonary pathology should be taken seriously and symptomatic treatment instituted before general anaesthesia if possible. Anaesthetic drugs with a short duration of action and rapid recovery phase should be chosen, for example, short-acting opioids, midazolam, propofol and isoflurane.

CHAPTER TWENTY ONE

Trauma Patients

Tanya Duke

INTRODUCTION

Traumatized patients can make up 10% of the caseload in small animal veterinary practice. Most of the injuries are sustained during road traffic accidents, but occasionally a patient with gunshot wounds may be seen (Norman *et al.*, 1989; Pavletic, 1996). Each type of injury has its own impact on the body, which must be assessed and treated.

The key to giving an anaesthetic successfully to a traumatized patient is in prompt evaluation and stabilization, so that the body can compensate for the pathophysiological changes due to anaesthesia. This chapter, therefore, initially discusses patient stabilization followed by methods of anaesthesia.

INITIAL PATIENT EVALUATION

The forces of impact on the body during road traffic accidents can cause such severe injury that death occurs within moments. Death results from serious damage to the central nervous system (CNS) and/or massive haemorrhage from rupture of the heart or large blood vessels.

In other patients with injuries caused by road traffic accidents, survival is highly dependent on the quality of care they receive in the hour after the accident (Kovacic, 1994). Failure to provide the injured animal with appropriate treatment during this time results in failure of the body's compensatory mechanisms, and death may occur as a result of cardiopulmonary collapse. Occasionally, a traumatized patient can show signs of initial resuscitation, but ischaemic or reperfusion injury at the cellular level results in systemic inflammatory response syndrome (SIRS) and multiple organ dysfunction syndrome (MODS). The CNS, myocardium, kidneys, gastrointestinal tract and liver become progressively underperfused, resulting in lipid peroxidation from released iron, progressive pulmonary oedema, protein malnutrition, failure of the immune response and disseminated intravascular coagulation. Appropriate triage, and initiation of fluid, oxygen and ventilatory therapy may reduce the number of animals that die from the effects of tissue ischaemia.

All patients with injuries caused by high energy impact should be regarded as being at high risk and should be admitted to hospital. The initial survey of injuries should be rapid and centre on the provision of life support. Vital signs should be assessed:

- Level of consciousness since the accident
- Adequacy of airway, breathing and circulation.

Trauma centres for humans use patient severity scales as a triage tool and these have been adapted for use in the veterinary setting (Martin, 1996). After the urgent problems have been addressed, a more detailed and thorough examination of the patient can follow to ensure nothing has been missed.

INITIAL TREATMENT

The patient should have at least two large-bore catheters placed into accessible veins. A surgical cut down to the jugular vein may be necessary in collapsed animals to allow catheterization for intravenous fluid therapy and measurement of central venous pressure. Crystalloids such as Hartmann's (lactated Ringer's) solution can be delivered initially at 90 ml/kg/h in dogs and 60 ml/kg/h in cats. Colloids such as dextran 70, starch- or gelatin-based colloids can be given initially at rates of 20 ml/kg/h (up to a maximum of 20 ml/kg/day). Colloidal fluids are particularly indicated if administration of crystalloids dilutes total protein concentration to ≤35 g/l. Improvement in circulation is vital to preserve tissue perfusion, and fluids should be given even if haemorrhage is not evident. Peripheral pulse quality, heart and respiratory rate, mucous membrane colour and level of consciousness should improve towards normal with aggressive treatment. Inotropes and/or vasopressors may be necessary in severely shocked patients (Figure 21.1).

Traumatized patients incur an oxygen debt due to a hypermetabolic state driven by catecholamine release and anaerobic respiration at the cellular level, and this must be repaid during resuscitation. The respiratory and cardiovascular system must therefore be functioning adequately for optimal oxygen delivery to tissues.

Vasopressor/Inotrope	Dosage	Comments
Dopamine	2–10 µg/kg/min (infusion)	Dopaminergic effects with 2–5 µg/kg/min; β_1 receptor stimulation with 5–10 µg/kg/min; α_1 receptor stimulation with 10–15 µg/kg/min
Dobutamine	2–15 µg/kg/min (infusion)	β_1 receptor stimulation
Phenylephrine	1–3 µg/kg/min (infusion)	α_1 receptor stimulation (limit use of potent α_1-adrenergic stimulants as continuous use can decrease blood flow through splanchnic viscera)
Noradrenaline	0.1–0.2 µg/kg/min (infusion)	Mixed α and β receptor stimulation
Ephedrine	0.05–0.1 mg/kg bolus	Mixed α and β receptor stimulation (effects last approximately 15–20 minutes)

Figure 21.1: *Dosages of inotropes and vasopressors used for haemodynamic support in dogs and cats.*

VENTILATION AND OXYGENATION OF TRAUMATIZED PATIENTS

The incidence of thoracic injury in dogs with fractures as a result of road traffic accidents has been reported to range from 38.9% to 59.5% (Spackman *et al.*, 1984; Tamas *et al.*, 1985; Selcer *et al.*, 1987). Thoracic injuries should always be at the forefront of the clinician's mind when examining traumatized patients.

The severity of pulmonary dysfunction can be assessed by observation of the patient's breathing pattern:

- Noisy respirations indicate upper airway obstruction (foreign body, laryngeal trauma)
- Prolonged expiration indicates small airway obstruction or pleural adhesions (asthma, bronchial obstruction)
- Rapid and shallow breathing indicates fluid or air in the pleura, or diaphragmatic hernia
- Laboured inspiration/expiration indicates lung oedema, pneumonia or aspiration
- Abnormal chest movement may indicate the presence of a flail chest (Murtaugh, 1994).

Oxygen is not contraindicated and should always be given. Oxygen can be given by face mask, nasal catheter, head tent (Figure 21.2) or oxygen cage. Unconscious patients should be intubated orotracheally and oxygen given from an anaesthetic machine or Ambu bag using oxygen-enriched air.

Upper airway obstruction due to severe head and neck injury may require a tracheotomy (see Chapter 13). Severely cyanotic and decompensating patients may require such a procedure without aseptic preparation. A transtracheal catheter (over-the-needle type, 18–14 gauge) can be used to supply oxygen in an emergency. Wherever possible, however, the patient should be intubated orotracheally with an endotracheal tube (ETT) that is smaller than usual, and then a tracheotomy should be performed with surgical precision. If tracheotomy tubes are not available, an ETT can be used.

If pleural air or pleural effusions are suspected, percussion of the chest should reveal hyper-resonance with pleural air and hyporesonance with pleural effusions. Thoracocentesis (with local anaesthetic infiltration) aids diagnosis and allows drainage of the pleural space. Stressed cyanotic animals can suffer cardiac arrest during positioning for radiography (Murtaugh, 1994).

The most sensitive means for assessing a patient is by arterial blood gas analysis. In dogs and some cats, the dorsal pedal artery is an easy site from which to obtain an arterial blood sample without risk of contamination with venous blood. The alveolar to arterial oxygen gradient (A–a) can be calculated if the patient is breathing room air at sea level:

$$A\text{–}a \text{ (kPa)} = (20^* - PaCO_2/0.8) - PaO_2$$

*For mmHg substitute 150 (1 kPa = 7.5 mmHg)

Where $PaCO_2$ is the partial pressure of carbon dioxide in arterial blood, and PaO_2 is the partial pressure of oxygen in arterial blood.

An A–a gradient of more than 2 kPa (15 mmHg) indicates severe mismatch of lung ventilation and perfusion. Another method to check for shunting of

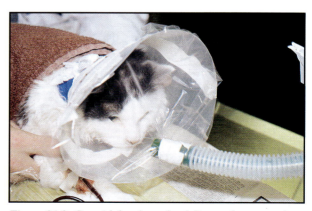

Figure 21.2: *Cat with head tent for delivery of oxygen using Bain breathing circuit.*

blood is to assume that the PaO_2 (in mmHg) should be almost five times the inspired oxygen (in percent) in healthy unanaesthetized individuals. If blood gas analysis is not available (local hospitals may help), clinical observation, auscultation, radiography and the use of a pulse oximeter may help guide treatment and decisions on whether to anaesthetize a patient. If anaesthesia can wait until the patient has had more time for recovery, then it should be postponed.

Pulmonary contusions account for 50% of thoracic injuries in cats and dogs (Tamas *et al.*, 1985). Contusions occur due to rapid compression–decompression forces during the traumatic event. On impact, the sudden increase in thoracic pressure may reach several hundred millimetres of mercury because the glottis limits emptying of air. Intra-alveolar, interstitial and interalveolar haemorrhages occur. Secondary oedema collapses pulmonary capillaries further, causing pulmonary hypertension. The distance over which oxygen has to diffuse increases, lowering PaO_2, and hypoventilation from chest pain further exacerbates hypoxaemia. Initially, a state of hypocarbia occurs as the hypoxic drive mechanism triggers ventilation, but hypercarbia follows as pulmonary damage progresses, and the respiratory muscles become tired from the extra work of breathing and concurrent poor oxygen delivery. The patient eventually dies from ventilatory failure. If pulmonary contusions are severe enough to cause hypoxaemia and hypercarbia, the patient will require ventilation (see below). Lesions worsen in the first 24–36 hours, and they may initially be missed. Radiographs may not accurately predict the presence of contusions for 4–6 hours after the injury. Resolution generally occurs within 3–7 days in patients that survive. Management of pulmonary contusions is supportive and depends on the severity. Mild cases may be managed by cage rest alone, but more severe cases require oxygen therapy and analgesics with little sedative effect, such as buprenorphine or butorphanol. Frusemide should be given if oedema is present, and antibiotics should be given on the basis of culture and sensitivity tests.

In a patient with a flail chest, there is a paradoxical movement of the chest wall (the wall moves in during inspiration), which may be associated with lung collapse on the affected side and hypoventilation resulting from pain. Dogs and cats with flail chests may have underlying lung injuries due to blunt trauma and sharp ends of fractured ribs. Treatment involves rest, oxygen therapy and analgesics. Surgical stabilization may be deferred until the patient has recovered from other injuries.

Patients with an open pneumothorax may have hidden damage to lung parenchyma. During inspiration, there is preferential intake of air through the rupture in the thoracic wall. The lung on the injured side will collapse, especially during inspiration, and expand slightly on expiration. Movement of air between the two lungs is called pendulum air and can cause hypoxaemia. A temporary seal can be placed over the hole using petroleum jelly-impregnated dressings, and as much air as possible should be evacuated from the pleural space. Oxygen therapy should be provided, and the patient stabilized before anaesthesia prior to wound treatment. Collapsed animals should be intubated promptly and ventilated. If the patient is stable, a wound can be surgically debrided under inhalational anaesthesia. Chronically collapsed lungs should not be re-expanded vigorously under anaesthesia as this may promote oedema formation.

A closed pneumothorax can be diagnosed by dullness on auscultation and hyper-resonance on percussion. Thoracocentesis confirms diagnosis, and as much air as possible should be evacuated using a butterfly needle, stopcock and syringe. Continuous formation of pleural air may necessitate continuous suction. Rapidly deteriorating patients usually have a tension pneumothorax. The patient collapses because lung expansion becomes limited and venous return to the heart is reduced. Orotracheal intubation, ventilation of lungs and placement of a chest tube and its connection to a continuous suction device should be performed. If the patient is stable, the damage may heal without surgical intervention. Surgical correction should be performed if the pneumothorax is unresponsive to management with continuous suction over several days.

Anaesthesia for the patient with pulmonary dysfunction

Respiratory emergencies may require fast sequence induction techniques. Drugs with reliable anaesthetic action in one injection site-to-brain circulation time should be used, to allow rapid intubation and connection to a source of oxygen and ventilation. Halfway measures, such as sedation with intravenous acepromazine or diazepam in cyanotic restless patients, do not work. Figure 21.3 lists suitable drugs. Caution should be taken when using propofol, alphaxolone/alphadolone and the barbiturates because of their hypotensive side effects. For rapid intubation, the following should be available:

- A good light source
- A range of ETT sizes
- A stylette
- Suction
- A tracheotomy kit.

For stable patients, light premedication can be used. Heavy sedation, however, should be avoided as drugs may depress the respiratory centre and the patient can adopt positions that limit good ventilatory movement. A low dose of acepromazine can be used in combination with pethidine (meperidine), butorphanol or buprenorphine.

Agent	Dogs	Cats	Comments
Propofol	6 mg/kg i.v.	8 mg/kg i.v.	No premedication
Propofol and diazepam	Propofol 6 mg/kg i.v. Diazepam 0.2 mg/kg i.v.	Propofol 8 mg/kg i.v. Diazepam 0.2 mg/kg i.v.	Give half the propofol, immediately follow with diazepam, wait 20 seconds, then titrate propofol until intubation is possible (flush between injections)
Thiopentone and diazepam	Thiopentone 15 mg/kg i.v. Diazepam 0.2 mg/kg i.v.	Thiopentone 15 mg/kg i.v. Diazepam 0.2 mg/kg i.v.	Give half the thiopentone, immediately follow with diazepam, wait 20 seconds, then titrate thiopentone until intubation is possible (flush between injections)
Diazepam and ketamine	Diazepam 1.0 mg/kg i.v. Ketamine 10 mg/kg i.v.	Diazepam 1.0 mg/kg i.v. Ketamine 10 mg/kg i.v.	Mix just before administration. Give half, then titrate rest to effect (results are variable)
Alphaxolone/ Alphadolone	Not applicable	12 mg/kg i.v.	Respiratory depressant. Preoxygenation advised

Figure 21.3: Injectable induction agents recommended for rapid sequence induction of dogs and cats with respiratory emergencies. Maintenance of anaesthesia is with inhalational techniques.

Cats may be either induced in a chamber or given rapid sequence induction, depending on their temperament. In cats, intramuscular administration of anaesthetic drugs such as ketamine combinations may cause hypoxaemia and cardiac arrest.

Inhalation with halothane or isoflurane should be used to maintain anaesthesia. Isoflurane may be the better choice of anaesthetic in the presence of myocardial contusions (see below). Nitrous oxide should not be used in the presence of a closed pneumothorax or where good oxygenation is questionable owing to pulmonary pathology.

If there is any doubt that a pneumothorax will develop intraoperatively, a chest drain should be preplaced on the non-dependent side after induction. This allows rapid evacuation of air.

Surgical procedures under regional anaesthetic techniques, such as extradural (epidural) or brachial plexus nerve block, may require patient sedation and compromise gaseous exchange, but can be considered in some quiet animals if oxygen is provided and controlled ventilation is not required.

HAEMORRHAGE

Left untreated, mortality has been found to be 50% with acute blood loss of 42–47% and 100% with >48% loss (Brasmer, 1984). Many patients may not have visible signs of haemorrhage, but blood loss should be suspected after blunt trauma. Blood loss may be confined to body cavities, and fractured bone ends often form large haematomas. In a patient with multiple fractures and pulmonary contusions, blood loss may be significant.

Compensation by the body can enable blood pressure to be maintained, although cardiac output decreases with a 10–20% volume deficit. Heart rate increases but may not be a reliable indicator of blood loss as the rate may not become tachycardic until the terminal stages. Respiratory rate has been found to increase dramatically after haemorrhage and this is thought to be due to decreased cerebral blood flow resulting in the accumulation of carbon dioxide and hydrogen ions in the respiratory centre. Packed cell volume (PCV) measurement is not a reliable indicator of haemorrhage owing to splenic contraction and fluid shifts. Total protein concentration has been found to increase initially as new plasma protein enters from lymphatics and extravascular albumin reserves. Lactic acid measurement is a sensitive indicator of survival in shock; if lactic acid persistently stays above 8 mM/l (72 mg/dl) the mortality rate is 90% (Brasmer, 1984).

Blood transfusions, including autotransfusion techniques in some cases, should be undertaken in patients with an acute decrease of PCV to <25%, or loss of >35% of blood volume (see Chapter 11). A PCV of 30% should be the goal during transfusion. Oxygen should still be given, as increasing the amount dissolved in plasma may make the difference between life and death. Ongoing bleeding can be treated by external counterpressure, ligation of blood vessels, pressure on arteries or inflation of a blood pressure cuff around a limb. Diagnosis of abdominal bleeding is best detected by peritoneal lavage (Crowe and Devey, 1994).

Anaesthesia for patients with unstable haemodynamics

Treatment of haemorrhage may require surgical management and thus anaesthesia. An attempt must be made to stabilize the patient as much as possible with fluid therapy and blood transfusions. Severe hypotension should be prevented with appropriate anaesthetic agents. Acepromazine and α_2-adrenergic agonists should be avoided, as should high doses of barbiturates, propofol and alphaxolone/alphadolone. If a rapid sequence induction is required in a hypovolaemic dog, thiopentone is preferable to propofol, although it should be borne in mind that both drugs are hypotensive (Ilkiw *et al.*, 1991, 1992). If etomidate is available, however, it can safely be given to hypovolaemic dogs for induction of anaesthesia (Pascoe *et al.*, 1992).

After preoxygenation for 5 minutes in dogs without respiratory difficulties, neuroleptanalgesic combinations can be given intravenously to induce anaesthesia (Figure 21.4) (Haskins *et al.*, 1991). Neuroleptanalgesic inductions are slow to administer and are not ideal for rapid sequence induction. They can also make dogs sensitive to noise but seem to cause little disruption of cardiovascular function. Bradycardia should be treated with an anticholinergic, preferably glycopyrrolate.

Opioids can also be used to provide some sedation before mask induction in cats and dogs (Figure 21.5). Benzodiazepine/ketamine combinations can be used in dogs and cats, either alone or after premedication with an opioid.

Despite their hypotensive effects, both isoflurane and halothane can be used to induce and maintain anaesthesia in hypovolaemic dogs (Pascoe *et al.*, 1994). In theory, a longer induction with an inhalational agent gives time for the body to adjust to changes without decompensating and provides oxygen by nature of the technique. Inhalational induction occurs more rapidly in depressed hypovolaemic patients because low cardiac output increases uptake of anaesthetic agents. During the maintenance period, further administration of analgesic agents allows the amount of halothane and isoflurane to be decreased.

Further circulatory support may be required in the form of blood, crystalloids, synthetic colloids, inotropes and vasopressors (see Figure 21.1). The mean blood pressure can be kept at a minimum 60 mmHg (systolic blood pressure 80 mmHg) until haemorrhage is controlled.

Agent	Dogs	Cats	Comments
Oxymorphone and diazepam	Oxymorphone 0.1–0.2 mg/kg i.v. Diazepam 0.25 mg/kg i.v.	Not applicable	Give opioid first, wait for sign of sedation, then give benzodiazepine. May need mask induction to allow intubation. Noise sensitive. Variable results (anticholinergic may be necessary for bradycardia)
Oxymorphone and midazolam	Oxymorphone 0.1–0.2 mg/kg i.v. Midazolam 0.25 mg/kg i.v.	Not applicable	As above
Fentanyl and diazepam	Fentanyl 0.01–0.02 mg/kg i.v. Diazepam 0.2 mg/kg i.v.	Not applicable	As above
Sufentanil and diazepam	Sufentanil 0.005 mg/kg i.v. Diazepam 0.2 mg/kg i.v.	Not applicable	As above
Hydromorphone and diazepam	Hydromorphone 0.2–0.3 mg/kg i.v. Diazepam 0.2 mg/kg i.v.	Not applicable	As above
Methadone and diazepam	Methadone 0.1–0.6 mg/kg i.v. Diazepam 0.2 mg/kg i.v.	Not applicable	
Etomidate and diazepam	Etomidate 1 mg/kg i.v. Diazepam 0.2 mg/kg i.v.	Etomidate 1 mg/kg i.v. Diazepam 0.5 mg/kg i.v.	May cause muscle tremors, reduced by diazepam (given as with thiopentone or propofol; see Figure 21.3)
Diazepam and ketamine	Diazepam 1 mg/kg i.v. Ketamine 10 mg/kg i.v.	Diazepam 1 mg/kg i.v. Ketamine 10 mg/kg i.v.	Mix just before use, give half, then titrate the rest to effect

Figure 21.4: *Injectable induction agents recommended for haemodynamically unstable dogs and cats. Maintenance of anaesthesia is with inhalational techniques.*

Agent	Dogs	Cats	Comments
Morphine and midazolam	Morphine 0.4-0.8 mg/kg i.m. Midazolam 0.2 mg/kg i.m.	Morphine 0.1-0.2 mg/kg i.m.	May vomit (best results in depressed or geriatric patients)
Pethidine (meperidine)	Pethidine 2-5 mg/kg i.m.	Pethidine 2-5 mg/kg i.m.	Light sedation
Methadone	Methadone 0.1-0.6 mg/kg i.m	Methadone 0.2 mg/kg i.m.	
Oxymorphone and midazolam	Oxymorphone 0.1-0.2 mg/kg i.m. Midazolam 0.2 mg/kg i.m.	Oxymorphone 0.1-0.2 mg/kg i.m. Midazolam 0.2 mg/kg i.m.	Best results in depressed or geriatric patients Cats may become dysphoric
Oxymorphone	Oxymorphone 0.1-0.2 mg/kg i.m.	Oxymorphone 0.1 mg/kg i.m.	
Hydromorphone	Hydromorphone 0.1-0.3 mg/kg i.m.	Hydromorphone 0.1-0.2 mg/kg i.m.	

Figure 21.5: Sedative agents recommended for haemodynamically unstable dogs and cats before induction by mask with an inhalational agent. Maintenance of anaesthesia is with inhalational techniques.

MYOCARDIAL CONTUSIONS

Blunt trauma to the myocardium can result in arrhythmias such as ventricular premature contractions and ventricular tachycardia. These arrhythmias are commonly observed in dogs and usually manifest 12-24 hours after trauma, but are often refractory to treatment. The patient's circulation should be assessed and hypovolaemia and electrolyte imbalances treated (especially hypokalaemia and hypomagnesaemia) (Wong *et al.*, 1993). If ventricular tachycardia or ventricular premature contractions are compromising the patient's circulation, anti-arrhythmic drugs can be used (Figure 21.6).

Anaesthesia for patients with myocardial contusions

Most patients can be stabilized and surgery delayed until myocardial arrhythmias have resolved. If treatment of open hindlimb fractures is required, local anaesthetics with opioids can be given extradurally. For procedures below the elbow, a brachial plexus nerve block can be performed. If general anaesthesia is indicated, arrhythmogenic drugs such as xylazine, thiobarbiturates and halothane should be avoided where possible, and neuroleptanalgesic combinations (see Figure 21.4) used for induction after preoxygenation. Mask induction can be used after premedication with a low-dose acepromazine/opioid combination. Maintenance of anaesthesia should be provided with isoflurane. Antiarrhythmic treatment may need to be continued during the anaesthetic period. The cardiovascular system should be monitored by electrocardiography and measurement of blood pressure.

INJURY TO THE CNS

Animals with head trauma may have increased intracranial pressure (ICP) due to swelling within the cranium. As ICP rises there is initial displacement of cerebro-

Anti-arrhythmic drug	Dogs
Lignocaine (lidocaine)	2 mg/kg slow i.v. bolus up to total 8 mg/kg. Infuse at 25-80 µg/kg/min
Procainamide	10-20 mg/kg slow i.v. bolus. Infuse at 10-50 µg/kg/min or give 6-20 mg/kg i.m. every 4-6 hours

Figure 21.6: Anti-arrhythmic agents for ventricular arrhythmias due to traumatic myocarditis in dogs.

spinal fluid, but there is little room for further expansion. Pressure increases markedly and eventually areas of the brain become ischaemic, or herniation occurs. A neurological examination should be performed at regular intervals to assess whether ICP is increasing. Sluggish perfusion of blood through the medulla of the brain is manifested by bradycardia, hypertension and changes in breathing pattern, such as tachypnoea, bradypnoea and Cheyne-Stokes or apneustic respiration. Systemic hypertension and bradycardia are a result of the body's attempt to maintain cerebral perfusion. Although rare, neurogenic pulmonary oedema may develop during increases in ICP (Diringer, 1993.) Deterioration in physical status is heralded by decreasing mental alertness and either anisocoria, constricted pupils or fixed and dilated pupils.

If head injury is suspected, treatment should be initiated to decrease ICP. Treatment includes giving mannitol (0.5-2.0 g/kg i.v. over 5-30 minutes), frusemide (0.7 mg/kg i.v., 15 minutes after mannitol) and hyperventilation to a $PaCO_2$ of 30-35 mmHg (Hopkins, 1996). The intravenous fluid rate should be decreased to 1-2 ml/kg/h as soon as possible, as crystalloids may exacerbate CNS oedema. Hypertonic saline (4-5 ml/kg 7% NaCl over 3-5 minutes) can help restore circulation yet limit increases in ICP, if there are no other contraindications such as dehydration, uncontrolled haemorrhage into the cranium, hypernatraemia, ketoacidosis and heart or renal failure (Dewey *et al.*, 1993).

Intermittent positive-pressure ventilation for head trauma

Hyperventilation requires endotracheal intubation. Administration of 100% oxygen for longer than 24 hours may damage the pulmonary system. In order to minimize this damage, humidified oxygen/air mixtures should be used for ventilation. The fraction of oxygen should be the minimum necessary to produce normoxia. This procedure is labour-intensive and requires investment in suitable equipment and technology. Long-term ventilation of a patient may not be feasible in some practices.

Patients can be sedated with pentobarbitone and placed on an infusion drip during the period hyperventilation is required. This technique should not be used for surgery because it does not produce analgesia, and high doses of pentobarbitone are required, which can cause cardiovascular depression. The initial bolus of pentobarbitone is 2–5 mg/kg i.v. given at an infusion rate of 1–2 mg/kg/h. The rate may need to be increased up to 6 mg/kg/h, but should be reduced if there are signs of deepening anaesthesia.

Pentobarbitone can be given in 5% dextrose solution, but greater accuracy can be achieved with a syringe driver. Non-depolarizing muscle relaxants can be used to supplement sedation and prevent extubation or resistance to intermittent positive-pressure ventilation.

Anaesthesia for patients with head injury

Anaesthesia for patients with stable haemodynamics can be induced with thiopentone/diazepam, propofol/diazepam or etomidate/diazepam. These induction agents lower cerebral metabolic rate and ICP. Neuroleptanalgesic combinations (see Figure 21.4) can be used to induce anaesthesia in dogs. Isoflurane, rather than halothane, is best used to provide maintenance of anaesthesia, as it does not disrupt autoregulation of cerebral

vasomotor tone when $PaCO_2$ is controlled. During anaesthesia, cerebral perfusion pressure should be maintained by ensuring that systemic blood pressure is normal to slightly above normal, and that the jugular veins are not compressed. In extreme hypertensive states, vasodilators such as nitroprusside should be avoided as they can increase ICP. If necessary, labetalol should be used (Diringer, 1993). Ketamine, α_2-adrenergic agonists and suxamethonium (succinyl choline) should not be used, as these drugs can increase ICP. Nitrous oxide may increase ICP, but this can be overcome by hyperventilation. Opioids can be used as long as $PaCO_2$ remains within normal limits (Cornick, 1992). Further details may be found in Chapter 20.

RUPTURE OF THE URINARY TRACT

Ruptured bladders are present in 62% of patients with injuries to the renal system caused by road traffic accidents. Unless there is another reason for anaesthesia, patient stabilization is possible. Leakage of urine into the abdomen produces hyperkalaemia, hyponatraemia, hypochloraemia and uraemia. Hyperkalaemia produces weakness, bradycardia and poor myocardial contractility. Patients should not be anaesthetized until potassium levels are within the normal range. Figure 21.7 outlines the treatment for hyperkalaemia. Uraemia causes CNS depression and a change in ionization of thiopentone, making it more potent. Patients are often in shock and require volume replacement. Catheterization of the bladder may enable urine to be drained from the abdomen through the bladder rupture. Direct peritoneal catherization may also be used to remove urine from the abdomen.

Anaesthesia for patients with rupture of the urinary tract

Anaesthesia can be performed using haemodynamically stable techniques, such as neuroleptanalgesic techniques in dogs, low doses of injectable agents/mask induction and inhalational anaesthesia for maintenance. Further details can be found in Chapter 17.

Treatment	Dosage	Comments
Crystalloids	Rapid infusion	Volume expansion. Promotes diuresis
10% calcium gluconate	0.5–1.0 ml/kg i.v. over 10–15 minutes	Reverses effects of life-threatening hyperkalaemia (effect is not long lasting: 15 minutes)
Sodium bicarbonate	1–2 mmol/kg over 10–15 minutes	Reverses acidosis. Drives potassium ions (K^+) into cells
Soluble insulin and dextrose	Dog: 2–5 IU insulin i.v. (with 2 g/IU dextrose i.v.) Cat: 0.5 IU insulin i.v. (with 2 g/IU dextrose i.v.)	Drives K^+ into cells. Hypoglycaemia possible

Figure 21.7: Treatment of hyperkalaemia in cats and dogs before anaesthesia.

THERMAL INJURIES

Hypothermia/frostbite

Avascular necrosis is a feature of areas exposed to sub-zero temperatures, and it may be accompanied by hypothermia. In cats, hypothermia commonly affects the ear pinnae, the tail and footpads, and in dogs the external genitalia and footpads. The affected areas should be thawed in warm water at 39-40°C. The areas should not be allowed to refreeze as this increases the area of necrosis. Thawed areas become erythematous over 2-3 days. Over several days, shrinkage and discoloration occur, and in 20-30 days demarcation and slough occur. During this time the patient may require analgesics, such as opioids and non-steroidal anti-inflammatory drugs. Concurrent hypothermia and shock must be treated. Dextran 40 has been recommended to prevent sludging in the peripheral circulation, but overhydration should be avoided as this may promote further oedema formation within the injured site.

Anaesthesia can be delayed until the patient is stable and demarcation is complete, allowing surgical removal of affected areas. Standard techniques for anaesthesia can be used in these patients.

Burn injuries

Above 50°C, denaturation of cellular proteins results in cell death. Hypovolaemic shock, caused by increased permeability of capillaries to substances with molecular weights <125,000 kDa, results in loss of circulating volume. In patients with >40% of the total body surface area affected, 50% of plasma can be lost to extravascular areas. The myocardium is depressed owing to circulating interleukins and complement, and is refractory to inotropic drugs during this time. Crystalloids should be given to replace fluid losses (kg (bodyweight) x % burn x 4 = ml required). Colloids can be given (0.3-0.5 ml/kg x % burn = ml), but preferably after 12 hours, once permeability of the capillaries has returned to near normal. Corticosteroids are not effective at decreasing permeability and may promote sepsis. In 3-5 days diuresis occurs, producing thirst and restlessness. Hyperkalaemia occurs initially and hypokalaemia during the diuretic phase. Sepsis is another possible sequel, as opportunistic bacteria can multiply in devitalized tissues. Anaemia occurs due to blood loss from the injury and surgical debridement, and there is poor regeneration because of bone marrow depression from sepsis. An increased metabolic rate up to twice that of the resting rate results in an increased oxygen demand and substrate requirement (30-80 kcal/kg/day). Energy is required to evaporate water from wounds, for increased work by the kidneys and for anabolism. After the first 24 hours, when ambient temperatures should be 24°C, energy requirements can be decreased by increasing ambient temperatures to 34°C.

Anaesthesia for patients with burn injuries

Anaesthesia may be required in patients with burn injuries, for applying dressings and debridement of injuries. An assessment of the airway should be made visually and by endoscopy if available. Endoscopy requires anaesthesia. Burns around the head and neck can make intubation difficult and alternative routes, such as tracheotomy, may need to be used.

Treatments for burn injuries are painful, and opioid analgesics should be used as part of the anaesthetic protocol. In haemodynamically stable patients, induction can be achieved with low-dose injectable agents, and maintenance of anaesthesia can be achieved with inhalational agents. The regimens outlined in Figure 21.4 should be used in hypovolaemic patients. Intramuscular sedation with tranquillizer/opioid combinations can be used for dressing changes but the patient should be closely monitored and oxygen given.

Patients with burn injuries are sensitive to suxamethonium (succinylcholine) and resistant to non-depolarizing muscle relaxants. Nitrous oxide may be contraindicated if pulmonary pathology is present or oxygen saturation decreases.

SMOKE INHALATION

Smoke contains gases that limit oxygen utilization (carbon monoxide, carbon dioxide, hydrogen cyanide) and gases that irritate the airway (aldehydes, hydrogen chloride, ammonia, sulphur dioxide). Lung damage can take a few days to manifest its full effects. Hot air or steam inhalation can result in oedema of the airways, and it can take up to 24 hours until peak effect is observed. Bacterial pneumonia is a common complication of smoke inhalation. Radiographs may be normal for the first 16-24 hours. If possible, arterial blood gas analysis and carbon monoxide concentrations should be measured. A normal PaO_2 may, however, be misleading as the oxygen-carrying capacity of haemoglobin may be reduced by carbon monoxide. A haemoximeter should be used to measure oxygen saturation of arterial blood, rather than a pulse oximeter. Treatment to reduce bronchospasm should be implemented using aminophylline, theophylline or terbutaline, and oxygen given by nasal insufflation, head tent or oxygen cage (Beasley, 1990).

Anaesthesia for patients with smoke inhalation injury

Anaesthesia may be required in patients with smoke inhalation injuries for bronchoalveolar lavage (BAL) or bronchoscopy to obtain samples for biopsy, culture or sensitivity tests. Such patients pose a risk of severe hypoxaemia during anaesthesia, and procedures should be kept as short as possible. Patients should receive oxygen at all times. Drugs with rapid elimination times should be used to minimize the period in which the pathophysiological changes due to anaesthesia compound those changes due to smoke inhalation. In dogs, the method of anaesthesia the author has used for BAL comprises premedication with glycopyrrolate (0.01 mg/kg i.m. or i.v.) followed by sufentanil (5 μg/kg i.v.). Once the dog has been narcotized, intubation is possible using a sterile ETT. The catheter for lavage should be placed through the ETT and the wash fluid passed through the catheter. Naloxone 0.04 mg/kg i.v. reverses the sufentanil. When the dog immediately coughs, the sample can be aspirated. Once extubation is accomplished, the dog is allowed to regain consciousness. If a slightly longer period of anaesthesia is required for bronchoscopy, anaesthesia can be maintained using inhalational techniques, but reversal can still be accomplished with naloxone. In cats the best method may be to induce anaesthesia with an inhalational agent using a chamber or mask, as this technique uses oxygen supplementation and recovery from anaesthesia is rapid.

OCULAR TRAUMA

Increased systemic blood pressure causes an increase in intraocular pressure and may produce further damage. Drugs such as ketamine and suxamethonium (succinylcholine) should be avoided. The patient should not be intubated during light planes of anaesthesia as coughing during tube placement can also increase blood pressure. Lignocaine (2 mg/kg i.v. in dogs and 0.25 mg/kg i.v. in cats) can be used before intubation to reduce coughing. Postoperatively, appropriate sedation and analgesia may be required to prevent the patient inflicting self-trauma and destroying delicate repairs. If muscle relaxants were used during surgery, appropriate measures should be taken to ensure the patient has been adequately reversed and that ventilation is optimal.

PREGNANT PATIENTS

If a pregnant animal is injured in a road traffic accident, the hypovolaemic shock resulting from severe injuries and haemorrhage may cause loss of the fetuses. Once the mother's injuries have been dealt with, fetal viability should be assessed with ultrasonography.

Abdominal injuries can cause rupture of the uterus, and life-saving surgery may be required. Hypovolaemia should be treated, as outlined above, before anaesthesia is induced. Emergency ovariohysterectomy, using local anaesthetics administered into the lumbosacral epidural space (1 ml/4.5 kg 2% lignocaine),

may result in hypotension due to vasomotor nerve block. Sedation of the mother with opioids/tranquillizers is often required, making surgery using epidural techniques more haemodynamically depressive than a well managed general anaesthetic technique. In pregnancy, the MAC of halothane is reduced by 25% and that of isoflurane by 40%, and anaesthetic uptake during mask/chamber induction enhanced (Palahniuk *et al.*, 1974).

REFERENCES

Beasley VR (1990) Smoke inhalation. *Veterinary Clinics of North America: Small Animal Practice* **20**, 545–555

Brasmer TH (1984) The physiologic response to trauma. In: *The Acutely Traumatized Small Animal Patient, vol 2*, pp.15–44. WB Saunders, Philadelphia

Cornick JL (1992) Anaesthetic management of patients with neurologic abnormalities. *Compendium of Continuing Education* **14**, 163–170

Crowe DT and Devey JJ (1994) Assessment and management of the hemorrhaging patient. *Veterinary Clinics of North America: Small Animal Practice* **24**, 1095–1121

Dewey CW, Budsberg SC and Oliver JE (1993) Principles of head trauma management in dogs and cats. Part II. *Compendium of Continuing Education* **15**, 177–192

Diringer MN (1993) Intracerebral hemorrhage: pathophysiology and management. *Critical Care Medicine* **21**, 1591–1603

Haskins SC, Copland VS and Patz JD (1991) The cardiopulmonary effects of oxymorphone in hypovolemic dogs. *Veterinary Emergency and Critical Care* **1**, 32–38

Hopkins AL (1996) Head trauma. *Veterinary Clinics of North America: Small Animal Practice* **26**, 875–889

Ilkiw JE, Haskins SC and Patz JD (1991) Cardiovascular and respiratory effects of thiopental administration in hypovolaemic dogs *American Journal of Veterinary Research* **52**, 576–580

Ilkiw JE, Pascoe PJ, Haskins SC and Patz JD (1992) Cardiovascular and respiratory effects of propofol administration in hypovolemic dogs. *American Journal of Veterinary Research* **53**, 2323–2327

Kovacic JP (1994) Management of life-threatening trauma. *Veterinary Clinics of North America: Small Animal Practice* **24**, 1057–1093

Martin DD (1996) Trauma patients. In: *Lumb and Jones Veterinary Anaesthesia, ed. Thurmon JC et al.,* pp. 829–843. Williams and Wilkins, Baltimore

Murtaugh RJ (1994) Acute respiratory distress. *Veterinary Clinics of North America: Small Animal Practice* **24**, 1041–1055

Norman WM, Dodman NH, Court MH and Seeler DC (1989) Anaesthetic management of the traumatized small animal patient. *British Veterinary Journal* **145**, 410–425

Palahniuk RJ, Shnider SM and Eger EI (1974) Pregnancy decreases the requirement for inhaled anaesthetic agents. *Anesthesiology* **41**, 82–83

Pascoe PJ, Haskins SC, Iliw JE and Patz JD (1994) Cardiopulmonary effects of halothane in hypovolaemic dogs. *American Journal of Veterinary Research* **55**, 121–126

Pascoe PJ, Ilkiw JE, Haskins SC and Patz JD (1992) Cardiopulmonary effects of etomidate in hypovolemic dogs. *American Journal of Veterinary Research* **53**, 2178–2182

Pavletic MM (1996) Gunshot wound management. *Compendium of Continuing Education* **18**, 1285–1299

Selcer BA, Buttrick M, Barstad R, *et al.* (1987) The incidence of thoracic trauma in dogs with skeletal injury. *Journal of Small Animal Practice* **28**, 21–27

Spackman CJA, Caywood DD, Feeney DA, *et al.* (1984) Thoracic wall and pulmonary trauma in dogs sustaining fractures as a result of motor vehicle accidents. *Journal of the American Veterinary Medical Association* **185**, 975–977

Tamas PM, Paddleford RR and Krahwinkel DJ (1985) Thoracic trauma in dogs and cats presented for limb fractures. *Journal of the American Animal Hospital Association* **21**, 161–166

Wong KC, Schafer PG and Schultz JR (1993) Hypokalemia and anaesthetic implications. *Anaesthesia Analgesia* **77**, 1238–1260

CHAPTER TWENTY TWO

Paediatric Patients

Daniel Holden

INTRODUCTION

Newborn cats and dogs are considered neonates until they are 4 weeks old; thereafter paediatric considerations apply until about 12 weeks of age. Anaesthesia may be required in these individuals for the urgent surgical correction of congenital abnormalities, or to allow other therapeutic and diagnostic procedures to be undertaken. In order to give a safe and effective anaesthetic, not only should technical considerations be borne in mind, but the anatomical, physiological and pharmacological differences that exist between paediatric and adult cats and dogs should also be recognized (Figure 22.1).

COMPARATIVE ANATOMY, PHYSIOLOGY AND PHARMACOLOGY

Respiratory system
One of the most striking physiological differences between paediatric and adult animals is the two- to

Parameter (units)	Normal value	
Rectal temperature (°C (°F))	35.4–36 (96–97) Increases to 37.7 (100) after 4 weeks of age	
Heart rate (beats per minute)	210+	
Arterial blood pressure (mmHg)	Systolic 70 Diastolic 45 Mean 60	
Haematocrit (%)	35–45 25–35	at birth at 28 days
Haemoglobin concentration (g/dl)	11–14 8–9	at birth at 28 days
Respiratory rate (breaths per minute)	20–36	

Figure 22.1: Normal values for selected physiological parameters in puppies and kittens.

threefold increase in tissue oxygen demand; this demand is met in part by a higher resting respiratory rate. Anatomical differences are also marked: in the paediatric patient the tongue is large relative to the size of the oral cavity, airway diameter is narrow (increasing resistance and therefore the work of breathing) and functional residual capacity (volume remaining in the lungs after expiration of normal tidal volume) may be lower than closing volume (critical lung volume at which small airways close) in some patients. These factors, together with high thoracic wall and airway compliance, lead to small and large airway closure and hypoventilation, especially in the presence of potent respiratory depressants such as volatile anaesthetic agents. The high oxygen demand also means that hypoxia under anaesthesia may be common. It is therefore desirable (if circumstances permit) to institute intermittent positive-pressure ventilation (IPPV) in all patients less than 6–8 weeks of age. Care should be taken not to induce barotrauma with excessive airway pressures.

Cardiovascular system
Immediately after birth, a marked fall in pulmonary vascular resistance occurs. Filling of the alveolae with air creates physical support for pulmonary vasculature, and vascular tone decreases as the alveolar oxygen tension increases. The abrupt cessation of placental blood flow increases the neonate's systemic vascular resistance. These factors combine to effectively reverse blood flow through the patent ductus arteriosus. Passage of blood with a high oxygen tension through the ductus causes its muscular wall to contract, and functional closure occurs. Left atrial pressure then increases, resulting in closure of the foramen ovale. As closure is initially functional and not anatomical, changes in oxygen tension or acid-base status due to respiratory disease may increase pulmonary vascular resistance and re-open fetal circulatory pathways.

Cardiac output in the paediatric patient is primarily dependent upon heart rate. This is due to the relatively large percentage of non-contractile cardiac mass and low ventricular compliance. As a result, stroke volume is effectively fixed, and increases in preload and afterload are poorly tolerated. The parasympathetic dominance that exists in the immature heart also means that the bradycardic influence of drugs such as opioids may induce severe hypotension. Due to these factors, paediatric patients are less able to endure blood loss than adults and losses of as little as 5 ml/kg may cause significant hypotension.

Haematopoiesis does not effectively commence until 2–3 months of age; before this time haemoglobin concentrations are lower than those of adults, further reducing the tolerance to surgical haemorrhage.

Hepatic function

Of main relevance to the anaesthetist with paediatric patients is the immaturity of the hepatic microsomal enzyme systems responsible for the metabolism and transformation of many anaesthetic and analgesic drugs. These systems are not considered fully functional until the animal is at least 8 weeks of age, and therefore drugs undergoing extensive hepatic metabolism should be avoided; failing this, doses should be reduced, and significantly longer elimination half-lives should be expected.

Glycogen storage in the neonatal and paediatric liver is minimal, and any excessive fasting or delay in feeding after anaesthesia results in rapid exhaustion of stores.

Renal function and fluid balance

Adult plasma albumin concentrations are not fully attained until an animal is about 8 weeks; therefore highly protein-bound drugs will exert a greater effect due to the greater proportion of free drug in circulation. Total body water content and extracellular fluid volume is higher than in adult animals, resulting in an increased volume of distribution of many drugs.

Renal function is also reduced in the first 6–8 weeks of life; paediatric patients cannot tolerate large volumes of fluid administered rapidly and are less well able to concentrate urine than adults. Solute loads are tolerated poorly, and all intravascular fluids should be administered carefully via a syringe pump or burette infusion set.

Temperature regulation

Low subcutaneous fat reserves, a high surface area: bodyweight ratio, poor thermoregulatory ability, less ability to shiver and a higher critical temperature (temperature at which metabolic activity is required to maintain a normal core temperature) all mean that paediatric and neonatal patients are at major risk of developing hypothermia during and after anaesthesia and surgery. Every attempt should be made to minimize anaesthetic and surgical time, and the importance of insulating materials, warming devices, minimal use of surgical preparation solutions and the maintenance of a high ambient temperature cannot be overemphasized.

PREOPERATIVE PREPARATION AND PREMEDICATION

It is both unnecessary and inadvisable to withhold food from unweaned puppies and kittens before anaesthesia. Excessive fasting may promote hypoglycaemia and predispose to hypothermia. Patients over 6 weeks old may require fasting for a maximum of 3 hours; withdrawal of water is not necessary.

The decision as to whether or not to give a premedicant depends upon many factors (such as underlying disease, duration of surgery, familiarity of drugs used), but in general the potential reduction in dose of induction and maintenance agents, as well as the benefit of providing intra- and postoperative analgesia, make some form of premedication seem a sensible option.

Three main classes of drug may be considered for use as premedicants: sedative-tranquillizers, opioid analgesic agents and anticholinergics (Figure 22.2).

Sedative-tranquillizing agents

In contrast to their variable sedative effects in adult animals, the benzodiazepines can provide consistently effective sedation in paediatric animals, although some paradoxical excitement may occasionally be seen. Cardiovascular depression is minimal with good muscle relaxation, but some respiratory depression does occur, and apnoea may be a problem if other depressant drugs are given. As these agents undergo extensive hepatic metabolism, care should be taken to avoid overdosage in patients less than 8 weeks of age. Of the available agents (none of which are licensed for use in veterinary species in the UK), diazepam and midazolam are the most common. Injectable diazepam exists in two forms in the UK: one with a propylene glycol carrier; and one as an emulsion. The former preparation may cause pain on injection (even intravenously), but can be given intramuscularly and is immiscible with other drugs (with the exception of ketamine). The emulsion form is only effective via the intravenous route and should only be diluted with normal saline. Midazolam is a water-soluble compound that can be administered by any route. Its potency is greater than that of diazepam, but its effects are shorter acting. Neither agent has any proven analgesic properties. Flumazenil is a specific benzodiazepine antagonist available for human use; its short duration of action (about 1 hour) may mean that repeat doses (0.1 mg/kg i.v.) may be required to reverse the effects of the initial drug.

Acepromazine is probably the most common routine premedicant in use in veterinary practice and can be used effectively to sedate healthy paediatric patients at doses of no more than 0.03 mg/kg. In very young (less than 8 weeks of age) or debilitated patients, acepromazine can cause profound and long-lasting sedation, together with cardiovascular collapse and hypothermia due to peripheral vasodilation; its use is contraindicated in these circumstances.

The α_2-agonist agents are very effective sedatives with some analgesic properties but can produce dramatic cardiovascular and respiratory depression. These agents are also extensively metabolized in the liver and their use should probably be avoided in anything other than fit healthy adult patients.

Opioid analgesic agents

Opioid analgesic agents are capable of providing profound analgesia both intra- and postoperatively and will also reduce the doses of other agents required to induce and maintain anaesthesia. The onset and duration of drug effects will vary considerably according to which agent is used. The two most serious side effects of opioids in paediatric patients are bradycardia, which can result in marked falls in cardiac output and blood pressure due to the rate-dependency of these variables in neonates, and respiratory depression, which may be compounded by administration of other agents. Partial agonists such as buprenorphine may be less potent respiratory depressants but may only provide moderate analgesia. Partial agonists may, however, be used to partially reverse the effects of pure agonist opioids while maintaining some analgesic effects – so-called

sequential analgesia. In any case, it may be prudent to have pure antagonists such as naloxone available in case excessive respiratory depression occurs.

Opioids are most commonly administered by intramuscular injection, but the use of subcutaneous, extradural or even intra-articular routes should be considered to provide analgesia while minimizing side effects.

Anticholinergics

The parasympathetic dominance and the high rate dependency of cardiac output make the preanaesthetic administration of an anticholinergic a sensible option, although there is some evidence to suggest that these agents may not be effective in puppies and kittens less than 2 weeks of age due to autonomic immaturity. Glycopyrrolate and atropine are the commonest agents in use and, in addition to reducing the incidence and severity of bradycardia, will also reduce respiratory tract secretions thereby lowering the incidence of potential airway obstruction. In spite of its slower onset of action, glycopyrrolate may be preferable to atropine due to its longer duration and lesser tendency to produce sinus tachycardia, although both drugs may be used intravenously to treat acute bradyarrhythmias.

Drug	Dose (mg/kg)	Route	Remarks
Acepromazine	0.01–0.03	s.c., i.m., i.v.	Avoid in patients under 8 weeks or in dehydration
Diazepam	0.1–0.4	i.m., i.v. (lipid preparation is i.v. only)	Uptake from i.m. is variable
Midazolam	0.1–0.25	s.c., i.m., i.v.	Shorter duration than diazepam
Flumazenil	0.1	i.v.	Reversal agent; short duration (60 min)
Xylazine	1–2	s.c., i.m.	Marked side-effects; avoid if under 12 weeks
Medetomidine	0.01–0.04	s.c., i.m.	More potent and longer acting then xylazine
Atipamezole	0.2–0.4	i.m., i.v. (not cats)	α_2-Antagonist
Pethidine (merperidine)	1–4	s.c. i.m.	Rapid onset; lasts approx. 2 hours
Morphine	0.05–0.2 (extradural: 0.1 in 0.25 ml/kg NaCl)	s.c. i.m.	Causes bradycardia; use with an anticholinergic
Butorphanol	0.05–0.3	s.c., i.m., i.v.	Useful sedative; analgesic effects uncertain
Buprenorphine	0.005–0.01	i.m.	Slow onset of action; useful for moderate pain
Naloxone	0.01–0.1	i.m., i.v.	Opioid reversal agent; will reverse analgesia. Short duration (30–60 min)
Atropine	0.02–0.04	s.c., i.m., i.v.	Rapid onset; used as therapy for bradycardia
Glycopyrrolate	0.01–0.02	i.m., i.v.	Slower onset; does not cross blood–brain barrier
Ketamine	1–3 5–10	i.v. i.m.	Very useful with benzodiazepines

Figure 22.2: Drugs used for sedation, chemical restraint and analgesia in paediatric patients.

INDUCTION OF ANAESTHESIA

In the vast majority of neonatal patients, the accepted induction method of choice is by face mask using a volatile agent such as isoflurane or halothane. Intravenous catheter placement in these individuals is often technically challenging and is usually most easily accomplished after induction and endotracheal intubation. Induction of anaesthesia with volatile agents is rapid due to the low functional residual capacity and relative increase in alveolar ventilation compared to adults. The ideal face mask should conform reasonably to the patient's face as ill-fitting masks effectively increase dead space and may prolong induction of anaesthesia. Of the two agents, isoflurane is the more popular due to its potential for rapid induction and recovery. It is characterized by a relative lack of myocardial depression and minimal myocardial sensitization to catecholamines. The less pleasant smell of isoflurane may mean that mask inductions with this agent are not significantly quicker than those with halothane. Of the new volatile agents, sevoflurane is used extensively in human paediatric anaesthesia due to its rapid kinetics, and it may well gain popularity in veterinary species for the same reasons. It should also be remembered that mask or chamber inductions with any agent considerably increase atmospheric pollution with anaesthetic gases.

Patients with significant dyspnoea or other evidence of hypoxia, or patients at increased risk of regurgitation and subsequent aspiration upon induction, are best induced with a rapidly acting intravenous induction agent and intubated quickly. Regardless of the induction technique employed, a wide range of endotracheal tube (ETT) sizes and an effective laryngoscope or light source should be readily available in order to establish a patent airway. Commercially available ETTs down to 2.0 mm internal diameter are available; smaller ETTs can be constructed from an intravenous catheter or similar material. All intubations should be performed with the utmost care, as damage to delicate structures and subsequent laryngeal oedema and spasm are easily induced.

Intravenous anaesthetic agents

Of the available intravenous anaesthetics, probably the most commonly used in paediatric patients in practice are propofol and ketamine. Because of their low muscle and fat masses, relatively low plasma protein concentrations and immature hepatic enzyme pathways, neonatal animals may show increased sensitivity to, and prolonged recovery from, barbiturate anaesthesia, and these drugs are best avoided in animals less than 8-10 weeks.

Propofol is an ultra-short-acting hypnotic that may be used for induction and maintenance of anaesthesia. Profound respiratory depression and hypotension may occur on induction, especially after rapid intravenous injection, and the effects of propofol on the baroreceptors may mean that the normal reflex tachycardic response to hypotension may be depressed or absent. To avoid these hazards, propofol is best administered slowly to effect rather than as a precalculated dose. Unconsciousness can be maintained by incremental dosage or infusion, although prolongation of recovery may be a problem with neonates, as the drug is highly lipid soluble and requires hepatic metabolism (although extra-hepatic sites have been described).

Although ketamine is licensed for sole use in cats, it should be used in combination with some form of sedative agent, the benzodiazepines being the most suitable in paediatric patients. Ketamine is an attractive agent for use in these individuals due to its analgesic properties and relative lack of cardiopulmonary depressant effects, but the drug does undergo extensive hepatic metabolism (with active metabolites) and renal elimination, and should therefore be used with care in neonates. Although laryngeal reflexes are maintained under ketamine anaesthesia, marked salivation can occur, and aspiration is therefore a risk. Its use should probably be restricted to induction of anaesthesia, or, in lower doses together with benzodiazepines, to provide immobilization for minor procedures.

MAINTENANCE OF ANAESTHESIA

Constant and meticulous attention should be paid to maintenance of a patent airway and adequate ventilation in paediatric patients, as drug-induced respiratory inadequacy and airway obstruction are common complications. Oxygen should be provided even if anaesthesia is being maintained intravenously. Nitrous oxide can be used to hasten induction via the second gas effect (see Chapter 9), but the higher oxygen consumption of the neonatal animal may mean that its use throughout the surgical procedure may not be desirable due to the reduction of inspired oxygen concentration. If nitrous oxide is used it should not constitute greater than half of the inspired gas mixture and should be avoided altogether if an absorber system with soda lime is being used.

The anaesthetic breathing system used should have minimal apparatus dead space, a low circuit volume and minimal internal resistance to gas flow. The Jackson-Rees modification of Ayre's T-piece is usually suitable; around 20 to 30 variations of the T-piece have been described, but the valveless models are most suitable. Scavenging from the open-ended bag can be difficult, and torsion of the bag about its long axis can lead to occlusion and pulmonary barotrauma; the bag should therefore be in constant view of the anaesthetist and taped in a safe position if necessary. Use of the T-piece requires high fresh gas flows (2.5–3 times minute volume to completely avoid rebreathing in spontaneous ventilation), which may precipitate hypothermia. Patients weighing over 5 kg can be maintained using other non-rebreathing systems such as the Bain, Lack or Magill or human paediatric circle absorber systems. Effective positive-pressure ventilation cannot be performed with the Lack or Magill systems for long periods, as marked rebreathing can occur. If automatic ventilators are being used, pressure-cycled systems are more suitable for paediatric patients to avoid the risk of barotrauma. Preset airway pressures should not exceed 20 cmH$_2$0.

Every effort should be made to conserve body temperature. Insulating blankets, bubble wrap and warmed cotton wool can all be wrapped around the patient and a surgical window prepared. Surgical preparation solutions should be applied with sterile swabs to minimize evaporative heat loss. The ambient temperature of the surgical area should be kept as high as possible, and all intravenous fluids should be warmed. Heat and moisture exchangers can be used but may increase the work of breathing in small subjects, as well as adding to apparatus dead space.

Intraoperative fluid administration is desirable in order to replace insensible losses, as well as to provide haemodynamic support. Puppies and kittens are relatively intolerant of an acute fluid load, and therefore rates of administration should not exceed 10 ml/kg/h. The use of syringe drivers or infusion pumps greatly facilitates accurate fluid therapy in these patients, although burette-giving sets are equally effective. Dextrose-containing low salt solutions (e.g. 0.18% saline in 4% glucose or 5% dextrose in water) are the most suitable for maintenance during anaesthesia, although in the event of significant blood loss (more than 10% of blood volume), an equal volume of colloid or fresh whole blood is indicated for restoration of circulating volume. Surgical swabs can be weighed to assess blood loss; 1 ml of blood weighs about 1.3 g. Although isotonic crystalloid fluids can be administered subcutaneously, the intravenous or intraosseous routes are preferable for longer-term, or more rapid, administration.

MONITORING DURING ANAESTHESIA

Monitoring of the paediatric patient should be attentive, and adverse trends should be identified and acted upon immediately. Although an increasing array of sophisticated electronic monitoring equipment is available for veterinary anaesthesia, there is no substitute for the constant physical presence of an attentive knowledgeable individual actively monitoring the patient's vital signs.

It should also be remembered that total anaesthetic time could be significantly increased due to the setting up of various monitoring systems and introduction of invasive monitoring lines, particularly if the anaesthetist is unfamiliar with the monitoring modality being used.

Monitoring of respiratory and cardiac sounds is best achieved with a precordial or oesophageal stethoscope, and an electrocardiograph will allow assessment of cardiac rhythm. Several devices are available for the non-invasive oscillometric measurement of arterial blood pressure (see Chapter 5). Invasive monitoring of arterial blood pressure is not only technically demanding (requiring cannulation of an undoubtedly small peripheral artery) but potentially expensive due to the equipment required. Assessment of the adequacy of the circulation in practice is therefore often somewhat qualitative and relies on subjective assessment of pulse pressure, capillary refill time, urine output and mucous membrane colour. This can be difficult in a small patient draped up for surgery, so preparation should ensure that adequate visibility under the drapes is maintained.

Basic monitoring of respiratory function consists of assessing respiratory rate and depth by visualization of chest wall excursions (the surgeon should be actively discouraged from leaning on the patient or leaving surgical instruments resting on the patient's chest or abdomen) and movement of the breathing system bag, together with sounds heard via the oesophageal stethoscope. Simple respiratory monitors that detect temperature changes or movement of gases in the airway are available; false values may be registered due to passive movement of air caused by manipulation of the patient's thorax. A more detailed description of respiratory monitoring equipment (pulse oximeters and capnographs) may be found in Chapter 5.

As previously mentioned, maintenance of adequate body temperature is essential and core temperature should be monitored frequently via a deep rectal or oesophageal probe. Soil temperature probes or thermistor probes designed for catering can often be purchased cheaply and adapted for use at minimal cost. Comparisons can be made with peripheral (e.g. interdigital) temperature readings in order to assess the adequacy of peripheral perfusion; a core–periphery gradient of greater than 6°C is indicative of inadequate peripheral perfusion.

POSTOPERATIVE CARE

As with any postoperative patient, constant attention should be paid to the airway, breathing and circulation. Human neonatal incubators are ideal for recovery of paediatric animals as they allow constant visualization of the patient and enable a warm humid and oxygenated environment to be maintained without the need for physical restraint. If necessary, the airway should be cleared and extubation performed as late as possible. Oxygen supplementation should be provided until recovery from anaesthesia is complete and normal body temperature is achieved. If respiration seems inadequate or there is evidence of hypoventilation or desaturation, positive-pressure ventilation with 100% oxygen should be instituted until the patient is capable of maintaining normal ventilation.

The danger of postoperative hypothermia and its attendant complications in paediatric and neonatal patients have already been emphasized; however, rewarming of the hypothermic neonate should be done slowly, as aggressive external heating may not only cause thermal injury but may also precipitate a hypotensive crisis due to rapid peripheral vasodilation. Instillation (and removal after 5 minutes) of 10 ml/kg warmed isotonic fluids into the rectum may be useful to raise core temperature; lavage of the urinary bladder with warm fluids has also been described and seems clinically effective. Thermal support should be maintained after normal body temperature has been reached, as relapse into hypothermia can occur in young patients.

Postoperative analgesia is a major concern in neonates, as any significant pain is not only morally and ethically unacceptable but may also inhibit normal feeding behaviour and therefore adversely affect food and fluid intake. Treatment of pain in very young animals is also complicated by the fact that neonatal pain behaviour patterns are different from those of adult animals and may not be as obvious. This may make recognition of the characteristic signs of pain difficult, but does not mean that the pain is experienced to a lesser degree. The preoperative use of opioids such as pethidine, morphine or buprenorphine will provide excellent analgesia postoperatively, but excessive or supplemental doses may produce respiratory depression; this is not a contraindication to their use, but means that doses should be carefully calculated and administered. Consideration should also be given to other techniques, such as local anaesthesia; the use of intra-articular, extradural, intercostal or other regional blocks should be considered where appropriate. Local anaesthetic solutions should be diluted by 50% to avoid the potential for overdosage. Bupivicaine is a longer-acting local anaesthetic agent with a duration of up to 8 hours, which can be used for effective regional anaesthesia. Care should be taken not to exceed a total dose of 2 mg/kg. Non-steroidal anti-inflammatory drugs are used extensively for relief of postoperative pain in animals; their extensive hepatic metabolism may make toxic effects more likely in paediatric or neonatal animals and doses should be reduced in neonates.

Every effort should be made to restore normal feeding and behaviour as soon as possible after anaesthesia. Unweaned neonates should be returned to the mother as soon as they are able to maintain respiratory and cardiovascular function. Excessive surgical skin preparations should be removed, as strong unfamiliar odours may precipitate rejection of the neonate by its mother. Any surgical dressings or supports applied should not inhibit the patient's ability to feed or drink. Early nutritional support should be instituted if any evidence of failure to feed within 24 hours of surgery is observed. Parenteral fluid administration should continue at maintenance rates until voluntary fluid intake has returned to normal levels.

CHAPTER TWENTY THREE

Geriatric Patients

Robert E. Meyer

INTRODUCTION

Anaesthesia for geriatric patients is not very different from anaesthesia for younger patients, except that it takes less agent for equivalent effect and the effect tends to last longer. Increasing age, by itself, does not necessarily increase the risk for adverse outcome during or after anaesthesia. Age-related concurrent disease, and not the ageing process, is primarily responsible for the progressive increase in morbidity and mortality observed in the elderly human surgical population, and the same is probably true for elderly dogs and cats. Thus, biological or physiological age, as assessed by preoperative physical examination and relevant laboratory testing, will be much more important than chronological age in formulating an appropriate anaesthetic plan that meets the specific needs of the elderly patient.

DEFINING THE GERIATRIC PERIOD

Seventy five to 80% of the anticipated natural life span has been suggested as the beginning of the geriatric phase of life for dogs; others have recommended that dogs over 10 years of age, and cats older than 12 years, may need special anaesthetic considerations.

PATHOPHYSIOLOGICAL CONSIDERATIONS

Changes in body composition and tissue atrophy associated with ageing combine to reduce anaesthetic requirements in elderly patients. Age by itself minimally increases the free fraction and activity of anaesthetic drugs that bind to plasma proteins, although concurrent age-related disease may significantly influence plasma protein levels and thereby influence drug effect.

Total distribution volume for lipophilic substances is increased in elderly patients due to decreasing skeletal muscle mass, combined with an increase in adipose tissue. Because the larger distribution volume acts as a reservoir for lipophilic anaesthetics, recovery can be prolonged to a greater extent than would be expected simply from reduced hepatic and renal drug clearance.

Controversy exists as to whether the clinically apparent increase in injectable anaesthetic drug potency in aged patients is a pharmacodynamic phenomenom, or a result of differences in early phase redistribution kinetics. Regardless of the actual mechanism involved, clinical experience and traditional measurements show significant age-related decreases in the dose requirement for nearly all injectable anaesthetics in elderly patients.

The minimum alveolar concentration (MAC) for inhaled anaesthetics progressively decreases by 30% from young adult values with increasing age. Similar decreases in MAC have been observed for desflurane, sevoflurane, halothane and isoflurane. This decrease in anaesthetic requirement parallels the reduction in brain neurotransmitter activity that occurs with increasing age.

Microsomal and non-microsomal hepatic enzyme activity remains relatively unchanged with increasing age. Total hepatic mass and blood flow are reduced, however, which leads to extended elimination half-lives for agents primarily eliminated by the liver.

Renal tissue mass and perfusion, particularly of the cortex, is reduced in elderly patients and results in decreased renal functional reserve. Due to reduced skeletal muscle mass, serum creatinine usually remains within the normal range. The awake glomerular filtration rate (GFR) is usually sufficient to avoid uraemia and maintain normal plasma osmolarity and electrolyte concentration.

Cardiac performance progressively decreases with age in response to reduced requirements for perfusion of skeletal muscle and metabolically active organs. Myocardial contractility remains relatively unchanged until late in life. Short-term increases in cardiac output are met through moderate increases in heart rate, stroke volume and left ventricular end-diastolic volume. Relatively small decreases in venous return, as occur during dehydration, haemorrhage, vasodilation or positive-pressure ventilation can compromise stroke volume and worsen perioperative hypotension. On the other hand, rates of intravenous fluid administration suitable for young patients may precipitate congestive heart failure and pulmonary oedema by increasing atrial and pulmonary artery pressures.

Chronic valvular disease occurs in 25% of dogs between 9 and 12 years of age, and in 33% of dogs 13 years and older. In cats, the incidence of hypertrophic cardiomyopathy due to hyperthyroidism also increases with age.

Ageing is associated with decreased clinical efficacy of β-adrenergic agonists. Vascular smooth muscle contractile responses, muscarinic cholinoceptor and α-adrenoreceptor activities are unchanged. Integrated autonomic reflex responses, such as baroreceptor responsiveness or vasoconstrictor responses to cold, are slower in onset, less in magnitude and less effective overall in maintaining tight cardiovascular homeostasis.

Lung changes in elderly animals include decreased elasticity and small airway closure. Greater portions of tidal ventilation occur at lung volumes below closing volume, resulting in increased residual volume, diffuse ventilation/perfusion (V/Q) mismatching and lower resting partial pressure of oxygen in arterial blood (PaO_2). Diffusion capacity and pulmonary capillary blood volume are decreased in aged animals, such that hypoxaemia is more likely to occur following sedation or anaesthesia without administration of supplemental oxygen. Costochondral ossification makes the thorax more rigid and decreases chest wall compliance, and geriatric spayed female cats with feline asthma are at risk from pathological rib fractures.

ANAESTHETIC RECOMMENDATIONS

The best anaesthetic agent or technique for the elderly patient will take into account remaining physiological reserves, and avoid imbalances in homeostasis. Ideally, anaesthetic plans should be pharmacologically simple for these patients and based on drugs that either do not require extensive metabolism for termination of action, or for which specific antagonists exist.

Preoperative evaluation
Particular attention should be given to auscultation of the heart and lungs. The owner should be questioned about the animal's activity and exercise tolerance. An in-hospital exercise challenge, such as a run down the hall or up a flight of stairs, can be useful in determining exercise tolerance in ambulatory patients. Any reports from the owner of periodic dyspnoea or night coughing in their pet warrant further investigation.

A haematocrit, total plasma protein, blood glucose and blood urea nitrogen should be considered as the minimum for preanaesthetic laboratory testing in this age group. Any concurrent disease should be noted and carefully considered for its potential effect on anaesthetic management.

Premedication
Opioids have mild sedative properties in most animals and minimal effects on cardiac contractility and pro-

vide excellent analgesia. They can reduce the amount of subsequent anaesthetic required for anaesthetic induction and maintenance and reduce postoperative analgesic requirements by preventing 'upregulation' of pain pathways in response to surgical manipulation (pre-emptive analgesia). Choices include oxymorphone 0.05–0.1 mg/kg i.m., butorphanol 0.2–0.5 mg/kg i.m., or pethidine (meperidine) 1–2 mg/kg i.m.

If additional sedation is required, acepromazine 0.025–0.05 mg/kg i.m. can be administered in combination with an opioid. The α_2-agonists should be used very carefully in this age group, and only in those patients without signs of valvular cardiac disease or pulmonary hypertension. Low doses of ketamine (5–8 mg/kg i.m.), can also be safely used in uncooperative cats, even in the presence of cardiomyopathy.

Antimuscarinic drugs should not be routinely administered to geriatric animals. These agents increase myocardial workload, can cause tachyarrhythmias and eliminate heart rate as an indicator of anaesthetic depth and sympathetic activity. Glycopyrrolate 0.005–0.01 mg/kg i.v., is preferred for treatment of vagally induced bradycardia, haemodynamically significant bradycardia resulting in hypotension or opioid-mediated second degree heart block. Glycopyrrolate is also the preferred anti-sialogue; however, since saliva production has both sympathetic (thick) and parasympathetic (thin) components, it will have little effect on the thick ropey saliva produced by anxious animals.

Induction
Suitable short-acting intravenous induction agents include thiopentone, propofol and etomidate. Ketamine increases both sympathetic activity and myocardial work and should be used cautiously in this age group. As a general rule of thumb, the doses of intravenous agents should be reduced by 10–40% to avoid possible overdose and to assure rapid recovery, and given more slowly than usual to allow for the delaying effect of prolonged circulation time (Figure 23.1). As thiopentone, propofol and etomidate provide little or no analgesia by themselves, they should be supplemented with opioids, α_2-agonists or inhalational anaesthetics for painful or noxious procedures. Supplemental oxygen should be given by mask or through an endotracheal tube to prevent hypoxia.

In some cases, it may be preferable to induce anaesthesia after premedication using a mask and an inhalational anaesthetic. This method provides excellent control of anaesthetic depth in sick or very old animals. Close attention to pedal withdrawal reflexes before endotracheal intubation will help avoid inadvertent overdose. Nitrous oxide in oxygen (2:1) can be added, if desired, to reduce the amount of inhalational anaesthetic required.

Local anaesthetic techniques can be useful for minor procedures, especially combined with sedation or neuroleptanalgesia. Regional anaesthetic techniques

Agent	Adjustment
Antimuscarinics (glycopyrrolate, atropine)	Same or slight increase in dose for equivalent heart rate response; central anticholinergic syndrome possible with atropine
Opioids	Reduce initial dose; anticipate increased duration of systemic and extradural effects
Phenothiazines, benzodiazepines	Reduce initial dose; anticipate increased duration (except midazolam)
α_2-agonists	Reduce dose; use with caution in patients with decreased cardiac reserve
Injectable induction agents (thiopentone, propofol, etomidate)	Moderate decrease (10–40%) in induction dose; decrease maintenance infusion rate
Inhalational anaesthetic agents	Reduce inspired concentration 30% (more with nitrous oxide/oxygen mixtures)
Spinal or extradurally administered local anaesthetics	Small to moderate decrease in segmental dose requirements; anticipate prolonged effects
Non-depolarizing muscle relaxants	Same or slight increase in initial dose; anticipate prolonged effect (except atracurium)
Anticholinesterases (edrophonium, neostigmine)	No change in dose or efficacy; slightly prolonged effect
β-agonists (dobutamine, isoprenaline)	Increase dose for equivalent cardiovascular responses

Figure 23.1: *Recommendations for dose adjustment of anaesthetic agents in geriatric patients.*

in elderly animals require lower doses (Figure 23.1), and intravenous fluids should be administered in the event of sympathetic blockade accompanied by hypotension. There is no clear evidence that regional anaesthesia confers any advantage over general anaesthesia in terms of overall outcome, although one or the other may be preferred for use in certain procedures or in some patients for other medical reasons.

Maintenance and recovery

Supplemental oxygen (at least 30–40% inspired concentration) should be administered throughout the anaesthetic and recovery periods to prevent hypoxia. Inhalational anaesthetics are preferred for procedures lasting longer than 15–20 minutes because of their controllability and ease of administration. Propofol can be administered for prolonged maintenance during non-invasive diagnostic procedures at a constant infusion rate of 0.2–0.6 mg/kg/min; an opioid can be added to provide additional analgesia for surgical procedures. Spontaneous ventilation is tolerated well by most patients; if controlled ventilation is necessary, a rate of 4–6 breaths per minute should provide adequate expiratory time in the event of delayed emptying of alveolar gases, with minimal effects on venous return.

To avoid hypotension, anaesthesia should be kept as light as possible. Balanced isotonic crystalloid solutions, e.g. lactated Ringer's solution, can be administered intravenously at 5–10 ml/kg/h. Fragile patients with poorly compensated heart failure may benefit from a loop diuretic after anaesthesia.

Since hypothermia will reduce anaesthetic requirement as well as prolong recovery from anaesthesia, body temperature should be monitored throughout the procedure. It is best to avoid hypothermia by a quick technique and the judicious use of circulating water blankets, towels or disposable aluminized paper space blankets to insulate the patient from conductive and radiation heat losses.

Although rapid return to consciousness is desirable, postoperative analgesia should not be withheld in order to speed recovery. Additional opioids may be required in animals with severe pain.

FURTHER READING

Thurmon JC, Tranquilli WJ and Benson GJ (1996) Neonatal and geriatric patients. In: *Lumb and Jones' Veterinary Anesthesia, 3rd ed*, ed. JC Thurmon *et al.*, pp. 844–848. Williams and Wilkins, Baltimore

CHAPTER TWENTY FOUR

Anaesthetic Emergencies and Complications

Ralph C. Harvey

INTRODUCTION

Anaesthesia is intended to be a controlled, benign and reversible process. Unfortunately, anaesthetic drugs produce their effects primarily by limited depression of vital physiological processes. The inherent dangers of anaesthesia and the debilitation of injuries and illness that require anaesthesia and surgery predispose the patient to the risks of serious complications and emergencies. Most anaesthetic complications and emergencies can be related to human error, equipment problems, ventilatory problems or circulatory problems. Most anaesthetic emergencies and complications can be prevented or adequately managed.

HUMAN ERROR

Human error is ultimately responsible for the majority of problems encountered with anaesthetic management. The importance of vigilance in anaesthetic care cannot be overemphasized. It has been noted that hundreds of errors are made through not looking, for every one error made through not knowing.

It should be recognized that there is a significant degree of safety with familiarity. Errors are more common when the anaesthetist is not familiar with either the drugs or the equipment being used. Miscalculation of anaesthetic drug doses is a common error; the narrow therapeutic index of most anaesthetic drugs makes correct dose determination or titration crucial. An absolute or relative overdose of anaesthetic can cause many problems from minimally excessive physiological depression to death.

An overdose of barbiturates should be managed by physiological support of ventilation, continuous monitoring of cardiopulmonary function, and intravenous fluid therapy, to speed recovery and improve cardiopulmonary function. Administration of bicarbonate at 0.5–1.0 mEq/kg can speed recovery from barbiturate overdose by favouring elimination. Overdoses of other anaesthetics are also managed with supportive care, which is often adequate in situations of mild to moderate overdose.

Fortunately there are specific antagonist drugs available to counteract the effects of some anaesthetic drugs. For μ-opioids, the pure antagonist agent naloxone will reverse the effects of an overdose. With a large overdose or with a long-lasting opioid, renarcotization can occur because naloxone has a relatively short half-life. For the α_2-agonist xylazine, there are specific antagonists available. One of these, yohimbine, has been developed and approved in the USA for use in dogs. Safe use of medetomidine, another powerful α_2-agonist, is similarly improved through the availability of a specific antagonist, atipamezole. Further details of the above antagonists may be found in Chapters 6 and 7.

Non-specific partial reversal of anaesthetic depression is possible by administration of the non-specific stimulant-antagonist drug, doxapram, which can be valuable in treating depression due to barbiturate overdose and is administered intravenously at a dose of 1.0–5.0 mg/kg. Although the net effect can be life saving, non-specific reversal has been associated with residual undesirable effects related to CNS stimulation. Other stimulants have been advocated to correct excessive depressant effects of various anaesthetics, but the benefits are usually very limited.

Errors in administration of anaesthetics also include the misidentification of drugs and accidental use of the wrong medication.

Anaesthetics administered by an incorrect route can also have very adverse effects. The extravascular injection of barbiturates can cause severe irritation and sloughing of surrounding tissue. Extravasation should be treated by infiltration of the site with lignocaine (lidocaine) and saline, followed by warm compresses.

EQUIPMENT PROBLEMS

Among the most serious of anaesthetic complications is the failure to deliver oxygen to the patient. This can be caused by respiratory obstruction, or misused or defective anaesthetic equipment. Empty cylinders or misconnected gas lines and breathing systems prevent the delivery of oxygen. Such problems must be recognized and corrected immediately. Delivery of nitrous oxide in combination with too little oxygen should be carefully avoided and is not always prevented by the fail-safe systems incorporated into modern machines. Empty anaesthetic vaporizers, vaporizers filled with the wrong agent or overfilling are also common problems. A more detailed discussion of anaesthetic equipment can be found in Chapter 4.

Kinked or plugged endotracheal tubes (ETTs) cause respiratory obstruction. Improper cuff inflation can result in obstruction, tracheal injury or aspiration pneumonitis. Improper placement of ETTs is very common, even in species that are easily intubated. Correct placement should always be verified.

An inability to fill the rebreathing bag adequately or to provide positive-pressure ventilation by squeezing the bag often indicates major leaks or disconnections. These can result in a failure to deliver anaesthetics and can substantially contribute to anaesthetic gas pollution of the veterinary hospital. Stuck valves in the anaesthetic machine or breathing system can cause difficulty in ventilation, inappropriate rebreathing of exhaled gases or the accumulation of excessive pressure. Patients that consistently seem to be anaesthetized too deeply or too lightly may indicate that vaporizer output is inaccurate as a result of wear and tear, the accumulation of deposits within the vaporizer, or other factors. These common problems emphasize the importance of regular inspection and maintenance of equipment.

Electrical problems with monitoring or supportive equipment risk injury to staff as well as to patients. Inadequately earthed or protected equipment can cause electrical burns, electrocution or fires. Unsafe or substandard equipment should be repaired or replaced. The risk of thermal injury is so great with electric heating pads that their use in anaesthetized patients is considered extremely hazardous. Warm water bottles or surgical gloves filled with warm water have been shown to be rather ineffective in raising the body temperature of hypothermic patients while at the same time constituting a significant risk of causing thermal burns at the site of contact. Circulating warm-water or hot-air blankets are much better alternatives.

VENTILATORY PROBLEMS

Hypoventilation due to anaesthetic overdose is one of the most frequently encountered and serious complications in anaesthesia, and may occur with either relative or absolute overdoses of many anaesthetics. Weakened debilitated animals are more susceptible to ventilatory depression, which may occur secondary to circulatory depression and inadequate perfusion of CNS respiratory centres, electrolyte imbalances, muscle relaxant drugs or thoracic injury. Support of ventilation requires endotracheal intubation and intermittent positive-pressure ventilation, preferably with an oxygen-enriched gas mixture. Identification and correction of the primary problem is then undertaken.

Hyperventilation is often due to inadequate anaesthetic depth and represents an excessive response to surgical stimulation. It is important to rule out the possibility of carbon dioxide accumulation, due to exhausted absorber granules, improper connection of the breathing circuit or insufficient gas flow. Panting can occur with opioids and thereby decrease effective ventilation. Panting may also represent an inconvenience to the surgeon. A less common cause of panting is hyperthermia. Erratic or jerky breathing patterns usually indicate improper anaesthetic depth. As before, airway obstruction and the various causes of carbon dioxide accumulation should be ruled out.

PALLOR AND CYANOSIS

Pallor of mucous membranes is a complex sign in that it may occur as a compensatory response to either excessively light or deep planes of anaesthesia. Reduced cardiac output and hypotension due to anaesthetic depression or increased sympathetic tone in response to pain can cause pallor. It is important to identify the cause to treat the problem appropriately. Incorrect management may compound the problem and cause decompensation and immediate deterioration.

Cyanosis rarely occurs in anaesthetized patients breathing oxygen. In order for cyanosis to develop, haemoglobin must be present in sufficient quantities and in the reduced (non-oxygenated) state. Hypoxaemia that accompanies anaemia, therefore, will not become evident through cyanosis. When cyanosis of either mucous membranes or blood in the operative field does occur, oxygen should be administered and adequate ventilation and pulse quality assured.

CIRCULATORY PROBLEMS

Hypotension
Either decreased cardiac output, or increased capacitance of the vasculature or inadequate blood volume causes hypotension. Intraoperative crystalloid therapy at a rate of 10 ml/kg/h is often appropriate for replacement in many surgical patients, but increased rates may be necessary. Clinical evaluation to distinguish between hypovolaemia and reduced cardiac output as causes of hypotension can be based on patient history and evaluation, including measurement of central venous and arterial pressures.

Vasodilation is a very common side effect of many anaesthetic drugs. The tranquillizer acepromazine can cause vasodilation and hypotension, particularly at high doses. The volatile anaesthetics also cause significant vasodilation. Most anaesthetics are also potent cardiac depressants, again particularly at high doses. Hypotension under anaesthesia is, therefore, most appropriately managed by reducing anaesthetic delivery and by fluid administration as primary management. Vasoactive drugs may also be required (see Chapter 14).

Bradycardia

Bradycardia is often associated with procedures or drugs that cause increases in vagal parasympathetic tone. Difficult endotracheal intubations, deep abdominal surgical procedures, intraocular surgeries and some surgeries on the neck or in the thorax can all cause vagally mediated bradycardia. Atropine or glycopyrrolate administration is effective for prevention of most vagal effects. Treatment after the vagal effects become evident is often less rewarding. Nonvagal bradycardias may result from excessive anaesthetic depth, hypoxia, hypothermia or hyperkalaemia. Bradycardia can be a very serious sign of a significant anaesthetic emergency. Administration of atropine and attention to possible causes are imperative.

Tachycardia

Heart rates above 180 bpm in dogs and above 200 bpm in cats are associated with decreased cardiac efficiency and increased cardiac workload. Tachycardia can be due to fear, pain, inadequate depth of anaesthesia, preanaesthetic excitement (or a rough induction of anaesthesia) or hypotension. These causes of supraventricular tachycardia should be recognized and treated.

Compensatory tachycardia in response to hypovolaemia and hypotension results in decreased coronary artery blood flow and increased myocardial work load. If other conditions contribute to hypoxia there is significant risk of development of more serious arrhythmias. Fluid therapy for hypovolaemia, adjustment of anaesthetic depth and supportive measures to avoid cardiovascular deterioration are necessary.

Ventricular tachycardia is a much more serious emergency. An occasional ventricular ectopic beat is cause for concern, but not necessarily indicative of patient distress. When ventricular arrhythmia becomes frequent, or progresses to ventricular tachycardia, immediate treatment is required, because it indicates an irritated, hypoxic or diseased myocardium.

Ventricular tachycardia should be treated with an intravenous bolus injection of 2% lignocaine at a dose of 0.5, 1, or 2 ml for small, medium or large dogs, respectively. This rule of thumb will allow for immediate therapy without an accurate dose calculation that could contribute to a life-threatening delay. It has been recommended that propranolol (0.04 mg/kg i.v.) is the drug of choice for treating ventricular arrhythmias in cats, but lignocaine is also effective. Total dose limitation is more important in cats because of their smaller body size and blood volume.

Bolus injections of lignocaine can be repeated to a total accumulated dose of about 10 mg/kg without significant risk of overdose. When two or three injections are required over a period of 15–20 minutes, it is necessary to convert to a continuous intravenous infusion of lignocaine at 30–80 µg/kg/min. Success in emergency management of ventricular arrhythmias is evaluated by continuous ECG monitoring. Refractory arrhythmias may require conversion with therapy based on procainamide and/or quinidine (see Chapter 14).

CARDIOPULMONARY ARREST AND CARDIOPULMONARY RESUSCITATION

Specifically with regard to cardiopulmonary resuscitation (CPR), there has been little improvement in methods and prognosis over the past 5 years. Recent reviews of clinical experience in CPR, and ongoing research in clinical and experimental CPR, makes it clear that success rates are never high. Complete recovery from asystolic cardiac arrest is extremely rare, particularly if the patient has serious underlying disease. However, early and aggressive resuscitation can be successful.

A cardiopulmonary arrest is always a true emergency situation. A rapid concise and well directed intervention is imperative to save the patient's life. It is extremely difficult for one person to provide successful CPR, and well coordinated action by a team of trained staff is necessary to realize the best chance for recovery. The entire staff of every veterinary clinic should be trained in the basic life support techniques of veterinary CPR and should be ready at all times to respond to the crisis of a cardiopulmonary arrest.

Preparation for emergency management requires more than acquisition of knowledge based on fundamental CPR technique and emergency drug therapy. Equally important is the training of associates and technical staff to facilitate a reasonably smooth team effort during a crisis situation. Optimally, there would be sufficient staff available so that individuals could be assigned to:

- Assessment of pulse quality
- Ventilation
- Chest compression
- Preparation and administration of drugs
- Maintenance of a record or flow sheet representing the time-course of events and progression of the resuscitation effort.

Supplies and drugs that might be needed for resuscitation and support should be stored in the immediate area. Preparation of a crash box and the training of staff in the use of its contents are an excellent and easy first step. A ready source of emergency supplies and drugs can be quite useful in prevention of cardiopulmonary arrests by the early treatment of less desperate complications and emergencies. Figure 24.1 shows the suitable contents of a crash box.

Careful patient monitoring, particularly under conditions of anaesthesia, surgery and post-operative recovery, is of paramount importance in avoiding cardiopulmonary arrest. Although it may not be possible to identify correctly all patients that have an increased risk of arrest, animals showing signs of respiratory depression or haemodynamic instability should receive special attention. Other groups of patients that should be considered to be at an increased risk are very young and very old animals, those debilitated by disease or injury, and those who have conditions or histories that might predispose to cardiopulmonary instability.

The signs of a cardiac arrest include:

- No auscultatable heartbeat
- No palpable arterial pulse
- Grey or cyanotic discoloration of mucous membranes
- Dilated pupils
- No ventilatory attempts (agonal gasps notwithstanding)
- Unconsciousness.

Certainly there are other signs of cardiac arrest, and some of those mentioned above may be absent or obscured in certain circumstances.

Little time exists between the moment of cardiac arrest and the time at which definitive support and resuscitation must begin. If treatment is not initiated immediately, irreversible and often fatal changes occur within 3 to 4 minutes. This time period may be much shorter in debilitated animals.

For those animals identified as being at very high risk, a thorough discussion with the owners of the prognosis and risk factors is particularly valuable. When faced with a grave situation, presented unexpectedly, many clients are often unprepared to make life and death decisions concerning their pet. With prior preparation, however, owners may be more able to consider the medical options available; whether to accept a recommendation for euthanasia if the prognosis becomes grave, or to request a 'do not resuscitate' (DNR) order if the likelihood of arrest is anticipated. Expressions by the client of such wishes can help to:

- Relieve the sense of anguish in making the decision of whether or not to attempt resuscitation in such animals
- Relieve the animal of further suffering and pain due to chronic disease or debilitation
- Avoid inappropriate resuscitation.

By prior discussion with owners concerning the potential for sudden deterioration, the veterinarian will also know when the clients wishes are for everything possible to be done.

Basic life support CPR

The first step indicated when an arrest is suspected is to make a quick assessment of the patient's condition. If the previously mentioned signs are noted, verifying cardiopulmonary arrest, the second step is to discontinue anaesthetic drug administration and call for help. This should ideally summon all members of the team who can provide assistance in resuscitation.

The treatment priorities are known as the ABCs of CPR.

Emergency drugs	
Atropine (0.6 mg/ml)	25 ml
Dexamethasone (2 mg/ml)	100 ml
Calcium gluconate 10%	10 ml
Doxapram hydrochloride (20 mg/ml)	20 ml
Dobutamine hydrochloride (12.5 mg/ml)	20 ml
Dopamine hydrochloride (200 mg/5 ml)	5 ml
Dextrose 50%	50 ml
Adrenaline (epinephrine) 1:1000	10 ml
Adrenaline (epinephrine) 1:10 000	10 ml
Heparin 1000 IU/ml	10 ml
Heparinized saline (4 IU/ml)	50 ml
Propranolol injection (1 mg/ml)	1 ml
Isoprenaline (1 mg/ml)	5 ml
Frusemide (40 mg/ml)	100 ml
Lignocaine 2%	100 ml
Naloxone (0.4 mg/ml)	10 ml
Potassium chloride 20%	10 ml
Sodium bicarbonate 8.4%	50 ml
Sodium chloride 0.9%	50 ml
Hydrocortisone sodium succinate 100 mg (2)	
Hydrocortisone sodium succinate 500 mg (2)	
Edrophonium chloride (10 mg/ml)	1 ml
Syringes and needles	
A variety of sizes, as available	
Intravenous catheters	
A variety of sizes, as available	
Miscellaneous	
Infusion plugs	
Five T-pieces for intravenous catheters	
3/0 monofilament nylon suture with straight needle	
Sterile lubricant packs	
Artificial tears	
Roll narrow gauze	
Three alligator clips (for ECG)	
Laryngoscope (long and short blades)	
Intravenous fluid set: 60 drops/ml	
15 drops/ml	
Intravenous fluid extension tubing	

Figure 24.1: Suggested contents for a crash box.

Airway

A represents the patient's airway. The oral cavity and laryngeal opening should be visually inspected to rule out obstruction by food or foreign material. The airway is then secured, if possible, by the placement of an ETT. Occasionally emergency surgical tracheostomy is required.

Breathing

B represents breathing, the second priority in initiating CPR. Artificial ventilation is most satisfactorily provided by the use of an anaesthetic breathing system with provision of oxygen rather than room air. Alternatively, a self-refilling or Ambu-type resuscitation bag may be used. Mouth-to-ETT or even mouth-to-muzzle techniques may be effective, although certainly less efficient for providing artificial ventilation.

Circulation

C represents circulation, which is provided by cardiac massage. Chest compressions are provided most often in non-surgical patients with the animal in lateral recumbency, usually with one hand on either side of the thorax. Positions of the resuscitator's hands for effective cardiac massage will vary with size and conformation of the patient, but correct position is of paramount importance to provide effective circulation and avoid irreparable damage to the liver, lungs and other vital organs (see below). The compressions should be quick, yet slightly sustained and at a rapid rate of 90–120 per minute.

Effective cardiac massage must be monitored throughout the resuscitation effort by palpation of the peripheral pulse. A palpable pulse must be detected, usually over the femoral or lingual artery. Observation of the plethysmographic waveform, as displayed on a pulse oximeter, is a very useful means of pulse evaluation. If a pulse is not detected, changes in the CPR technique must be made quickly to provide a pulse.

A simple change in hand placement or a change in position of the patient (both modified based mainly on the size of the animal) allows for optimal external massage in a variety of veterinary patients. For example, one hand may encircle the sternum and provide massage by opposing force of the thumb and fingers for cats and very small dogs, whereas the large breeds of dog will usually require both hands over the heart on one side of the thorax. Other technical modifications that may provide improved cardiac massage might include changes in patient position, abdominal binding and simultaneous ventilation and cardiac compression. While such adjustments may be necessary for effective CPR, it should be noted that there may be a greater risk of damage to vital organs with these techniques and they should be reserved for selected cases in which the standard approach is not effective.

Open chest cardiac massage: Open chest cardiac massage may be indicated in arrest victims that are anaesthetized for surgical procedures of the thorax or abdomen. When arrest occurs during a thoracotomy, the surgeon should immediately begin direct cardiac massage at the rate of 60–100 compressions per minute. If cardiac arrest occurs during a laparotomy, the surgeon should immediately enter the thorax by opening the diaphragm to reach the heart.

Even though open chest cardiac massage is so much more effective than closed chest CPR in providing cardiac output and cerebral and coronary blood flow, emergency thoracotomy is not associated with an increased chance of survival. The considerable disadvantages of emergency thoracotomy create reasonable reluctance to perform this procedure. If direct massage of the heart is to be performed for CPR, the decision should be made early and the procedure performed quickly.

Drug therapy in CPR

D stands for drug therapy, the fourth priority in CPR. Emergency drugs should be injected intravenously and circulated by cardiac massage. Intracardiac injections are to be avoided if possible. Intratracheal injection or intraosseous injections of some emergency drugs are acceptable and valuable alternatives when necessary. Figure 24.2 lists suggested drug doses for CPR in dogs and cats. The indications for each medication and the appropriate doses will depend upon individual circumstances in each arrest situation, including such factors as underlying disease and duration of cardiac arrest. The veterinary surgeon directing the resuscitation should customize drug therapy.

It must be recognized that rapid fluid administration is of crucial importance in most cases. Cats should generally receive 20 ml/kg and dogs 40 ml/kg of a balanced electrolyte solution by rapid intravenous administration through a large bore catheter. However, although inadequate circulating volume is the most frequent cause of unsuccessful resuscitation, excessive fluid load and resultant pulmonary oedema may be the second most common cause of failure. Therefore, once the recommended fluid load has been given, the need for further fluid therapy must be considered carefully.

Definitive therapy: ECG classification

Other drugs used in resuscitation are selected according to the type of cardiac arrest. Cardiac arrest may be classified into one of three types by ECG evaluation: ventricular or complete asystole; ventricular fibrillation; or electromechanical dissociation (EMD). The absence of all electrical activity or the absence of ventricular activity on the ECG indicates complete or ventricular asystole. Grossly irregular electrical activity is typical of ventricular fibrillation. Electro-

Emergency drug	Dose	Bodyweight (kg)								
		2.5	5	10	15	20	25	30	40	50
Arenaline (epinephrine) 1:1000, 1 mg/ml	0.1 mg/kg	0.25	0.5	1	1.5	2	2.5	3	4	5
Atropine 0.54 mg/ml	0.025 mg/kg	0.1	0.2	0.4	0.6	0.8	1	1.2	1.6	2
Lignocaine (lidocaine)* 20 mg/ml	1.0 mg/kg	0.125	0.25	0.5	0.75	1	1.25	1.5	2	2.5
Sodium bicarbonate 1 mEq/ml	1.0 mEq/kg	2.5	5	10	15	20	25	30	40	50
Hydrocortisone sodium succinate	30 mg/kg	75 mg	150 mg	300 mg	450 mg	600 mg	750 mg	900 mg	1200 mg	1500 mg
Counter-shock External Internal	1-10 J/kg 0.1-1 J/kg	25 J 2.5 J	50 J 5 J	100 J 10 J	150 J 15 J	200 J 20 J	250 J 25 J	300 J 30 J	400 J 40 J	500 J 50 J

Figure 24.2: *Cardiopulmonary resuscitation quick reference chart. Doses for adrenaline, atropine, lignocaine and sodium bicarbonate are in ml and are suitable for intravenous administration. Use double this i.v. dose if giving adrenaline, atropine or lignocaine by the tracheal route.*

* This dose of lignocaine may be repeated up to three times in dogs.
Adapted from Robello and Crowe (1989).

mechanical dissociation is characterized by the presence of electrical signals that range from fairly normal complexes to wide and bizarre waveforms but are not accompanied by any cardiac contraction or arterial pulse.

In addition to continued CPR on the basis of the ABCs, definitive treatment of the specific type of arrest should be initiated immediately.

For asystole, the administration of adrenaline is recommended. A 1:1000 concentration (1 mg/ml) of adrenaline is injected in a central vein (a deep jugular catheter would be ideal). Doses of up to 1, 2 or 3 ml are recommended for small, medium and large dogs, respectively. This 'rule of thumb' avoids costly delays in calculating precise doses based on actual or estimated bodyweight and a recommended dose schedule. These doses are considerably higher than those recommended previously, because recent research data suggests that these higher doses are more effective in many arrest situations. Atropine administration is also often valuable to counteract vagal effects that may contribute to the arrest.

For ventricular fibrillation, external or internal electrical defibrillation with a DC defibrillator is the best option. Power settings are selected on the basis of patient size and response to previous attempts (see Figure 24.2). The use of lignocaine and/or adrenaline for ventricular fibrillation is controversial, but generally recommended. In the absence of an electrical defibrillator other therapies, including a pre-cordial chest thump or various drug combinations, have been successful on occasions. Fortunately, cats and dogs in some situations are capable of achieving spontaneous defibrillation.

Therapy for EMD is particularly unrewarding. This condition is indicative of a deteriorating hypoxic myocardium. The prognosis is grave. Recommended therapies include continued basic life support CPR and drug therapies that may include high doses of corticosteroids, intravenous dopamine infusion, calcium salts and sodium bicarbonate. It is currently recommended that bicarbonate administration in CPR be limited to situations with pre-existing hypoperfusion and in relatively prolonged resuscitations with poor circulation for extended periods of time. Calcium administration is generally contraindicated in CPR owing to a strong association with adverse cerebrovascular effects and post-resuscitation encephalopathy.

Cerebral resuscitation will always be a formidable challenge, but there are promising developments in the prevention and treatment of reperfusion injury to the brain and heart.

Patients that are successfully resuscitated require continued intensive monitoring and critical care support to optimize recovery.

DELAYED RECOVERY

Delayed recovery from anaesthesia is managed by recognition of different causes and the ruling out of individual possibilities. A systematic approach to potential causes will provide for balanced care with correction of multiple factors including: hypothermia; inadequate fluid support; reduced metabolism and clearance of drugs; and debilitation associated with the stress of anaesthesia and surgical trauma.

Deterioration due to a hypoxic episode must be considered.

HYPOTHERMIA

Hypothermia is among the most common of anaesthetic complications. Body heat is lost through preparation of the surgical site, contact with cool surfaces such as surgical tables, breathing of dry anaesthetic gases, and evaporation from the airways and the surgical field. Moderate hypothermia is a frequent problem even with attention to these factors. Body temperatures down to approximately 33 °C increase oxygen and energy requirements because of shivering during recovery but most patients can tolerate this level of hypothermia. More extreme hypothermia causes delayed recovery and reduces tissue oxygenation.

OTHER COMPLICATIONS

Many other complications and emergencies can occur either during, or associated with, anaesthesia. These include anaphylactic-like reactions, hyperthermia, biochemical imbalances and many surgical complications such as haemorrhage and pneumothorax. Avoidance of complications and effective management of emergencies requires continued vigilance and immediate appropriate actions. Although all anaesthetized patients are at risk of life-threatening complications, vigilance and individualized patient management contribute to anaesthetic safety and successful outcome.

REFERENCES AND FURTHER READING

Adams HR and Wingfield WE (1992) Circulatory shock and cardiopulmonary resuscitation: current perspectives and future directions. *Journal of the American Veterinary Medical Association* **200**, 1833–1834

Anon (1986) Standards and guidelines for cardiopulmonary resuscitation and emergency cardiac care. *Journal of the American Medical Association* **255**, 2905–2989

Eiker SW (1986) Complications in anesthesia. *Seminars in Veterinary Medicine and Surgery* **1**, 204–214

Evans AT (1996) Anesthetic emergencies and accidents. In: *Lumb and Jones Veterinary Anesthesia*, ed. JC Thurmon *et al.*, pp. 849–860. Williams and Wilkins, Baltimore

Fagella AM (1991) Cardiopulmonary cerebral resuscitation. *Proceedings of the Academy of Veterinary Cardiology meeting, April 13–14*, pp. 41–47

Haskins SC (1985) Principles of operating room emergencies. In: *Textbook of Small Animal Surgery*, ed. DH Slatter, pp. 389–412. WB Saunders, Philadelphia

Haskins SC (1992) Internal cardiac compression. *Journal of the American Veterinary Medical Association* **200**, 1945–1947

Henik RA (1992) Basic life support and external cardiac compression in dogs and cats. *Journal of the American Veterinary Medical Association* **200**, 1925–1931

King L and Hammond R (1999) *Manual of Canine and Feline Emergency and Critical Care*. BSAVA, Cheltenham

Muir WW (1987) Cardiopulmonary resuscitation. *Proceedings of the Veterinary Critical Care Society Meeting*, pp. 719–723

Muir WW and Hubbell JAE (1995) Respiratory emergencies and cardiac emergency and shock. In: *Handbook of Veterinary Anesthesia, 2nd edn*, ed. WW Muir and JAE Hubbell, pp. 388–447. Mosby, St Louis

Robello CD and Crowe DT (1989) Cardiopulmonary resuscitation: current recommendations. *Veterinary Clinics of North America* **19**, 1127–1149

Rush JE and Wingfield WE (1992) Recognition and frequency of dysrhythmias during cardiopulmonary arrest. *Journal of the American Veterinary Medical Association* **200**, 1932–1937

Skippen PW (1992) Cardiopulmonary resuscitation and cerebral outcome: is there any hope? *Anesthesiology Clinics of North America* **10**, 619–643

Trim CM (1988) Anesthetic emergencies and complications. In: *Manual of Small Animal Anesthesia*, ed. RR Paddleford, pp. 147–198. Churchill Livingstone, New York

Van Pelt DR and Wingfield WE (1992) Controversial issues in drug treatment during cardiopulmonary resuscitation. *Journal of the American Veterinary Medical Association* **200**, 1938–1944

PART FOUR

Anaesthesia and Analgesia
for Exotic Species

CHAPTER TWENTY FIVE

Fish

Hamish Rodger

INTRODUCTION

Anaesthetics are regularly used in fish to reduce stress or pain. Although it is still unclear whether fish sense pain as mammals do, they do perceive and react to their environment, which, if adverse, will induce stress. If fish are exposed to adverse stimuli there will be a series of reflex responses, which can be violent and harmful to the patient. It is, therefore, particularly important to provide either sedation or anaesthesia in situations of adverse stimuli.

Anaesthesia or sedation is required for procedures in fish where it would not be necessary in domesticated mammals, such as handling, immobilization, prolonged transport, minor surgery, biopsy, grading of juveniles, radiography and administration of topical or injectable treatments. In contrast to terrestrial animals, the external epidermal layers of fish are composed of living cells and hence delicate handling is essential. If unanaesthetized fish are handled, they usually struggle and, if restrained in this state, skin damage can occur easily. Such damage can be life threatening due to secondary bacterial infections and failure of osmoregulatory balance (Figure 25.1). The clinician who wants to examine a fish closely must therefore sedate or anaesthetize the patient. When examining anaesthetized fish, the hands should be wet and preferably gloved in smooth plastic. It is not advisable to hold anaesthetized fish out of water for more than a few minutes, and during this time they should be kept moist. After the clinical procedure and recovery from anaesthesia, the fish should be monitored for 2 hours and then checked regularly for up to 96 hours to screen for delayed stress problems.

Suitable anaesthetics for fish, that are both efficacious and safe, have been simply defined by Gilderhaus and Marking (1987) as those that:

- Induce a state in the fish whereby it can be manipulated and handled readily within 3 minutes or less
- Allow the fish to recover to normal swimming within 10 minutes or less
- Cause no mortality after 15 minutes exposure to the anaesthetic solution.

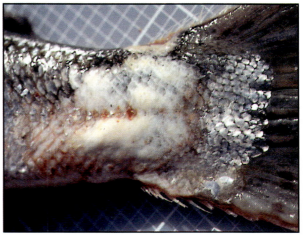

Figure 25.1: Epidermal necrosis and sloughing at the caudal peduncle of a salmon which had been hand held without sedation or anaesthesia.

In addition to these requirements, the ideal agent should render the patient insensible to pain and provide good muscle relaxation. Also, the agent should be easy to administer, stable, inexpensive and have a wide margin of safety.

SIGNS AND STAGES OF ANAESTHESIA IN FISH

As with mammals, the signs and stages of anaesthesia in fish vary markedly from species to species, according to the life stage, environmental temperature, condition of the patient and the drug used. As the majority of fish anaesthetics are given by bath, the signs relate to behaviour and body position in the water column. During slow inductions, fish can be seen to pass through planes of anaesthesia similar to those in mammals; these are outlined in Figure 25.2. In general, loss of balance occurs resulting in the ventrum being uppermost, and the fish either floats to the water surface or remains on the tank bottom. Fish in deep narcosis (stage II, plane 2) can be examined closely, can have external samples or fin or skin biopsies taken or can be given injections. At stage III, plane 1, fish can undergo minor surgical procedures.

Stage	Plane	Category	Behavioural response of fish
0		Normal	Swimming actively, reactive to external stimuli, equilibrium normal and muscle tone normal
I	1	Light sedation	Voluntary swimming continues, slight loss of reactivity to visual and tactile stimuli, respiratory rate normal, equilibrium and muscle tone normal
I	2	Deep sedation	Voluntary swimming stopped, marked loss of reactivity to visual and tactile stimuli, slight decrease in respiratory rate, equilibrium normal but muscle tone slightly decreased
II	1	Light narcosis	Excitement phase may precede increase in respiratory rate, loss of equilibrium with efforts to right itself, muscle tone decreased
II	2	Deep narcosis	Ceases to respond to positional changes, decrease in respiratory rate to near normal, total loss of equilibrium with no efforts to right itself but some reactivity to strong tactile stimuli
III	1	Light anaesthesia	Total loss of muscle tone, further decrease in respiratory rate
III	2	Surgical anaesthesia	Total loss of reactivity, respiratory rate very low
IV		Medullary collapse	Total loss of gill movement followed in several minutes by cardiac arrest

Figure 25.2: *Signs and stages of anaesthesia in fish (adapted from Brown, 1993).*

When performing minor surgery on an anaesthetized fish, the patient should be placed on a moist surface, such as a paper towel, for 3–4 minutes before being placed in the recovery tank. Anaesthesia can be maintained for longer periods but more complicated circulation systems need to be established (Stoskopf, 1993). Recovery can be assisted by holding the fish upright in the water column and moving it forward through the tank, thereby assisting fresh water flow over the gills.

If euthanasia is required this can be achieved by simply allowing the fish to remain in the anaesthetic bath for a prolonged period or by exposing the fish to a high concentration of the agent (usually 10 times the anaesthetic dose). In larger patients, such as sharks or conger eels, euthanasia can be achieved by giving pentobarbitone intravenously or intraperitoneally.

METHODS OF ADMINISTRATION

Administration of anaesthetics to fish is usually via a bath solution, but some workers have used spray or injections. The standard practice for bath anaesthetics is to have three containers or tanks filled with the water in which the patient is to be held; this avoids stresses such as sudden temperature or chemical changes. The first container is the original holding tank, the second is the anaesthetic bath and the third is the recovery tank (Figure 25.3). It is useful to have an anaesthetic tank that is premarked for a standard volume, and in which a predetermined amount of anaesthetic stock solution can be diluted. Factors for successful anaesthesia include:

- Aeration or oxygenation of all the tanks throughout the procedure
- Conducting a test bath on a small number of fish if larger numbers need anaesthetizing
- Starving the fish for 24 hours before anaesthesia
- Not disturbing the fish before the bath.

DRUGS AND DOSAGES

A large number of agents for fish anaesthesia are listed in the literature, ranging from xylazine to tobacco juice. However, only a few chemicals have proved their worth and these are the agents discussed in this section. Although non-chemical methods, such as electric shock, have also been used, chemical methods are preferred at present.

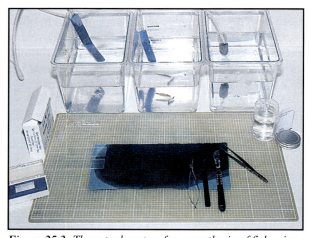

Figure 25.3: *Three-tank system for anaesthesia of fish using aeration and a prepared moist examination area.*

Benzocaine

Benzocaine (ethyl aminobenzoate) is used in several medical preparations, e.g. throat lozenges, haemorrhoid remedies, and it is a useful fish anaesthetic. It needs to be dissolved in ethanol or acetone, and such a stock solution should be stored in a brown bottle as it is light-sensitive. A stock solution of 10% (100 g/l) is easy to use, and for most species effective anaesthesia can be achieved with a bath concentration of 25–100 mg/l. Lower dosages are required for diseased fish or those in poor condition. The drug is more toxic in warm water, but higher doses are required for the same effect at a lower temperature. There is, therefore, a narrow margin of safety at high temperatures.

Precautionary notes with benzocaine are:

· Adequate aeration is necessary because respiration is rapidly depressed
· An alternative agent should be used if the patient is being treated with sulphonamides as benzocaine is hydrolysed to para-aminobenzoic acid in their presence
· It is highly fat soluble and therefore fat mature fish or gravid females may have prolonged recovery.

Tricaine

Tricaine methane sulphonate, or tricaine, was developed for fish anaesthesia, and it is the most commonly used drug for this purpose in North America. It is available as a soluble powder. A stock solution can be prepared (10 g/l) and stored in a brown bottle for up to one year. This will facilitate accurate dosage. For most species, practical anaesthesia can be achieved using a dosage of 50–100 mg/l, i.e. 5–10 ml of a 10 g/l stock solution for every litre of water.

Tricaine is acidic and when added to fresh water can significantly lower the pH. Buffering is usually necessary and sodium bicarbonate is commonly used at 200–250 mg per 100 mg tricaine. Buffering is not necessary in sea water. Tricaine is more toxic in young fish and in soft warm water. Dosage should therefore be adjusted accordingly. At lower dosages of 15–25 mg/l, sedation can be induced in salmonids, which is useful for transport or grading. Tricaine has also been given by spray at 150 mg/l over the gills of large broodstock.

Quinaldine sulphate

2-Methyl quinolone sulphate, or quinaldine sulphate, can be used alone or synergistically with tricaine. It is highly soluble in water but acidic and therefore requires buffering in fresh water, as with tricaine. A 10 g/l working solution can be stored in a brown bottle for up to one year. At 25 mg/l salmonids lose equilibrium in less than 4 minutes. Dosages range from 15 to 60 mg/l. The drug is less toxic in very soft water than in hard, but toxicity increases as water temperature rises.

In combination with tricaine, there is a faster induction than with either product alone, and the usual ratio of tricaine to quinaldine sulphate is 10:1.

Metomidate

There has been some renewed interest in the potential use of metomidate in fish species, predominantly in developing aquaculture species such as Cod, Halibut and Red Drum (Mattson and Riple, 1989; Malmstrøm et al., 1993; Massee et al., 1995). Induction is rapid, and fish should be removed from the anaesthetic solution after losing equilibrium. A dark skin coloration is often induced, probably as a result of the metabolic blockade of cortisol production, but normal colour returns upon recovery from anaesthesia. Dosages recorded vary for different species but are as follows:

· 10 mg/l for Halibut
· 5 mg/l for salmonids
· 1–2.5 mg/l for Channel Catfish
· 2.5–5 mg/l for marine tropicals and sharks
· 0.06–0.20 mg/l for transport sedation.

Phenoxyethanol

2-Phenoxyethanol is available as an oily liquid, and although a narrow margin of safety has been reported and adverse physiological effects considered likely to occur in fish, some workers rely on this chemical for routine use. A working dosage for slow induction of salmonids is 100 ppm (0.1 ml/l), although dosages of 0.2–0.6 ml/l can be used. Goldfish can be anaesthetized at 0.4–0.5 ml/l when temperatures are <25°C. Higher temperatures require higher dosages, as do larger fish. Hyperactivity is often recorded on induction and this usually takes the form of 'motorboating' around the water surface. For this reason, the drug is not used by many practitioners. Corneal damage may also be induced by this drug.

Clove oil

Clove oil has been widely used as a fish anaesthetic in South East Asia for many years, and it is only relatively recently that interest has developed in its use in other parts of the world (Munday and Wilson, 1997). Clove oil is familiar in Western countries as a topical dental anaesthetic. Commercially available clove oil comprises 85–95% eugenol, which has been shown to be a safe anaesthetic and sedative agent for a large range of fresh and sea water fish and some crustaceans. Recovery time from anaesthesia is longer than with tricaine or benzocaine and this can be advantageous depending on the species and clinical situation. Rapid induction, i.e. less than 60 seconds, can be achieved at dosages of 25 ppm

(0.025 ml/l), but slower induction can be achieved with lower dosages.

Non-chemical methods

Both hypothermia and electroanaesthesia have been used in fish, although these methods are not considered suitable at present.

CONCLUSION

As fish vary markedly in their sensitivity to various agents, it is advisable that the practitioner find one or two agents that work well for the species they are dealing with. Careful attention to detail will reduce both morbidity and mortality.

REFERENCES

Brown LA (1993) Anaesthesia and restraint. In: *Fish Medicine,* ed. MK Stoskopf, pp. 79–90. WB Saunders, Philadelphia

Gilderhaus PA and Marking LL (1987) Comparative efficacy of 16 anesthetic chemicals on rainbow trout. *North American Journal of Fisheries Management* **7**, 288–292

Malmstrøm T, Salte R, Gjøen HM and Linseth A (1993) A practical evaluation of metomidate and MS-222 as anaesthetics for halibut (*Hippoglossus hippoglossus L.*). *Aquaculture* **113**, 331–338

Massee KC, Rust MB, Hardy RW and Stickney RR (1995) The effectiveness of tricaine, quinaldine sulphate and metomidate as anaesthetics for larval fish. *Aquaculture* **134**, 351–359

Mattson NS and Riple TH (1989) Metomidate, a better anaesthetic for cod (*Gadus morhua*) in comparison with benzocaine, MS-222, chlorobutanol and phenoxyethanol. *Aquaculture* **83**, 89–94

Munday PL and Wilson SK (1997) Comparative efficacy of clove oil and other chemicals in anaesthetization of *Pomacentrus amboinensis*, a coral reef fish. *Journal of Fish Biology* **51**, 931–938

Stoskopf MK (1993) Surgery. In: *Fish Medicine,* ed. MK Stoskopf, pp. 91–97. WB Saunders, Philadelphia

CHAPTER TWENTY SIX

Reptiles

Dermod Malley

INTRODUCTION

In reptiles, anaesthesia may be necessary not only for reasons of humanity and technical efficiency but also for the safety of handlers, as some species are strong, quick, vicious or venomous. The diversity and large number of species within the order Reptilia complicate anaesthesia in these animals, make a comprehensive treatise difficult to achieve within the limit of one chapter, and underline the necessity of accurate identification of the species to highlight interspecies differences with particular regard to physiological status (e.g. health, gravidity, hibernation).

ANATOMICAL AND PHYSIOLOGICAL CONSIDERATIONS

There are many anatomical and physiological differences between reptiles and mammals, which are of importance to the anaesthetist.

Dependence on the environment

Preferred body temperature and humidity
Reptiles are incapable of generating their own body heat, but every species has a preferred body temperature (PBT) and an optimal temperature range (OTR) within which its metabolism functions. The PBT is defined by Brattstrom (1965) as 'the narrow range of temperature at which ... reptiles are found carrying on their normal activities' (this may be extended to include the metabolism of xenobiotic agents). The PBT is the optimal core temperature at which the auscultated heart rate should adhere to the following allometric formula:

$$\text{Heart rate (pulse) of reptiles} = 34 \, (W)^{-0.25}$$

Where W is the body weight in kg.

PBT may be related to the environmental temperature of the vivarium.

Humidity
Humidity is important for the proper functioning of reptilian body systems. The full effect of this is not completely understood, but dehydration will be discussed later.

Ultraviolet light
A source of ultraviolet light is important for diurnal species of the order Sauria and is used to compensate for basking in the sun. Most reptiles presented to the clinician are maintained in captivity and some are captive bred, so the length of exposure and the wavelength of the light concerned is of significant clinical importance. The full effect of ultraviolet radiation is not fully understood.

Skin sensitivity
Skin sensitivity is extremely well developed in reptiles and this becomes obvious to the clinician when restraint is required for completion of even the most simple stimulatory procedure (e.g. hypodermic injection).

Respiratory system
There is no muscular diaphragm in reptiles. To compensate, snakes, lizards and crocodilians use intrapulmonary and intercostal muscles to vary lung volumes, whereas chelonia use the muscles of the pectoral and pelvic girdles. As the action of these muscles is affected by the relaxant effect of anaesthetic agents, anaesthetists must be prepared to use intermittent positive-pressure ventilation (IPPV) throughout the maintenance of anaesthesia. IPPV is used to ensure that two-fifths of the coelom is inflated at each respiratory excursion.

Small amounts of oxygen are absorbed at sites in the pharyngeal and cloacal epithelia, in bladders off the dorsal wall of the cloaca and through the skin as well as at the main site, the faveolar epithelium of the lungs. This phenomenon may lead to the dilution of anaesthetic gases and may make inhalation anaesthesia difficult to maintain.

Tidal volume is variable in reptiles and is affected by external factors such as ambient temperature (and possibly humidity) and also by internal physiological and pathological factors such as gut and oviductular content (food and eggs) and hyperplasia of internal organs (e.g. ovarian follicles, neoplasia, abscesses).

The lungs of reptiles are fixed and shaped like a honeycomb with a large central space that acts as anatomical dead space as well as a reservoir for unexpired gases at the end of an anaesthetic session. The existence of an air sac in snakes must be considered during recovery from anaesthesia with volatile agents and may require prolonged flushing with air or an oxygen/carbon dioxide mixture postoperatively.

Mucus is not normally produced in great quantities by reptiles, so the administration of mucolytics or depressants of bronchial secretion should not be routinely necessary.

Anatomy of the upper respiratory tract

Reptiles breathe by inhaling boluses of air (gular gulping) and not by rhythmical inhalation. The anatomy of the reptilian upper respiratory tract is also distinctive:

- The glottis is kept closed at rest, and the aditus laryngis is opened by the dilator glottis muscle only during active respiration
- The carina of *Testudo* spp. is situated so close to the aditus laryngis that it is possible to intubate only one bronchus, an obvious and undesirable error that must be avoided
- The fleshy tongue of chelonians, crocodilians and some saurians often obscures the aditus laryngis and must be depressed in order to visualize the area during intubation
- The soft palate of crocodilians is long and must be raised to allow access to the aditus laryngis.

Circulatory system

The significance of the reptilian renal portal system has been a subject for discussion between physiologists and practising anaesthetists for decades. The renal portal system consists of bilateral valves in a vein which extends from the junction of epigastric and external iliac veins to the kidneys. These valves are opened by the action of acetylcholine and closed by adrenaline (epinephrine). Traditionally, clinicians have avoided injecting agents into the caudal half of the reptilian body to avoid loading the kidneys with nephrotoxic xenobiotics or with physiologically active agents that could be excreted before they exerted their effects elsewhere. The author has always relied on the extreme sensitivity of the reptile's skin to stimulate the production of adrenaline (and close the valves) and finds that the renal portal system does not seem to be of great practical importance. Recent research suggests that the valves may not be as pharmacologically important as previously considered (Beck *et al.*, 1995).

Reptiles can survive on anaerobic metabolism and can therefore hold their breath for long periods. This is because the cardiac ventricle is a single chamber from which blood can be pumped to the pulmonary and systemic circulation in differing proportions. During periods of apnoea (e.g. during a dive) flow favours the systemic circulation. This makes induction with volatile agents tedious and provides particular difficulties with aquatic and amphibious reptiles and necessitates tracheal intubation and IPPV.

Fluid homeostasis

Reptiles do not sweat but lose excessive body water by expiration. Although the epithelial area of the reptilian respiratory system is considerable, it may not be greater (when related to the bodyweight or surface area) than that of birds and mammals (P Zwart, personal communication). However, thought should be given to humidifying inspired gases during prolonged anaesthesia.

As with mammalian species it is important to understand the intricacies of reptilian fluid homeostasis, especially as many commonly used agents are nephrotoxic (e.g. non-steroidal anti-inflammatory drugs) or excreted by the kidneys (e.g. ketamine). Slightly more than 50% of reptilian body fluid is maintained in the intracellular compartment, and the circulating fluid volume percentage is lower than it is in mammals. In spite of a remarkable ability to cope with hypertonic solutions, reptiles are usually infused with replacement fluids of lower osmolarity than that used in mammals, especially when they are maintained at their preferred ambient temperature. Fluid replacement should be achieved with solutions that are isotonic with reptile body fluids (i.e. equivalent to 0.65% saline). Owing to the tendency of reptiles to produce lactic acid after simple activities such as feeding, excitement, handling, anaesthesia and even sudden changes in ambient temperature, it is best to avoid infusion with lactated fluids (Dessauer, 1970).

Tolerance to xenobiotics

Venomous reptiles in particular are remarkably tolerant to physiologically active agents (e.g. Gaboon Vipers tolerate muscle relaxants and Australian colubrids are tolerant of the effects of curariform drugs (Calderwood 1971; Bennett 1991)). The Indigo Snake (*Drymarchon corais cooperi*) shows no response to 0.015 mg/kg etorphine administered intramuscularly, and crocodilians are erratic in their response to etorphine (Bennett, 1991). Crocodilians and chelonians absorb and detoxify drugs very slowly. Anaesthesia in lizards may be induced very rapidly with propofol, alphaxolone/alphadolone or isoflurane, so care must be taken not to overdose these animals. Amphibious species require the addition of 10% carbon dioxide to gaseous induction mixtures.

Lack of eyelids

Snakes and geckos do not possess eyelids. Their corneas may desiccate under anaesthesia and this may be prevented by the use of artificial tears.

INJECTION SITES

Before any injections in reptiles, the veterinarian must scrub the skin thoroughly with a detergent-based povidone–iodine solution to ensure near aseptic conditions, as reptiles are notoriously susceptible to abscessation and septicaemia.

Intramuscular injections in all species should be truly intramuscular as inadvertent injection into fascia produces equivocal responses. Many species may develop a cutaneous slough after subcutaneous injection. This may be prevented by diluting the product with a suitable agent (refer to the manufacturer), by wiping the needle clean just before injection and by massaging the site thoroughly after injection (the author uses a soft toothbrush and scrubs the skin at the same time). As parasitism is so frequently encountered in vivarium-bound reptiles the warning is justified that ivermectin should not be used simultaneously with benzodiazapines, and at no time should ivermectin be administered to chelonians.

Chelonians (tortoises, turtles, terrapins)

Intravenous route

When administering drugs by the intravenous route in chelonians:

- The jugular vein is the favoured superficial blood vessel for blood sampling but is also useful for administration of intravenous agents (Figure 26.1). It is accessible and easily visible on both sides of the neck but its position varies from species to species. Recalcitrant animals can be immersed in tepid water (land tortoises) and the head grasped when the animal raises it to the surface to breathe. Gentle handling is imperative for this procedure. (The use of ketamine and medetomidine (see Figure 26.9) shows promise as a pre-induction sedative for all species.)
- To gain access to the subcarapacial vein the tortoise's head must be held within the shell. The needle, previously bent to an angle of 100 degrees, is inserted in the dorsal midline and passed under the nuchal scute dorsally until it hits bone. The needle is then withdrawn slightly and blood aspirated. Perivascular leakage and haematoma formation is frequently encountered at both the jugular and subcarapacial sites, so it is advisable to maintain pressure for 5 minutes after venepuncture
- The caudal vein is approached on the dorsal midline of the tail. This vessel is very small in many species and non-existent in others e.g. the Hermann's Tortoise (*Testudo hermanni hermanni*) in which the dorsal intravertebral sinus may be entered inadvertently (Ippen and Zwart, 1995)
- The brachial venous plexus can be approached from the ventromedial aspect proximal to the carpus (Willette Frahm, 1995), and the femoral venous plexus is approached at the plantar aspect of the femur.

Intracardiac route

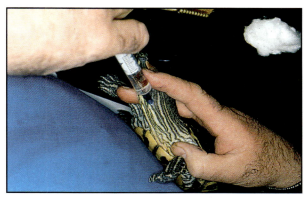

Figure 26.1: *Intravenous injection, into the jugular vein, in a Red-eared Terrapin* (Trachemys scripta elegans).

Intracardiac injections may be performed via the junction of the pectoral and abdominal scutes of the plastron. The site may have to be drilled before injection and sealed with cyanoacrylate afterwards (anaesthesia is required before drilling).

Intracoelomic route

Intracoelomic injections are performed in the notch of the plastron in the axillary and inguinal areas through the soft skin cranial to the front of the back legs. The plunger should be withdrawn before the fluid is administered to ensure that the bladder, bowel or lung have not been punctured. If this is the case, fluid will be aspirated and the needle must be withdrawn and the process repeated on the contralateral side.

Epicoelomic route

Epicoelomic injections are administered into the space bounded by the pectoral musculature, the pleuroperitoneum and the plastron. The entry site is ventral to the scapulohumeral joint and dorsal to the plastron (Jarchow, 1988).

Intramuscular route

Suitable sites for intramuscular injection in chelonians are the pectorals, quadriceps femoris or semimembranosus/semitendinosus group.

Intraosseous route

Fluids can be administered to chelonians by the intraosseous route into the tibia or the axillary bony pillar of the carapace. It may be necessary to drill a small hole in the carapace with a dental high-speed drill after aseptic preparations. The author uses a short spinal needle (Howard Jones 21 gauge, 3/4 inch) in both sites. A needle in the tibia can be bent against the carapace when the leg is retracted.

Subcutaneous route

When administering drugs by the subcutaneous route, the needle is inserted at the point at which the axillary or inguinal skin joins the carapace.

Saurians (lizards)

Intravenous route

When administering drugs by the intravenous route in saurians:

- The caudal vein can be accessed by the ventral approach with the animal in dorsal or ventral recumbency (Figure 26.2); a soft table covering is useful. The needle is inserted in the midline at an angle of 45 degrees to the frontal plane with the bevel of the needle facing cranially, thus the lumen of the needle avoids the dorsal wall of the blood vessel
- The ventral abdominal veins can be used: these paired midline veins can be injected with practice and good restraint
- The cephalic vein lies in a similar position to that of mammals. The transcutaneous approach requires surgical incision.

Intracoelomic route

The approach is to one side of the midline (to avoid the paired ventral abdomen veins), 80% of the way from the pectoral to pelvic girdle (to avoid the liver and intracoelomic fat body) with the needle directed towards the parietal pneumoperitoneum to avoid the viscera.

Intramuscular route

Intramuscular injections are given into the triceps and quadriceps femoris: the skin must be tensed firmly against the underlying muscle before insertion of the needle.

Intraosseous route

Fluid therapy by the intraosseous route is a surprisingly simple procedure in lizards, even in adult iguanas, and seems to the author to be relatively humane and free of pain. A spinal needle is inserted into the medullary cavity via the tibial crest.

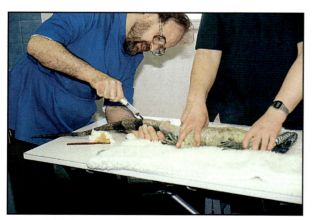

Figure 26.2: *Intravenous injection: ventral approach to the caudal vein of a Green Iguana (Iguana iguana).*

Subcutaneous route

Subcutaneous injections are usually administered along the back but, if performed in the belly, care must be taken to avoid the ventral abdominal vein.

Ophidians (snakes)

Intravenous route

Access to the palatine vein in the oral cavity is easily achieved for the administration of an intravenous induction agent. After withdrawal of the needle, pressure should be maintained with a damp cotton bud for 1–2 minutes to prevent perivascular leakage and haematoma formation.

Intracardiac route

The beating heart can be palpated in snakes at a point approximately 25–30% of the way from the nose to the vent. The snake is usually lightly restrained in ventral recumbency ('sternal recumbency in mid-air'), and the apex beat of the heart is localized by digital palpation at a point approximately 25–30% of the way from the nose to the vent. This is the author's preferred method of administering doxapram to snakes that are slow to recover from a prolonged anaesthetic.

Intramuscular route

Snakes can be injected deeply into the paravertebral muscles.

Subcutaneous route

Subcutaneous injections are given along the back where the skin is less tightly adherent to the underlying musculature than in the ventral region. Care must be taken not to lacerate muscle as this may lead to haematoma formation.

Crocodilians (crocodiles, alligators, caimans, gavials)

Intravenous route

For reasons of operator safety the most accessible vein is the (ventral) caudal vein.

Intracoelomic route

Refer to saurians above for approach to intracoelomic injections.

Intramuscular route

Intramuscular injections are given in the limbs and in the dorsal musculature at the base of the tail.

Intraosseous route

Intraosseous fluids can be administered into the tibial medullary cavity.

Subcutaneous route

Subcutaneous injections are administered in the axillary or inguinal regions where the skin is less tightly attached than elsewhere.

PHYSICAL RESTRAINTS

Reptiles must be handled deftly, confidently and carefully. Snakes are particularly prone to bruising which can lead to a fatal myositis. Rough handling can lead to cardiovascular problems, falling arterial oxygen tension (PaO_2), increased carbon dioxide tension ($PaCO_2$) and cardiac arrhythmias.

Once adequately restrained, further immobilization can be achieved by the following methods:

- Hypothermia. Owing to their dependence on PBT to maintain their metabolism, reptiles become quiescent at low temperatures. This has no analgesic effect, and extremely low temperatures create the risk of cerebral necrosis. Hypothermia has no place in the humane restraint of reptiles
- The vasovagal response is used in lizards. Pressure on the eyes causes hypotension and bradycardia and the resultant immobility may be sufficient for simple non-painful procedures such as radiography. Recovery is spontaneous after tactile or sonic stimulation. Some clinicians maintain this pressure by placing cotton pads on the closed eyelids, and holding the pads in place with a bandage
- As with other primitive creatures, darkness sedates reptiles and many remain immobile when covered. This may be achieved simply by covering the animal with a dark cloth or by bandaging or hooding the head to cover the eyes, ears and 'pineal eye', although the last procedure may exert its effect by the vasovagal response (see above).

Electroanaesthesia has been used in iguanas. A combination of low- and high-frequency sine waves is used. The frequencies should range from 1500 to 3000 cycles per second and the current up to 20 milliamperes (Bennett, 1991). Congestion of the brain seen in dogs at postmortem examination after electrical euthanasia and comments made by human patients after electroconvulsive therapy lead this author to believe that electroanaesthesia may be inhumane.

PREPARATION OF THE PATIENT

Preanaesthetic evaluation

Species identification of the subject may not be simple as the owner or keeper may not be aware of this important fact. Good reference books are essential. The need to know the species involved is important because each species has a differing response to anaesthetic agents, and also because it is very important to maintain a reptile at its PBT to allow its metabolism to optimize before, during and after the administration of

an anaesthetic. Acquisition of the optimal core body temperature can be verified by assessing the heart rate. It is imperative to weigh the subject so that doses may be calculated accurately. Digital metric electronic weighing scales are preferred for this purpose. Clinical assessment follows the same routine as with any other veterinary patient. A detailed clinical history of the subject, including particularly the ambient temperature at which it is maintained, is extremely important. As many anaesthetic agents used in reptiles are excreted by the kidneys, the hydration of the subject is important and may be assessed by measuring the PCV or blood urea concentration. The reader is referred to the *BSAVA Manual of Reptiles* for details on clinical assessment of reptiles.

Fluid therapy

Signs of dehydration

In snakes, signs include reduced dermal turgor and increased creasing of the skin. In chelonians (Figure 26.3) and lizards these signs are accompanied by enophthalmos, which is also seen in crocodiles. In all reptilian species, emaciation, inanition, lethargy and reduced bodyweight, although not specific, may be indicators of dehydration. Although much work needs to be done on the full significance of biochemical parameters in reptile blood, elevated PCV and increased concentrations of total proteins, uric acid and urea may also be indicative of dehydration.

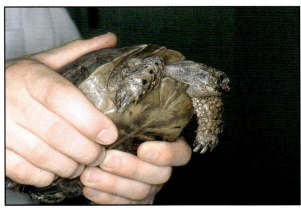

Figure 26.3: *Increased folding of the skin and enophthalmos in a dehydrated Spur-thighed Tortoise* (Testudo graeca).

Fluids that would be regarded as hypotonic in mammalian terms are used for replacement by both oral and parenteral routes in reptile clinics. Dehydration may be corrected by the following methods:

- Simple immersion in water at the PBT of the species concerned. Some Orders of reptiles (e.g. Chelonia) have the ability to absorb water through the cloaca. A bathing reptile may soon start to drink

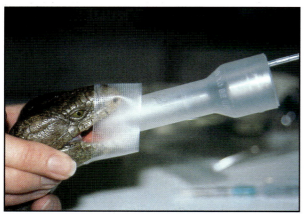

Figure 26.4: *Oral rehydration in a Prehensile Skink* (Corucia zebrata).

Courtesy of SJ Divers and In Practice.

- Oral administration of fluids is usually easily achieved by stomach tube (Figure 26.4). Proprietary fluids as used for mammals should be diluted by a further 10%
- Parenteral administration is performed by the infusion of a solution, which may be made by adding one part of 5% dextrose in 0.9% sodium chloride, one part of Ringer's or equivalent solution (preferably not lactated) and one part of water for injection
- Fluids should be warmed to the PBT of the species concerned, and great care should be taken to sterilize the injection site before infusion. Preferred routes are intraosseous (lizards, chelonians and crocodilians), intracoelomic (all Orders) and epicoelomic (i.e. into the space bounded by the pectoral musculature, the pleuroperitoneum and the plastron of chelonians). In snakes the intracardiac route is sometimes used, debilitated specimens tolerating the implantation of a cardiac catheter. The amount of fluid to be infused depends on the requirement. Traditionally, 3% of the bodyweight is administered daily by intravenous, intracardiac or intraosseous routes as maintenance, with 50% of the estimated fluid loss being replaced daily over 48 hours. The author has frequently administered the estimated replacement dose in chelonian and saurian subjects as a single bolus by the intracoelomic route without ill effect.

Fasting

Fasting is usually necessary in preanaesthetic preparation of the reptilian patient. The main aim of fasting is to avoid the compression of lung tissue that follows large meals, especially in carnivorous species. Feeding live food should be avoided in insectivorous species as insects may irritate the gastrointestinal canal of a comatose reptile, even to the point of injury. Lawton (1992) recommends fasting chelonians and lizards for 18 hours and snakes 72 to 98 hours before anaesthesia. Regurgitation is seldom a problem in reptile anaesthesia, except in snakes that have recently fed and in Mediterranean tortoises that have consumed large amounts of bulky vegetables.

Preoperative drugs

The use of antibiotics preoperatively is routine in some practices. A reptile may need a course of antibiotics to clear an underlying infection (as indicated by an increased total white blood count, with heterophilia or monocytosis) before the administration of an anaesthetic.

The use of sedative agents can also be considered (Figure 26.5). It is important for the clinician to be aware that sedation can often carry the same risk as the injection of an anaesthetic.

The use of analgesics may be considered preoperatively, especially if surgery of the skin, coelomic cavity or skeletal system is involved. The non-steroidal anti-inflammatory drugs carprofen and ketoprofen, are particularly useful (Figure 26.6).

Anticholinergic premedication is seldom used routinely in reptiles (see Introduction and Figure 26.7).

Drug	Dose and route	Comment
Phenothiazine derivatives	Acepromazine 0.1-0.5 mg/kg i.m. (Frye, 1991a) Chlorpromazine 10 mg/kg i.m. (Bennett, 1991)	Acepromazine was shown to have no effect on Garter Snakes (*Thamnophis sirtalis*) (Zwart and Lagerweij, 1971)
Benzodiazepines	Diazepam 0.22-0.62 mg/kg (Bennett, 1991) before use of suxamethonium Midazolam 2 mg/kg i.m. or s.c. with ketamine at 20-40 mg/kg i.m. or s.c. (Bennett, 1991)	Potentiated by ivermectin (Do not use ivermectin in Chelonia)

Figure 26.5: *Sedatives agents used in reptiles.*

properly (a snake should be able to move its full body length, a tortoise should be able to walk with its plastron clear of the ground and a lizard should be able to run). Even after this time, regular postoperative checks should be maintained in case residues of anaesthetic agents recirculate from various sites (lipid stores, gas pockets). Excretion of ketamine may be aided by the use of intraosseous or intravenous fluids.

The animal should not be subject to changes in its ambient temperature, which should be maintained at the PBT and OTR for the species concerned. Monitoring of temperature is important as increased ambient temperatures lead to an increased oxygen requirement.

Peace, quiet, and privacy are essential during hospitalization of reptiles, and all stress factors must be kept to a minimum.

Ventilation of the vivarium should be maintained in case there is a build up of exhaled anaesthetic gases, which could contribute to a prolonged recovery.

Hygiene of the vivarium is of paramount importance. Povidone–iodine solutions are recommended for vivarium hygiene, particularly as bacteria of the family Enterobacteriaceae are frequently implicated in postoperative infections.

Postoperative analgesia is usually managed with NSAIDs, particularly ketoprofen and carprofen. Doses of these agents are listed in Figure 26.5.

The use of analgesics is just as important in reptiles as in other species. Repeat doses are based on clinical observation and experience. The author has had unpleasant experiences with the use of flunixin meglumine in reptiles so no longer uses it for these animals.

ACKNOWLEDGEMENT

The author thanks Professor Emeritus Peer Zwart for his encouragement, advice and support in the compilation of this chapter.

REFERENCES AND FURTHER READING

Beck K, Loomis M, Lewbart G, Spelman L and Papick M (1995) Preliminary comparison of gentamicin injected into the cranial and caudal limb musculature of the eastern box turtle, *Terrapene carolina carolina*. *Journal of Zoo and Wildlife Medicine* **26(3)**, 265–268

Bennett RA (1991) A review of anaesthesia and chemical restraint in reptiles. *Journal of Zoo and Wildlife Medicine* **22(3)**, 282–303

Bennett RA (1994) Current techniques in reptile anaesthesia and surgery. In: *Proceedings of the American Association of Zoo Veterinarians and Association of Reptilian and Amphibian Veterinarians Annual Conference*. Pittsburgh, pp. 36–44

Blood DC and Studdert VP (1988) *Baillière's Comprehensive Veterinary Dictionary*, ed. RCJ Carling. Baillière Tindall, London

Boever WJ and Caputo F (1982) Telazol(Cl-744) as an anaesthetic agent in reptiles. *Journal of Zoo Animal Medicine* **13**, 59–61

Bonath K (1979) Halothane inhalation anaesthesia in reptiles and its clinical control. In: *International Zoo Year Book*, ed. PJS Olney. Zoological Society of London, London

Brattstrom BH (1965) Body temperatures of reptiles. *American Midlan. Naturalist* **73**, 376–422

Brogard J (1987) Anesthésie et chirurgie. In: *Les Maladies des Reptiles*. Editions du Point Vétérinaire, Maisons Alfort

Calderwood HW (1971) Anaesthesia for reptiles. *Journal of the American Veterinary Medical Association* **159(11)**, 1618–1625

Cooper JE (1974) Ketamine hydrochloride as an anaesthetic for East African reptiles. *Veterinary Record* **95**, 37–41

Cooper JE (1976) Veterinary attention for reptiles. In: *Veterinary Annual, 16th edn.*, ed. CS Grunsell and FWG Hill p.232. John Wright and Sons, Bristol

Dessauer HC (1970) Blood chemistry of reptiles. In: *Biology of the Reptilia, vol 3*, ed. C Gans and TS Parsons. Academich Press, London

Divers SJ (1996) Basic reptile husbandry, history taking and clinical examination. *Journal of Veterinary Postgraduate Clinical Study – In Practice*, **18(2)**, 51–65

Faulkner JE and Archambauet A (1993) Anaesthesia and surgery in the green iguana. *Seminars in Avian and Exotic Pet Medicine* **2(2)**, 103–108

Frye FL (1991a) Captive husbandry. In: *Biomedical and Surgical Aspects of Captive Reptile Husbandry, vol 1, 2nd edn*, p31. Krieger, Florida

Frye FL (1991b) Anesthesia. In: *Biomedical and Surgical Aspects of Captive Reptile Husbandry, vol 2, 2nd edn*, pp.423–437. Krieger, Florida

Frye FL (1994) *Reptile Clinician's Handbook. A Compact Clinical and Surgical Reference*. Krieger, Florida

Goebel T and Spoerle H (1991) Blood-collecting technique and selected reference values for the Hermann's Tortoise (*Testudo hermanni hermanni*). *Fourth International Colloquium on Pathology and Therapy of Reptiles and Amphibians*. pp.129–134, Bad Neuheim

Heard DJ (1993) Principles and techniques of anaesthesia and analgesia for exotic practice. Exotic Pet Medicine 1. *Veterinary Clinics of North America: Small Animal Practice* **23(6)**

Holt PE (1981) Drugs and dosages. In: *Diseases of the Reptilia vol.2*, ed. JE Cooper and OF Jackson. Academic Press, London

Ippen R and Zwart P (1995) Histological study of the tail vein of Hermann's tortoise (*Testudo hermanni*) *Proceedings of the 5th International Colloquium on Pathology of Reptiles and Amphibians*, April 1995. Alpen a/d Rijn

Jarchow JL (1988) Hospital care of the reptile patient. In: *Contemporary Issues in Small Animal Practice, vol 9: Exotic Animals* ed. ER Jacobson and GV Kollias Jr, pp.28–30. Churchill Livingstone, New York

Lawton MPC (1992) Anaesthesia. In: *Manual of Reptiles*, ed. PH Beynon. p.170. British Small Animal Veterinary Association, Cheltenham

Mader DR (1996) *Reptile Medicine and Surgery*. WB Saunders, London

Millichamp NJ (1988) Surgical techniques in reptiles. In: *Contemporary Issues in Small Animal Practice: Exotic Animals*, ed. ER Jacobson and GV Kollias Jr, pp.49–59. Churchill Livingstone, New York

Page CD (1993) Current reptilian anaesthesia proceedures. In: *Zoo and Wild Animal Medicine: 3. Current Therapy*, ed. ME Fowler, pp.140–143. WB Saunders, Philadelphia

Pokras MA, Sedgwick CJ and Kaufman GE (1992) Therapeutics. In: *Manual of Reptiles*, ed. PH Beynon, p.197. British Small Animal Veterinary Association, Cheltenham

Richter AG and Benirschke K (1977) Venipuncture sites defined and chromosome count in two giant tortoises. *Zoonooz* **50(2)**, 129–134

Richter AG, Olsen K, Fletcher K, Benirschke K and Bogart M (1977) Techniques for collection of blood from Galapagos tortoises and box turtles. *Veterinary Medicine Small Animal Clinician* **72(8)**, 1376–1378

Rival F (1993) Anaesthésie et réanimation des reptiles. *Proceedings of the Annual Congress CNVSPA*, pp.311–322. CNVSPA, Paris

Samour HJ, Risley D, March T, Savage B, Nieva O and Jones DM (1984) Blood sampling techniques in reptiles. *Veterinary Record* **144**, 472–476

Schobert E (1987) Telazol – use in wild and exotic animals. *Veterinary Medicine*. pp.1080–1088

Willette Frahm M (1995) Blood collection techniques in amphibians and reptiles. In: *Current Veterinary Therapy XII. Small Animal Practice*, ed. RW Kirk. pp.1344–1348. WB Saunders, Philadelphia

Zwart P and Lagerweij E (1971) Premedication and narcosis in garter snakes (*Thamnophis sirtalis*). *Verhandlungsbericht des XIII Internationalen Symposiums über die Erkrankungen der Zootiere. [Proceedings of the 13th International Symposium on the Diseases of Zoo Animals.]* Helsinki. pp.237–240

CHAPTER TWENTY SEVEN

Birds

Neil A. Forbes

INTRODUCTION

Anaesthesia of avian patients presents many challenges to the practitioner, not least of which is the great interspecies variation compared to mammals. This means that there are significant differences in response to a number of anaesthetic and analgesic drugs. Birds may also mask signs of illness until late in the disease process, when rapid decompensation can occur; a thorough preanaesthetic examination is therefore vitally important. The avian respiratory system is markedly different to that of mammals, with separate ventilatory and gas exchange components, making it the most efficient vertebrate respiratory system.

THE AVIAN PULMONARY SYSTEM

The avian pulmonary system is different from that of mammals in ways that are very important to the anaesthetist. Not least important of these differences is the fact that gas exchange is 10 times more efficient in birds than in mammals (James *et al.*, 1976) and hence overdose with inhaled anaesthetics is more likely.

The avian lung, although not rigid, is fixed to the roof of the thorax. It is less distensible than its mammalian counterpart and thus can function with a thinner blood–air barrier. In most species, there are eight air sacs - the unpaired cervical and unpaired clavicular, the paired cranial thoracic, the paired caudal thoracic and the paired abdominal sacs. Together, they account for 80% of the volume capacity of the avian respiratory system (Coles, 1985). The air sacs also have diverticulae, which extend into several bones, including the femur and humerus. Air sacs have poor vascularity, which prevents them from taking a significant part in gas exchange and may render them susceptible to certain infections e.g. *Aspergillus fumigatus*. The air sacs also host certain parasites, such as *Serratospiculum* spp. and *Cyathostoma* spp.

On inspiration, muscles cause ventral movement of the sternum; this creates a negative pressure in the air sacs within the thoracoabdominal cavity. In response to this negative pressure, air is drawn sequentially through the nares, the nasal cavity and the choana and through the rima glottidis into the trachea. The trachea of birds is inherently different from mammals as it is relatively wider and the tracheal rings are complete. The trachea generally divides at the level of the syrinx (voice box) into the primary bronchi. The location of the syrinx at the caudal end of the trachea explains why birds may vocalize while breathing through an endotracheal tube (ETT). After the primary bronchi, inspired air passes through a system of secondary bronchi and tertiary bronchi into the air sacs (Figure 27.1). Inspired air is divided so that some is directed to the cranial group of air sacs (cervical, clavicular and cranial thoracic) and some to the caudal group (caudal thoracic and abdominal). The tertiary bronchi are known as parabronchi and are surrounded by a mantle of air sacs and air capillaries. This mantle is also invested with a rich network of blood capillaries and is the site for gas exchange (Fedde, 1986). The typical avian lung consists primarily of palaeopulmonic parabronchi. Expiration is an active process initiated by muscles causing dorsal movement of the sternum (Figure 27.2). Aerodynamic valves at the junctions of bronchi ensure that airflow through the palaeopulmonic parabronchi is unidirectional in both inspiration and expiration (Figures 27.1 and 27.2). Most avian species (but not penguins and emus) also have neopulmonic parabronchi, which permit gas exchange with air passing to and from the caudal air sacs; air flow in neopulmonic parabronchi is bidirectional (Figures 27.1 and 27.2).

Because of the preponderance of unidirectional air flow and the cross-current relationship of air and blood flow in the parabronchi, there is minimal time lag in the absorption of oxygen. This arrangement enables a larger percentage of oxygen to be extracted from the inspired air than is normal in mammals. At sea level, inspired air has a partial pressure of oxygen (PO_2) of approximately 140 mmHg (18.7 kPa) while PO_2 in the cranial air sacs may fall to as low as 92 mmHg (12 kPa), suggesting that the efficiency of oxygen extraction in birds far surpasses that of mammals.

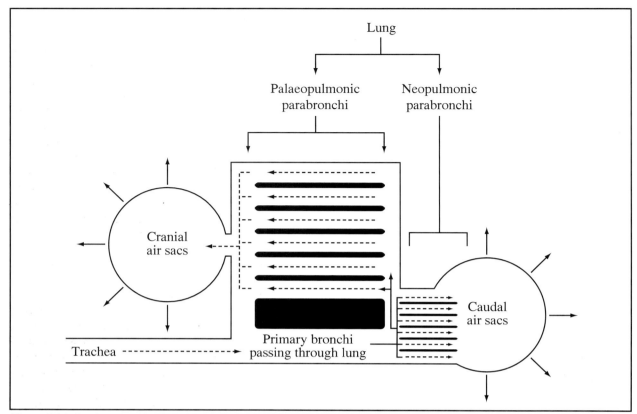

Figure 27.1: *Inspiration in birds.*

Adapted from Fedde (1986).

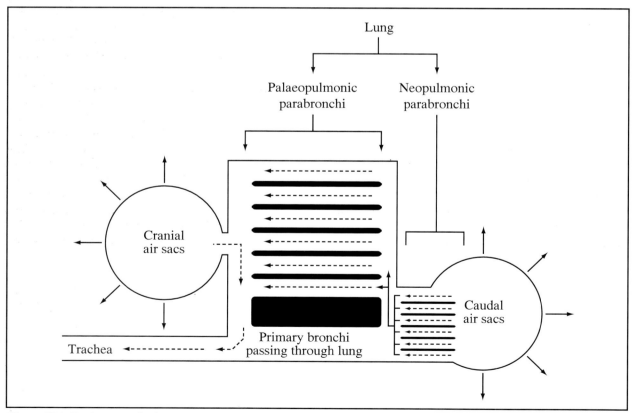

Figure 27.2: *Expiration in birds.*

Adapted from Fedde (1986).

SPECIAL CONSIDERATIONS

Age
Atheroma and arteriosclerosis are common in many avian species, particularly in older, inactive individuals that have been fed on an excessive or high fat diet. Clinical signs are not apparent before death, although such birds often have raised blood cholesterol concentrations. It should be remembered, however, that a high cholesterol concentration does not necessarily mean that atheroma is present.

Respiratory disease
Respiratory disease is common in many avian patients. If the disease is restricted to the air sacs, the primary signs may not include dyspnoea, but rather inappetence, general malaise or vomition. Disease may also affect the syrinx, situated at the bifurcation of the trachea. A change in a bird's voice is almost pathognomic for syringeal aspergillosis, which presents as a true emergency. If respiratory disease affects the lung parenchyma itself, dyspnoea is severe and often accompanied by cyanosis. Dyspnoea worsens on handling. Oxygen therapy is recommended before anaesthesia or handling of any dyspnoeic bird.

Body condition
Body condition may be assessed by palpating the amount of muscle covering the pectoral area. However, experience is required to accurately assess condition in this way, because normal muscle mass varies greatly between species and even within closely related groups.

Abdomen
The structure of the air sacs means that if ascites, or other space-occupying lesions are present in the abdomen, considerable respiratory embarrassment results. Preoxygenation is also recommended in such cases.

Dorsal recumbency
Dorsal recumbency during anaesthesia restricts movement of the sternum and reduces minute volume by 10–60%; hence, birds should not be kept on their backs for longer than is necessary. Movement of the sternum should never be compromised e.g. by restraint, heavy drapes or surgical instruments.

Hypothermia
Hypothermia is a significant problem with all but the briefest avian anaesthetics. All birds should be placed on a heated pad or under a heat lamp during surgery. If it does not interfere with surgery, the body may be enclosed in bubble wrap or an exposure blanket to conserve body heat. Feathers should not be clipped, otherwise they will not be replaced until the next moult. The minimum area necessary should be plucked and the skin prepared for surgery with minimum amounts of antiseptic soap. Excessive use of liquid antiseptics, especially alcohol, increases evaporative heat loss. Healthy avian skin carries a much smaller number of bacteria than mammalian skin, suggesting that exhaustive skin preparation is unnecessary in birds. Adhesive, transparent surgical drapes help to minimize the area of plucking and permit easy direct observation of the patient.

Endotracheal intubation
Endotracheal intubation is recommended for all anaesthetized birds, with the possible exception of those weighing under 100 g where the small diameter of the tube increases the risk of obstruction by dried secretions. Intubation enables effective intermittent positive-pressure ventilation (IPPV), facilitates scavenging of waste anaesthetic gases and minimizes the chance of aspiration of food material. The rima glottidis (opening to the trachea) is situated in the caudal part of the tongue. In some species (e.g. pigeons and raptors), it is readily visible, while in others (e.g. psittacines) the large fleshy tongue must be pulled forwards with atraumatic forceps to enable visualization before intubation. Figures 27.3, 27.4 and 27.5 show the tracheal openings of a raptor, a psittacine and a waterfowl, respectively. The crista ventralis (ventral crest) of the larynx has been described in penguins (Spheniscidae), *Anas* and *Apteryx* and may be seen in other species, such as some hornbills, some toucans and some gulls. This horn-like projection across the lumen of the glottis can prevent intubation. Birds with this structure should have anaesthesia induced by mask, and maintained by using air sac perfusion anaesthesia (see below). In birds, the tracheal cartilage rings are complete, in contrast to those in mammals. It has been recommended that the accessory cuffs on ETTs should not be inflated because the complete tracheal

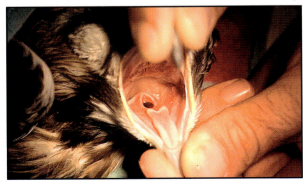

***Figure 27.3:** The rima glottidis of a raptor.*

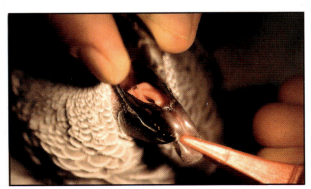

***Figure 27.4:** The rima glottidis of a psittacine.*

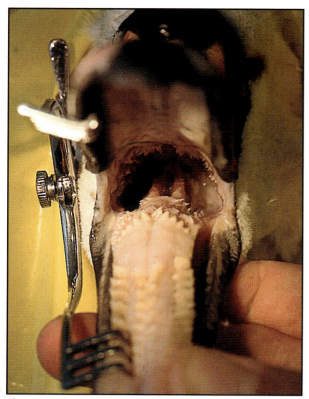

Figure 27.5: The rima glottidis of a swan.

rings are relatively non-compliant and cuff inflation may lead to pressure necrosis. However, Curro (1998) advises that cuffs should be inflated just enough to prevent gas leaking around the cuff. Suction equipment, such as a urinary catheter (Jackson's or male dog catheter) and syringe, should always be available to clear secretions from the trachea and ETT.

Air sac perfusion

The unique structure of the avian pulmonary system allows oxygen and anaesthetic gases to be delivered by air sac perfusion (or insufflation). This technique may be employed if access to the head, mouth or trachea is required e.g. for the surgical treatment of syringeal aspergilloma. Air sac perfusion anaesthesia induces pupillary dilation and hence is useful for ophthalmological examinations and surgery. Placement of the air sac tube is generally made after induction of anaesthesia. Air sac perfusion tubes should be prepared in advance; a 4 mm tube is used for a bird weighing 350 g and pro rata for larger or smaller birds. The section of tube which is to be within the body cavity should have not only an open end, but also a series of additional holes in the lateral walls, such that they cannot all become blocked (Figure 27.6). Soft tubing is less likely to become kinked. Two transfixion ligatures should be preplaced in the tube in preparation for suturing in place in the abdominal wall after placement. A number of sites have been recommended for air sac perfusion. This author favours using the left abdominal air sac entered through a prelumbar site that is ventrocaudal to the

ischium of the pelvis. In this method, the leg is pulled forward and an incision made ventral to the lumbar musculature (Figure 27.7). The perfusion tubing is then angled cranially, pushed in and sutured into the muscular body wall (either directly or with a tape butterfly). The other commonly used site involves penetrating the left caudal air sac between the last and penultimate ribs on the left side at the site commonly used for surgical sexing of birds. After placing the tube into an air sac, it is usually connected to the fresh gas flow from an anaesthetic machine. The anatomy of the avian pulmonary system causes gas infused into the caudal air sac to pass out of the trachea via the gas-exchanging parabronchi (see above and Figures 27.1 and 27.2); hence anaesthetic and respiratory gas exchange can occur while the patient is apnoeic. The fresh gas flow usually contains oxygen and anaesthetic vapour that may be warmed and humidified by bubbling the mixture through a chamber containing warm water. Gas flow rate may be regulated so that the bird just stops breathing; a flow of 0.5–1.0 l/min is usually a good starting point for medium-sized waterfowl. Excessive fresh gas flow rates should be avoided, otherwise a respiratory alkalosis may occur (Korbel, 1998). The vaporizer setting should be regulated to provide an adequate plane of anaesthesia. An ETT should be placed to allow removal of waste anaesthetic gas. Air sac perfusion tubes may be left in situ for 1 to 3 weeks, in order to enable repeated anaesthesia, surgery or treatment of tracheal lesions. Ducks and other diving birds are sometimes difficult to anaesthetize with a mask, and may also be difficult to

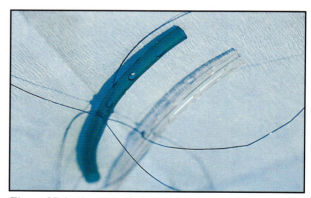

Figure 27.6: Air sac perfusion tube.

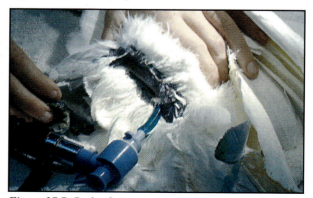

Figure 27.7: Prelumbar insertion site for air sac perfusion.

maintain under anaesthesia via an ETT. This may be due to stimulation of the diving reflex, by contact of the mask with the head, causing apnoea (Ludders and Matthews, 1996) or it may be associated with high inspired oxygen concentrations causing depression of respiratory drive (Seaman *et al.*, 1994). These problems may be circumvented either by positive-pressure ventilation or injectable induction followed by air sac perfusion anaesthesia.

PREPARATION OF THE PATIENT

Preanaesthetic evaluation
Assessment of the health status of the patient before anaesthesia is essential, but the stress resulting from examination and the collection of samples must be weighed against any potential advantages. Avian patients should be as fit as possible before administration of anaesthetics, and this may entail initial medical stabilization. Dehydration should be corrected. Preoperative data should include haematocrit and blood glucose concentration. In elderly birds, assessment of liver and kidney function is also desirable. If the haematocrit is <20%, either severe anaemia or haemodilution is present and anaesthesia should be delayed, if possible. Birds with impaired renal function should not receive ketamine because a large fraction of this drug undergoes elimination via the kidney. Halothane is contraindicated in birds with impaired liver function and in birds that are excited or distressed. Local anaesthetics are not advocated as sole anaesthetic agents in birds because physically restrained birds are usually fractious and distressed. The dose of most local anaesthetics that cause unwanted side effects, such as seizures and excitement, is often only a little more than the therapeutic dose. Therefore, local anaesthetics such as lignocaine (lidocaine), which are supplied in concentrations suitable for dogs and cats, should be used cautiously (or never) in small birds.

Bodyweight
Bodyweight is an important part of the preanaesthetic evaluation because it allows accurate calculation of the

Psittacine	Bodyweight (g)
Scarlet Macaw	1000
Lesser Sulphur Crested Cockatoo	300
Great Sulphur Crested Cockatoo	700
African Grey Parrot	250–500
Budgerigar	30–50
Lovebird	45–55
Cockatiel	80–120
Amazon Parrot	250–700

Figure 27.8: Average bodyweights of some commonly treated psittacines.

doses of any drugs that will be given. The average weights of some commonly treated psittacines are shown in Figure 27.8.

The weights should be used only as a general guide. Even experienced avian anaesthetists find difficulty in accurately estimating bodyweight; thus all birds that may receive injectable drugs should be weighed before anaesthesia.

Fluid therapy
All surgical cases should receive fluids, which should be warmed to 37–40°C before administration. Crystalloid preparations temporarily improve circulating volume, but generally pass into the extravascular compartment within 30 minutes. Colloidal preparations provide circulating volume expansion for several hours. Administration may be via a capped indwelling catheter in the basilic vein, although the medial tarsal, or jugular veins can also be used. Alternatively, subcutaneous, intramuscular or intraosseous (cranial tibiotarsus or ulna) routes may be used.

Fluids should be given at a dose rate of 20 ml/kg as a bolus before surgery and then at a rate of 15 ml/kg/h. In small birds, this may be achieved with a syringe pump, but in larger birds this may be accomplished by slowly giving boluses at intervals of 5 minutes, or by intraosseous infusion.

Surgical techniques to minimize haemorrhage, including diathermy, should be utilized. Avian blood does not require crossmatching, and unmatched transfusions can be repeated after a lapse of 1 week. Recent work (Degernes, 1997) suggested that erythrocyte survival was 9–11 days in homologous transfusions and 2–3 days in heterologous transfusions. Survival of erythrocytes was reduced to 24 and 12 hours in the heterologous group after sequential transfusions. Any bird with a haematocrit of <20% should receive a transfusion.

Fasting
Small birds (bodyweight <200 g) rarely require fasting. In most larger birds, the period from withdrawal of food to reintroduction of food after recovery from anaesthesia should not exceed 3 hours, to avoid the possibility of hypoglycaemia. Waterfowl and carnivorous birds should be fasted for 4–10 hours, depending on size and species. To minimize the risk of regurgitation and aspiration of food material, birds should not be anaesthetized if they have a full crop.

Parasympatholytic premedication
Premedication is generally not required. Atropine may be used at a dose of 0.04–0.1 mg/kg, but is rarely indicated. Although parasympatholytic drugs reduce the quantity of respiratory secretions, they also tend to make the secretions more viscous, which increases the risk of ETT obstruction.

Analgesic	Dose (mg/kg i.m.)
Butorphanol	2
Carprofen	2–4
Ketoprofen	2–4

Figure 27.9: Recommended analgesic agents for use in birds.

ANALGESIA

In the wild, any bird exhibiting weakness or illness is likely to be quickly dispatched by a predator. Birds therefore try to conceal any physical or mental disadvantage for as long as possible, so it rarely becomes evident that a bird is suffering pain. Analgesia is, however, essential in avian surgery, not only on welfare grounds, but also because relief of pain speeds the return to normal food consumption. Animals with high metabolic rates need to feed frequently, so a rapid return to feeding after surgery is vital. Analgesia should provide pre-, intra- and postoperative pain relief. Analgesics are more effective when they are given before the onset of pain.

Some anaesthetic agents have analgesic properties, while others require supplementation. Figure 27.9 shows some analgesics that have been safely and successfully used in birds.

Non-steroidal anti-inflammatory drugs

Flunixin meglumine (0.5 mg/kg i.m.; Heard, 1997) is safe and effective, but may produce gastrointestinal and renal side effects when used for a long time. Carprofen (2–4 mg/kg i.m.) and ketoprofen (2–4 mg/kg i.m.) have been safe and effective in the hands of many clinicians.

Opioids

Paul-Murphy (1997) has shown buprenorphine to be ineffective in psittacine birds, while butorphanol (2 mg/kg i.m. once daily) is safe and effective. Because the majority of the endogenous opioid receptors in birds are stereospecific for κ-agonists, rather than μ-agonists, it is to be expected that κ-agonistic drugs such as butorphanol are more likely to be useful in birds than conventional μ-agonists, such as morphine.

Steroids

Birds are very susceptible to the deleterious side effects of glucocorticoids, and doses should be kept to a minimum. The use of ultra-short-acting steroids such as hydrocortisone sodium succinate (10 mg/kg i.v.) or prednisolone sodium succinate (11–25 mg/kg i.v.) minimizes these risks. If dexamethasone is used, the dose should not exceed 2–4 mg/kg i.v. or i.m. once daily. Glucocorticoid therapy should not exceed 48 hours' duration.

INJECTABLE RESTRAINT AND ANAESTHESIA

Sedation is an undervalued technique for restraint and handling of large wild birds. The clinician must consider not only the ease of examination for him/herself, but also the effect of stress on the unsedated bird. The safest and most effective restraining drug is ketamine (see below). In highly excitable or distressed birds, low doses of diazepam (≥0.5 mg/kg i.m.) are useful.

The choice of anaesthetic agent often depends on availability of drugs and the experience of staff. Although most drugs can be given either by intramuscular or intravenous routes, the intravenous route is more reliable and a lower total dose can be used. The latter route is, however, technically more difficult and probably more stressful. Anaesthesia can be maintained by the intermittent administration of boluses. Intravenous injections

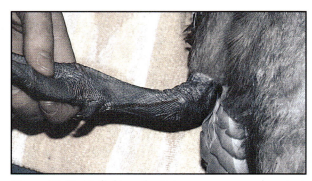

Figure 27.10: Medial tarsal vein in a swan.

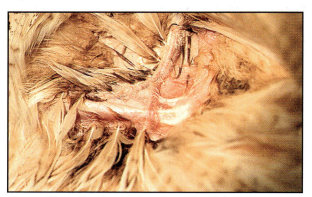

Figure 27.11: Basilic vein in a Peregrine Falcon.

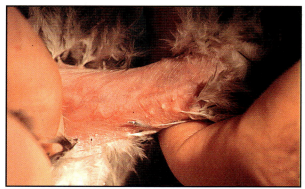

Figure 27.12: Right jugular vein in an African Grey Parrot.

Agent	Dose and route	Duration	Comments
Ketamine	5–30 mg/kg i.v. or i.m.	20–30 minutes	Duration is dose dependent. Recovery can be excessively long (3 hours). Poor muscle relaxation
Ketamine and diazepam	5–20 mg/kg and 1.0–1.5 mg/kg i.v. (slow) or i.m. (use separate syringes)	30 minutes	Good muscle relaxation
Ketamine and midazolam	5–20 mg/kg and 0.2 mg/kg i.v. or i.m. (mix in same syringe)	30 minutes	Good muscle relaxation
Ketamine and xylazine	5 mg/kg and 0.25–0.5 mg/kg i.m. or i.v.	30–45 minutes	Good muscle relaxation. Increased adverse cardiopulmonary effects. Xylazine may be reversed with atipamezole
Ketamine and medetomidine	3–6 mg/kg and 150–350 μg/kg i.m. or i.v.	20 minutes	Rapid reversal with atipamezole. Patient standing 10 minutes after reversal
Tiletamine/ zolazepam	5–10 mg/kg i.m.	30–45 minutes	Prolonged recovery (2–5 hours)
Alphaxalone/ alphadolone	36 mg/kg i.m. or 5–10 mg/kg i.v.	20–30 minutes	Some species show adverse reactions. Large administration volume
Propofol	14 mg/kg i.v.	2–7 minutes	Ultra-short-acting

Figure 27.13: Parenteral anaesthetic agents for use in birds.

may be given via the basilic vein, the right jugular vein or the medial tarsal vein. The most accessible vein varies somewhat with species (Figures 27.10, 27.11 and 27.12).

It is usually advantageous to fix a catheter with sutures in the vein; this facilitates administration of anaesthetics, fluid therapy and emergency treatments (e.g. doxapram and adrenaline).

A summary of commonly used parenteral anaesthetic agents is shown in Figure 27.13.

Although intubation is not required for delivering injectable anaesthetics, it is recommended to minimize the risk of aspiration of crop reflux and to facilitate positive-pressure ventilation to treat respiratory arrest.

Ketamine

Ketamine is a very useful drug in birds, but the dose should be computed carefully if prolonged recovery periods are to be avoided. When given intravenously, the effects of ketamine are dose dependent. Anaesthesia may be prolonged by giving extra doses of 30–50% of the induction dose as needed. Because small birds have high metabolic rates than larger birds, they tend to require larger doses based on bodyweight. Figure 27.14 lists satisfactory initial doses of ketamine for birds of different bodyweight.

Ketamine is ineffective in penguins, gallinules (coots, moorhens etc.), water rail, Golden Pheasant, toucans and hornbills. It requires hepatic biotransfor-

mation and renal excretion. It also causes dose-dependent respiratory and cardiac depression that varies somewhat with species. Recovery from ketamine anaesthesia is characterized by excitation, incoordination, head shaking and wing flapping.

In order to reduce these adverse side effects, ketamine is usually given in combination with diazepam (1.0–1.5 mg/kg), midazolam (0.2 mg/kg), xylazine (0.25–0.5 mg/kg) or medetomidine (0.15–0.35 mg/kg). These combinations provide greater muscle relaxation than ketamine alone and reduce the total dose of ketamine required. This, in turn, reduces the prolonged recovery time that can be a feature of ketamine anaesthesia. The action of all these adjuncts to ketamine anaesthesia may be abbreviated with specific antagonists. The benzodiazepines (diazepam, midazolam) may be reversed with flumazenil, while the α_2-agonists (xylazine and medetomidine) may be reversed with atipamezole.

Bodyweight	Dose (mg/kg)
100–150 g	30
200–400 g	20
750–1000 g	10
>2 kg	5

Figure 27.14: Satisfactory initial doses of ketamine for birds of different bodyweights.

Oesophageal stethoscope

An oesophageal stethoscope is a cheap and effective method of cardiac monitoring, and it may be linked either to ear pieces or to a microphone, amplifier and loudspeaker. An electrocardiogram (ECG) may be obtained by using atraumatic clamps, or disposable stick-on patches applied to the tarsometatarsus and carpal joints. In very small birds, an ECG can be conveniently obtained from a human paediatric cardiac pacing electrode inserted into the oesophagus. The R-wave counter on modern electrocardiographic units allows accurate measurement of the avian heart rate, which is usually too fast for counting by eye or ear. Insufficient depth of anaesthesia is signalled by the heart rate increasing immediately in response to surgical intervention. Ordinarily, heart rate should not fall below 120 beats per minute. Acceptable heart and respiratory rates for birds under anaesthesia are shown in Figure 27.16.

Blood gas analysis

Blood gas analysis is useful and now becoming a more affordable technique.

Pulse oximeters

Pulse oximeters should be used with care: oximeter probes should be placed close to a peripheral artery, because the aim is to detect insufficiency of the peripheral circulation before problems of the central (core) circulation. If a fall in core circulation is awaited, the bird is likely to be in circulatory collapse before anyone is aware of the problem. Some companies have now developed specific unidirectional cloacal probes. A peripheral arteriole should be monitored rather than the aorta or renal artery. Changes in SpO_2 should be considered as a trend rather than an accurate analysis (Schmitt *et al.*, 1998). If pulse oximetry is used with care and a full anatomical knowledge of the circulation, it can be invaluable. Used wrongly by the uninitiated, it will give a false sense of security and tempt a reduction in visual awareness of other indicators.

Capnography

Capnography (see Chapter 5) gives a very accurate indication of the patient's breathing pattern (Cruz *et al.*, 1997), although the relation between end-tidal carbon dioxide and arterial carbon dioxide tension has not been described in birds as it has in mammals.

ANAESTHETIC EMERGENCIES

Apnoea

- Turn off anaesthetic gas
- Increase oxygen flow rate to flush system
- Place bird in sternal recumbency
- Attempt respiratory stimulation by pulling tongue and depressing sternum

Bodyweight	Cardiac rate/minute	Respiratory rate/minute
40–100 g	600–750	55–75
100–200 g	450–600	30–40
250–400 g	300–500	15–35
500–1000 g	180–400	8–25
5–10 kg	60–70	2–20

Figure 27.16: Normal expected heart and respiratory rates in anaesthetized birds.

- IPPV once every 5 seconds
- Administer doxapram 5–7mg/kg i.v. (preferably), sublingually or i.m.
- Administer atipamezole if xylazine or medetomidine has been used in the anaesthetic protocol.

Fortunately there is a significant time lapse between apnoea and cardiac arrest when using isoflurane or sevoflurane (but not halothane). If apnoea is noticed promptly, cardiac arrest should always be avoidable when using isoflurane.

Cardiac arrest

- Turn off anaesthetic gas
- Give rapid external or internal cardiac massage
- Administer adrenaline 0.1–0.2mg/kg i.v.

Tracheal blockage

- Ensure oxygen flow from machine
- Clear pharynx and glottis
- Ensure ETT patency is not compromised
- Apply suction or remove ETT
- Place abdominal air sac breathing tube (if required).

Haemorrhage

- Increase rate of fluid administration, especially colloidal solutions
- Apply haemostasis
- Administer homologous (preferably) or heterologous blood transfusion intravenously or intraosseously.

POSTOPERATIVE PERIOD

In view of their high metabolic rates, it is very important that birds recover from anaesthesia quickly and eat soon after recovery. Birds weighing under 100 g should eat within 30 minutes of recovery, and if they do not they should be crop fed. All birds should recover in a warm environment, preferably 24–26°C. A darkened environment, away from excessive noise, will also improve quality of recovery.

Self-inflicted injuries during recovery may be minimized by wrapping the bird in a cloth or towel. Once the bird is awake enough to crawl out from the towel, it is usually conscious enough to stand without traumatizing itself.

REFERENCES AND FURTHER READING

Beynon PH, Forbes NA and Harcourt-Brown NB (eds) (1996) *Manual of Raptors, Pigeons and Waterfowl*. BSAVA, Cheltenham

Beynon PH, Forbes NA and Lawton M (eds) (1996) *Manual of Psittacine Birds*. BSAVA, Cheltenham

Coles BH (1985) *Avian Medicine and Surgery*. Blackwell Scientific, Oxford

Cooper JE and Frank LG (1973) Use of the steroid anaesthetic CT1341 in birds. *Veterinary Record* **92,** 474–479

Cooper JE and Redig PT (1975) Unexpected reactions to the use of CT1341 by red-tailed hawks. *Veterinary Record* **97,** 352

Cornick-Seahorn JL (1996) Anesthesiology of ratites. In: *Ratite Management, Medicine and Surgery*. pp. 79–94. Krieger, Florida

Cruz JI, Lopez J and Falceto V (1997) Capnography for anaesthetic monitoring in birds. In: *Proceedings of the European Association of Avian Vets Conference*. pp. 38–41. Association of Avian Vets, Florida

Curro TG (1998) Anaesthesia of pet birds. *Seminars in Avian and Exotic Pet Medicine* **7,** 10–21

Degernes LA, Crosier M, Harrison LD, Whitt Smith D, Dennis P and Gebhard D (1997) Investigation of homologous and heterologous avian blood transfusions. In: *Proceedings of the Association of Avian Vets Conference*. pp. 277–278. Association of Avian Vets, Florida

Fedde MR (1986) Respiration. In: *Avian Physiology, 4th edn*, ed. PD Sturkie, p. 191. Springer-Verlag, New York

Fedde MR (1993) Structure and function of the avian respiratory system. In: *Core Topics*. Association of Avian Vets Annual Conference, Florida

Forbes NA and Altman RB (1998) *Self Assessment in Avian Medicine and Surgery*. Manson, London

Frank LG and Cooper JE (1974) Further notes on the use of CT1341 in birds of prey. *Raptor Research* **8,** 29–32

Heard DJ (1997) Anaesthesia and analgesia. In: *Avian Medicine and Surgery*, ed. RB Altman, SL Clubb, GM Dorrestein and K Quesenberry, pp. 807–828. WB Saunders, Philadelphia

James AE, Hutchings G, Bush M, Natarajan TK and Burns B (1976) How birds breathe: correlation of radiographic with anatomical and pathological studies. *Journal of the American Radiological Society* **17,** 17

Korbel R (1998) Ophthalmoscopy in raptors. In: *Raptor Biomedicine II*, ed. Lumeij JT *et al.* Proceedings of the International Raptor Biomedical Conference, South Africa. August 9–11, 1998

Kreeger TJ, Degernes LA, Kreeger JS and Redig PT (1993) Immobilisation of raptors with tiletamine and zolazepam (Telazol). In: *Raptor Biomedicine*, ed. PT Redig, JE Cooper, JD Remple, DB Hunter and T Hahn. Minnesota University Press, Minneapolis

Ludders JW and Matthews N (1996) Birds. In: *Lumb and Jones' Veterinary Anesthesia, 3rd edn*, ed. JC Thurmon, WJ Tranquilli and GJ Benson, pp. 645–669. Williams and Wilkins, Baltimore

Paul-Murphy J (1997) Evaluation of analgesic properties of butorphanol and buprenorphine for the psittacine bird. In: *Proceedings of the Association of Avian Vets Annual Conference*. Association of Avian Vets, Florida

Samour JH, Jones DM, Knight JA and Howlett JC (1984) Comparative studies of the use some injectable anaesthetic agents in birds. *Veterinary Record* **115,** 6–11

Schmitt PM, Göbel T and Trautvetter E (1998) Evaluation of pulse oximetry as a monitoring method in avian anaesthesia. *Journal of Avian Medicine and Surgery* **12,** 91–100

Seaman GC, Ludders JW, Erb HN and Gleed RD (1994) Effects of low and high fractions of inspired oxygen on ventilation in ducks anesthetised with isoflurane. *American Journal of Veterinary Research* **55,** 395–398

Sinn LC (1994) Anesthesiology in Avian Medicine: Applications and Applications, ed. BW Ritchie, GW Harrison and LR Harrison, p. 1066. Wingers, Florida

Wheler C (1993) Avian anaesthetics, analgesics and tranquillisers. *Seminars in Avian and Exotic Pet Medicine* **2,** 17. WB Saunders, Philadelphia

Zenker W, Janovsky M, Kurzweil J and Ruf T (In Press) Immobilisation of the common buzzard (*Buteo buteo*) with oral tiletamine/zolazepam. In: *Raptor Biomedicine II*, ed. Lumeij JT *et al.* Proceedings of the International Raptor Biomedical Conference, South Africa. August 9–11, 1998

Animal (bodyweight)	Subcutaneous administration (ml)	Intraperitoneal administration (ml)
Mouse (30 g)	1–2	2
Hamster (100 g)	3	3
Gerbil (60 g)	1–2	2–3
Rat (200 g)	5	5
Guinea pig (1 kg)	10–20	20
Chinchilla (400–600 g)	10–20	20
Ferret (800 g female; 1500 g male)	10–20	20–30
Rabbit (3 kg)	30–50	50

Figure 28.2: Volumes and routes of fluid for routine administration in small mammals. Bodyweights are approximate.

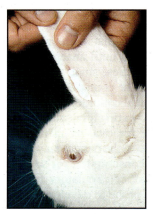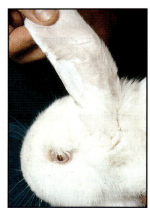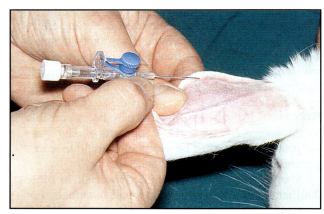

Figure 28.3: EMLA (Eutectic Mixture of Local Anaesthetics) cream can be applied to the ear vein or central ear artery to allow pain-free catheterization. The cream is applied quite thickly (left), covered in a waterproof dressing (e.g. clingfilm) (centre) and then protected with an adhesive bandage. (Right) After 45–60 minutes, the dressing and cream are removed and venepuncture carried out.

tion, subcutaneous administration of fluids may be ineffective until peripheral circulatory function is improved. Intravenous fluid therapy presents no particular difficulties in rabbits and ferrets, although the small size of the peripheral veins in dwarf rabbit breeds can present technical difficulties, as can the animal's tendency to flinch when venepuncture is attempted. Flinching can be overcome by applying a local anaesthetic cream over the marginal ear vein (Figure 28.3). After 45–60 minutes, full skin thickness anaesthesia is produced, enabling pain-free (and hence movement-free) venepuncture. In smaller mammals such as mice and hamsters, intravenous injection is difficult although placement of a 24 gauge over-the-needle catheter in the rat's lateral tail vein (Figure 28.4) is practicable. Guidelines for volumes and rates of replacement are no different from those in the dog and cat (see Chapter 11).

As an adjunct or alternative to parenteral fluid therapy, oral rehydration therapy should be considered, especially in rabbits and rats. It is not necessary to withhold food and water for prolonged periods from rodents and rabbits, as these species do not vomit. Removing water 1 hour before induction is sufficient. Food should be withheld from ferrets for 8–12 hours before induction, to minimize the risk of vomiting.

CHOICE OF ANAESTHETIC

After evaluation and stabilization of the patient, if required, an anaesthetic regimen can be selected. The majority of injectable and inhalational agents available for use in the dog and cat can be used in small mammals, but practical constraints such as the difficulties of intravenous injection may limit the use of some agents (e.g. propofol). Local anaesthesia is of less value in small mammals than in dogs and cats because of the difficulties of physical restraint – unlike dogs, few rodents can be persuaded by their owners to remain immobile while procedures such as skin suturing are carried out. However, use of local anaesthetic techniques to provide additional analgesia in conjunction with low doses of injectable anaesthetics or low concentrations of inhalants can be valuable.

The difficulty of giving anaesthetics by the intravenous route in small mammals has some important practical implications. When anaesthetics are given intravenously, the dose can generally be adjusted to provide the desired effect in a particular individual. Allowance can easily be made for individual and breed or strain variation, and over- or underdosing is easy to avoid. When giving anaesthetics by the intramuscular, intraperitoneal or subcutaneous routes, a calculated

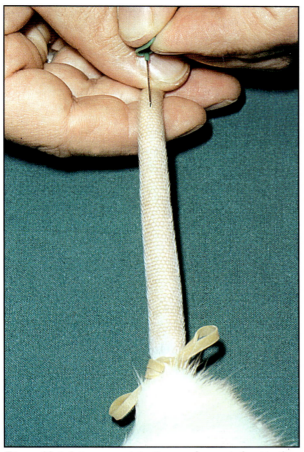

Figure 28.4: Intravenous injection can be carried out in the rat via the lateral tail veins. These vessels can also be catheterized percutaneously for fluid therapy using a 24 gauge over-the-needle catheter. An elastic band can be used as a tourniquet to dilate the vein and aid needle placement, then released before injection.

dose is given, and there is no opportunity to adjust it to the individual's requirements. Large variations in response (up to 150% difference in sleep times) related to genetic background, age and sex have all been documented in small rodents (Flecknell, 1996). For this reason it is advisable to select an anaesthetic regimen with a wide safety margin and, if possible, one that is completely or partially reversible.

A second consequence of administration by these routes is that relatively large doses of drug are given and recovery times tend to be prolonged. In small mammals this is undesirable because of the risks of hypothermia during recovery, the problems associated with prolonged respiratory depression and the potential metabolic effects of several hours unconsciousness or sedation. Once again, then, use of a reversible anaesthetic regimen can be advantageous.

Many of these problems can of course be overcome by using inhalational anaesthetics, and in many instances these are the agents of choice in small rodents.

INJECTABLE ANAESTHETICS

A number of commonly used anaesthetic regimens are described briefly below. If injectable, rather than inhalational, agents are to be used, the author's preference is to give either fentanyl/fluanisone and midazolam, or ketamine/medetomidine in rodents and rabbits, and ketamine/medetomidine or propofol in ferrets. Where possible, the anaesthetic regimen is partially reversed with the appropriate antagonist.

Dose rates for individual species are given in Figures 28.5 and 28.6. Most anaesthetic combinations are

Drug	Mouse	Hamster	Gerbil	Rat	Guinea pig	Chinchilla	Ferret	Rabbit
Acepromazine	2.5 mg/kg i.m.	2.5 mg/kg i.m.	2.5 mg/kg i.m.	2.5 mg/kg i.m.	2.5 mg/kg i.m.	0.5 mg/kg i.m.	0.2 mg/kg i.m. or s.c.	0.5 mg/kg i.m.
Atropine	40 µg/kg s.c. or i.m.	40 µg/kg s.c. or i.m.	40 µg/kg s.c. or i.m.	40 µg/kg s.c. or i.m.	50 µg/kg s.c. or i.m.	-	0.05 mg/kg s.c. or i.m.	40 µg/kg s.c. or i.m.*
Diazepam	5 mg/kg i.m. or i.p.	5 mg/kg i.m. or i.p.	5 mg/kg i.m. or i.p.	2.5 mg/kg i.m. or i.p.	2.5 mg/kg i.m. or i.p.	5 mg/kg i.p.	2 mg/kg i.m.	1-2 mg/kg i.m. or i.p.
Fentanyl/fluanisone 'Hypnorm'	0.5 ml/kg i.m. or i.p.	0.5 ml/kg i.m. or i.p.	0.5 ml/kg i.m. or i.p.	0.5 ml/kg i.m. or i.p.	0.5 ml/kg i.m.	-	0.5 ml/kg i.m.	0.5 ml/kg i.m.
Medetomidine	30-100 µg/kg s.c.	100 µg/kg s.c. or i.p.	100-200 µg/kg i.p.	30-100 µg/kg s.c. or i.p.	-	-	0.1 mg/kg s.c.	0.5 mg/kg i.m. or s.c.
Midazolam	5 mg/kg i.m. or i.p.	5 mg/kg i.m. or i.p.	5 mg/kg i.m. or i.p.	5 mg/kg i.p.	5 mg/kg i.m. or i.p.	-	1 mg/kg i.m.	2 mg/kg i.v., i.m. or i.p.
Xylazine	5-10 mg/kg i.p.	5 mg/kg i.m.	2 mg/kg i.m.	1-5 mg/kg i.m. or i.p.	-	-	1 mg/kg i.m. or s.c.	5 mg/kg i.m.

Figure 28.5: Suggested doses of preanaesthetic and other drugs for use in small mammals. Note that considerable individual variation in response can occur.

* Many rabbits have high levels of atropinase, and a more reliable anticholinergic effect is provided by glycopyrrolate 0.1 mg/kg s.c. or 0.01 mg/kg i.v.

Drug	Mouse	Hamster	Gerbil	Rat	Guinea pig	Chinchilla	Ferret	Rabbit
Alphaxalone/alphadolone	10–15 mg/kg i.v.	150 mg/kg i.p.	80–120 mg/kg i.p.	10–12 mg/kg i.v.	40 mg/kg i.p.	–	8–12 mg/kg i.v. 12–15 i.m.	6–9 mg/kg i.v.
Effect	zz	z	z	zz	z	–	z	z
Fentanyl/fluanisone + diazepam	0.4 ml/kg i.p. + 5 mg/kg i.p.	1 mg/kg i.m. or i.p. + 5 mg/kg i.p.	0.3 ml/kg i.m. or i.p. + 5 mg/kg i.p.	0.6 ml/kg + 2.5 mg/kg i.p.	1 ml/kg i.m. or i.p. + 2.5 mg/kg i.p.	–	–	0.3 ml/kg i.m. + 1–2 mg/kg i.m., i.v., i.p.
Effect	zz	zz	zz	zz	zz	–	–	zz
Fentanyl/fluanisone + midazolam	10.0 ml/kg i.p.	4.0 ml/kg i.p.	8.0 ml/kg i.p.	2.7 ml/kg i.p.	8.0 ml/kg i.p.	–	–	0.3 ml/kg i.m. + 1–2 mg/kg i.p. or i.v.
Effect	zz	zz	zz	zz	zz	–	–	zz
Ketamine/acepromazine	100 mg/kg + 5 mg/kg i.p.	150 mg/kg + 5 mg/kg i.p.	75 mg/kg + 3 mg/kg i.p.	75 mg/kg + 2.5 mg/kg i.p.	125 mg/kg + 5 mg/kg i.m.	40 mg/kg + 0.5 mg/kg i.m.	–	50 mg/kg i.m. + 1 mg/kg i.m.
Effect	z	z	z	z	z	zz	–	zz
Ketamine/diazepam	100 mg/kg + 5 mg/kg i.p.	70 mg/kg + 2 mg/kg i.p.	50 mg/kg + 5 mg/kg i.p.	75 mg/kg + 5 mg/kg i.p.	100 mg/kg + 5 mg/kg i.m.	20 mg/kg + 5 mg/kg i.p.	25 mg/kg i.m. + 2 mg/kg i.m.	25 mg/kg i.m. + 5 mg/kg i.m.
Effect	z	z	z	z	z	z	zz	zz
Ketamine/medetomidine	75 mg/kg + 1.0 mg/kg i.p.	100 mg/kg + 250 µg/kg i.p.	75 mg/kg + 0.5 mg/kg i.p.	75 mg/kg + 0.5 mg/kg i.p.	40 mg/kg + 0.5 mg/kg i.p.	–	8 mg/kg i.m. + 0.1 mg/kg i.m.	25 mg/kg i.m. + 0.5 mg/kg i.m.
Effect	zz	zz	zz	zz	z	–	zz	zz
Ketamine/xylazine	80–100 mg/kg + 10 mg/kg i.p.	200 mg/kg + 10 mg/kg i.p.	50 mg/kg + 2 mg/kg i.p.	75–100 mg/kg + 10 mg/kg i.p.	40 mg/kg + 5 mg/kg i.p.		25 mg/kg i.m. + 1–2 mg/kg i.m.	35 mg/kg i.m. + 5 mg/kg i.m.
Effect	z!	z!	z!	z!	zz!	zz	zz	zz
Pentobarbitone	40–50 mg/kg i.p.	50–90 mg/kg i.p.	60–80 mg/kg i.p.	40–50 mg/kg i.p.	37 mg/kg i.p.	40 mg/kg i.p.	25–30 mg/kg i.v. or 36 mg/kg i.p.	30–45 mg/kg i.v.
Effect	z!	z!	z!	z!	zz!	z!	zz!	z!
Propofol	26 mg/kg i.v.	–	–	10 mg/kg i.v.	–	–	–	10 mg/kg i.v.
Effect	zz	–	–	zz	–	–	–	z

Figure 28.6: Suggested doses of anaesthetic agents for use in small mammals. Note that considerable individual variation in response can occur.

z, light anaesthesia; zz, surgical anaesthesia; !, narrow safety margin.

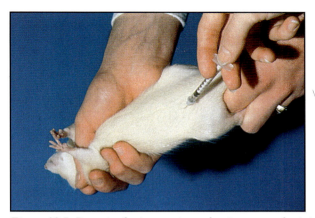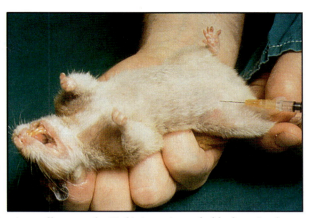

Figure 28.7: *Restraint for intraperitoneal or intramuscular injection in small mammals. (Left) An assistant holds the animal around the shoulders, with a thumb positioned under the patient's mandible. (Right) In mice and hamsters, the animal is simply restrained by the scruff.*

given as a single injection by the intramuscular or intraperitoneal route. Intraperitoneal injection is a relatively simple procedure in small mammals and the same general approach is adopted in all species. It is easier if an assistant restrains the animal (Figure 28.7), and the anaesthetist can then extend one hind limb and inject into the middle of the right posterior quadrant of the abdomen. This minimizes the risk of inadvertent puncture of the bladder, which lies in the midline just anterior to the pelvic brim. Injecting into the right side of the abdomen also avoids the caecum, which is large and thin walled in all rodents, and so may reduce the risk of injecting into the gastrointestinal tract. Intramuscular injections can be made into the quadriceps, with the animal restrained by an assistant in a similar manner. The anaesthetist immobilizes the limb and the muscle and injects into the middle of the muscle mass. Subcutaneous injections are made into the scruff.

In rabbits, it is often advantageous to give preanaesthetic medication by the intramuscular or subcutaneous route and to follow this with an intravenous induction agent or an inhalational agent. For example, administration of fentanyl/fluanisone produces analgesia and peripheral vasodilation, together with sedation. It is then relatively simple to place an intravenous catheter into an ear vein and induce surgical anaesthesia with midazolam or diazepam, injected intravenously, 'to effect.'

Neuroleptanalgesic combinations

When used alone, fentanyl/fluanisone produces sedation and sufficient analgesia for superficial surgery in most small mammals (see Figure 28.5). The degree of muscle relaxation is generally poor and the high doses needed for more major surgery produce marked respiratory depression. Combining this regimen with a benzodiazepine (midazolam or diazepam) produces surgical anaesthesia with only moderate respiratory depression. The combination has the advantage that it can be partially reversed with a mixed opioid agonist/antagonist such as butorphanol or a partial agonist such

as buprenorphine (Figure 28.8). This reverses the respiratory depression caused by the fentanyl, but maintains postoperative analgesia. The benzodiazepine antagonist flumazenil can be used to further speed recovery, but repeated doses are needed to avoid resedation. The dose needed depends upon the dose of benzodiazepine used.

In small rodents, a mixture of midazolam and fentanyl/fluanisone can be given as a single intraperitoneal injection. In rabbits it is preferable to give the latter agent first, by intramuscular injection. The midazolam or diazepam can then be given intravenously to effect as described above.

Other neuroleptanalgesics

Etorphine/methotrimeprazine can be used alone and in combination with midazolam in rats, and produces longer periods of anaesthesia, with similar effects to fentanyl/fluanisone or fentanyl/fluanisone/midazolam. In other species, the combination produces more severe respiratory depression and its use is not recommended.

When used alone, fentanyl/droperidol produces effects similar to fentanyl/fluanisone, but with a greater tendency to produce limb rigidity. In combination with midazolam its effects are unpredictable, and it is best used alone to provide immobility, sedation and analgesia for minor procedures.

Ketamine

When used alone, ketamine produces immobility but little analgesia in small rodents. Its effects are greater in rabbits, but the degree of analgesia is insufficient for any surgical procedure. In the ferret, immobilization and a degree of analgesia sufficient for superficial minor surgery is produced, but ketamine is best given in combination with other agents.

When combined with acepromazine, midazolam or diazepam, ketamine produces light to moderate surgical anaesthesia in ferrets, rabbits and chinchillas. In small rodents the effects of these combinations are less predictable and usually only light planes of anaesthe-

Analgesic	Mouse	Hamster	Gerbil	Rat	Guinea pig	Chinchilla	Ferret	Rabbit
Buprenorphine	0.1 mg/kg s.c.	0.1 mg/kg s.c.	0.1 mg/kg s.c.	0.05 mg/kg s.c.	0.05 mg/kg s.c.	??0.05 mg/kg s.c. 8-12 hours	0.01-0.03 mg/kg i.m., i.v. or s.c. 8-12 hours	0.01-0.05 mg/kg s.c.
Butorphanol	1-5 mg/kg s.c.	?	?	2 mg/kg s.c.	2 mg/kg s.c.	??2 mg/kg s.c. 4 hours	0.4 mg/kg i.m. 4-6 hours	0.1-0.5 mg/kg s.c.
Carprofen	?	?	?	5 mg/kg bid	?	?	?4 mg/kg s.c.	1.5 mg/kg orally bid ?1-3 mg/kg s.c.
Flunixin	2.5 mg/kg s.c. bid	?	?	2.5 mg/kg s.c. bid	?	?	0.5-2 mg/kg s.c. bid or uid	1.1 mg/kg s.c. bid
Ketoprofen	?	?	?	5 mg/kg i.m.	?	?	?1 mg/kg s.c.	3 mg/kg i.m.
Nalbuphine	4-8 mg/kg s.c.	?	?	1-2 mg/kg i.v.	?	?	–	1-2 mg/kg i.v.

Figure 28.8: *Suggested doses of analgesic agents for use in small mammals.*

sia, insufficient even for minor surgery, are produced. In contrast, administration of ketamine in combination with medetomidine or xylazine results in surgical anaesthesia in most small mammals. Its effects are slightly less uniform in guinea pigs, and some individuals may not become sufficiently deeply anaesthetized for major surgery. In these circumstances, it is preferable to deepen anaesthesia using an inhalational agent, or to provide additional analgesia using local anaesthetic drugs. Since ketamine alone has limited effects in small mammals, reversal of medetomidine or xylazine with atipamezole greatly speeds recovery. Since ketamine seems to have limited analgesic effects in small mammals, if atipamezole is used after surgery, then an analgesic should be given to provide postoperative pain relief (see below).

Barbiturates

Pentobarbitone has been used for many years to produce anaesthesia in small rodents and rabbits. It has a narrow margin of safety, the anaesthetic dose being close to the lethal dose in many animals. It is best used in low doses to provide light planes of anaesthesia, with inhalational agents used to deepen anaesthesia if required. In the rabbit, even careful administration of a diluted solution (6 mg/ml) is hazardous, and respiratory arrest may occur before surgical planes of anaesthesia are attained.

Thiopentone, methohexitone and thiamylal can all be used to produce short periods of anaesthesia when given intravenously. In rabbits and ferrets this can be useful both for short surgical procedures, and to allow intubation followed by maintenance with volatile agents.

Propofol

When given intravenously, propofol produces short periods of surgical anaesthesia in rodents and ferrets, and additional doses can be given to prolong the period of anaesthesia without unduly prolonging recovery. In rabbits, it can provide sufficient depth of anaesthesia for intubation, but respiratory arrest usually occurs before the onset of surgical anaesthesia.

Alphaxalone/Alphadolone

In rabbits, effects similar to those of propofol result after intravenous injection with alphaxalone/alphadolone, with respiratory arrest occurring before surgical anaesthesia is attained. Sufficient depth of anaesthesia for intubation can be produced. In small rodents, intravenous administration produces surgical anaesthesia, which can be prolonged with additional doses. It has been recommended for intramuscular injection in guinea pigs, but the high dose required to produce anaesthesia requires administration of large volumes of drug (3.3 ml for an animal weighing 1000 g). In ferrets, surgical anaesthesia is produced when the drug is given intravenously, and anaesthesia can be prolonged by administration of additional doses.

INHALATIONAL AGENTS

Halothane, isoflurane and methoxyflurane can all be used to produce safe and effective anaesthesia in small rodents and ferrets. Induction can be via a face mask, but it is often easier and may be less stressful

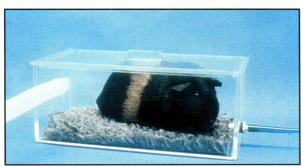

Figure 28.9: Induction of anaesthesia in the guinea pig using an anaesthetic chamber. Note that the gas is ducted in at the bottom of the chamber and excess gas removed from the top.

to use an anaesthetic induction chamber, filled from an anaesthetic machine using a calibrated vaporizer (see Chapter 4). These can be purchased commercially or can be constructed from clear plastic containers. It is important to fill the chamber from the bottom and to remove waste anaesthetic gas from the top (Figure 28.9), as the anaesthetic vapour is denser than air. Removal of gas from the bottom of the chamber can significantly increase the time taken to achieve an appropriate concentration for induction of anaesthesia (4% halothane, 5% isoflurane). Once the animal has become anaesthetized it can be removed from the chamber and very brief procedures (<1 minute) can be carried out. Anaesthesia can easily be maintained using a face mask (1.5–2.5% halothane, 1.5–2.5% isoflurane). Induction of anaesthesia is rapid in these small mammals, typically being complete in 2–3 minutes. Recovery is also rapid – rodents recover their righting reflex in 5–10 minutes after 30 minutes anaesthesia and have regained their co-ordination in a further 10 minutes.

Old-style anaesthetic chambers, in which liquid anaesthetic is placed on a cotton wool or gauze pad, must not be used with halothane or isoflurane as dangerously high concentrations (>20%) of anaesthetic vapour are produced.

In the rabbit, exposure to halothane or isoflurane is associated with breath holding, which may be prolonged (>2 minutes). Animals may struggle violently during induction and seem to resent the procedure. When placed in an anaesthetic chamber, they attempt to avoid inhaling the vapour. If mask induction is to be used, the mask should be briefly removed if apnoea occurs and replaced when the animal breathes. Alternatively, a sedative or tranquillizer can be given. Although this prevents struggling, breath holding may still occur, and the mask may need to be temporarily removed. Administration of oxygen is not associated with breath holding, and it is advisable to allow the animal to breath 100% oxygen for 1–2 minutes before adding halothane or isoflurane, to minimize the risk of hypoxia. It is generally preferable to induce anaesthesia with an injectable agent, intubate the rabbit, then maintain with a volatile agent.

INTRAOPERATIVE CARE AND ANAESTHETIC MONITORING

Whichever anaesthetic regimen is chosen, careful monitoring of the patient is important to allow early detection and correction of any problems that may arise. As with other species, respiratory and cardiovascular function are of primary importance, but in small rodents in particular, maintenance of body temperature is critical. It is also important to remain aware of the small size of these animals. Traction during surgery, placing instruments across the animal's chest, or steadying the surgeon's hand on the animal can seriously compromise respiratory movements, and must be avoided. Loss of small volumes of blood are of great significance. For example the total blood volume of a mouse is only 2–3 ml (70 ml/kg).

Monitoring and maintenance of body temperature is of particular importance. Small mammals have a higher surface area to bodyweight ratio than larger species such as the cat and the dog, and so lose heat more rapidly. Most anaesthetics depress thermoregulation, and this effect, coupled with use of cold fluids, shaving and preparation of the surgical site and use of cold anaesthetic gases can rapidly result in severe hypothermia. Small mammals should be placed on a heating pad (Figure 28.10) and, if necessary, covered in insulating material (e.g. bubble packing or aluminium foil). Body temperature should be monitored and, although this is difficult without specialist equipment in mice, suitable inexpensive thermometers for larger rodents can be obtained easily (Figure 28.10).

Respiratory function
Respiratory rate can be monitored relatively easily in animals weighing more than 200 g – the tidal volume of smaller animals is usually insufficient to trigger the thermistor sensors used in most respiratory monitors. A better indication of respiratory function can be

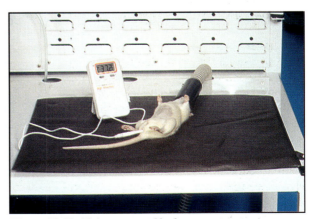

Figure 28.10: Maintenance of body temperature using a heating pad, and monitoring using an inexpensive electronic thermometer. The thermometer has upper and lower temperature alarms and, although not as accurate as more expensive devices, is usually adequate for detecting changes in body temperature during anaesthesia.

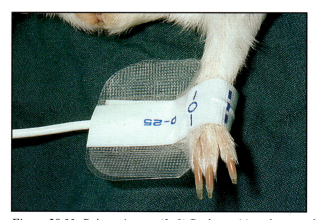
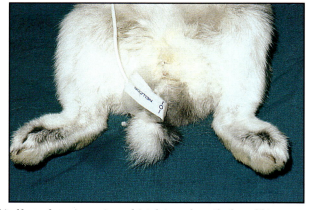

Figure 28.11: Pulse oximetry. (Left) Probe positioned across the hindfoot of a guinea pig and (right) on the tail of a rabbit.

gained by using a pulse oximeter (see Chapter 5). These generally work well in animals weighing more than 200 g. Probes can be placed on the feet of rats and guinea pigs and across the tail in rabbits (Figure 28.11), or on the tongue or toe pad in rabbits and ferrets. The probes generally function well, but in smaller animals they are particularly susceptible to signal loss caused by peripheral vasoconstriction. This is a common problem when anaesthesia is produced using ketamine/ medetomidine or ketamine/xylazine. Many instruments designed for use in man will have an upper heart rate limit of 250 beats per minute. This is frequently exceeded in many small mammals. Some instruments will continue to register an accurate oxygen saturation, but others may fail at high heart rates. If possible, it is helpful to assess an instrument before purchase, and in many instances instruments designed for veterinary use are to be preferred. Several of these have upper heart rate limits of 300–350 beats per minute or greater, and so can be used to their full potential with small mammals.

If respiratory depression occurs, as in large species, it can be treated by assisted ventilation and use of respiratory stimulants such as doxapram (5–10 mg/kg i.m., i.v. or i.p.). It is advisable to give oxygen immediately after induction of anaesthesia with injectable anaesthetics, since all of the agents used produce some degree of respiratory depression. In many instances severe hypoxia occurs, and if uncorrected this can lead to cardiac failure. A particular problem with small mammals is the difficulty of endotracheal intubation. Assisting ventilation by manually compressing the thorax, and providing oxygen by face mask, can be effective, but attempts to ventilate the lungs using a face mask are often relatively ineffective. In small rodents such as the rat, ventilation can be assisted temporarily by positioning the animal with its head and neck in extension and placing the barrel of a plastic syringe over the nose (Figure 28.12). Gently blowing down the tube will usually enable the lungs to be inflated. It is preferable to intubate rabbits, and this can be achieved relatively easily. Three approaches have been described and all can be used successfully. One option is to purchase suitable laryngoscope blades (Wisconsin size 0 (for animals weighing 2–3 kg) and 1 (3–5 kg)) and to intubate under direct vision. This is made easier if an introducer is used to straighten the ETT and guide it into the larynx. A similar technique can be employed using an otoscope to visualize the larynx (Figure 28.13). An introducer is passed down the speculum into the trachea, the otoscope is removed and the ETT is passed over the introducer and into the

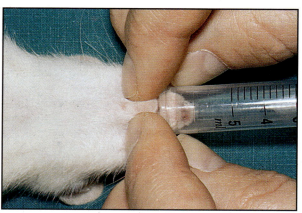

Figure 28.12: Assisting respiration in the rat by blowing gently down the barrel of a 5 ml syringe (a 2 ml syringe is a suitable size for mice and hamsters).

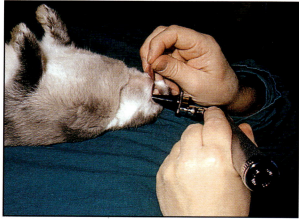

Figure 28.13: Intubation of the rabbit, using an otoscope to visualize the larynx.

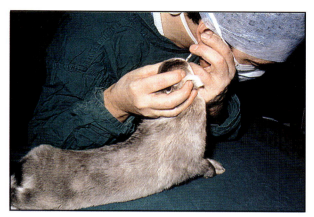

Figure 28.14: *Intubation in the rabbit using a 'blind' technique.*

trachea. The introducer is then removed and the tube tied in place. Either a specially designed introducer can be purchased or a bitch or cat urinary catheter, with the luer fitting removed (so that it can fit through an otoscope speculum), can be used. Endotracheal tube outer diameters (OD) should be 3–5 mm for large rabbits (>2.0 kg). Smaller rabbits require an ETT of ≤2.5 mm OD. Very small rabbits need purpose-designed tubes or home-made tubes manufactured from suitable tubing. An alternative intubation technique requires no special equipment. The rabbit is held with its head and neck extended (Figure 28.14) and the tube advanced slowly down the pharynx. The anaesthetist listens at the end of the tube for breath sounds, which gradually increase in volume as the tube tip approaches the larynx. If the tube enters the larynx, the animal will often give a soft cough and the breath sounds will continue to be heard. Placement in the oesophagus results in loss of breath sounds. If this occurs, the tube can be withdrawn and advanced again. This technique is surprisingly simple to master, but when used with small rabbits (<2 kg), it may be difficult to detect breath sounds. Although a modified stethoscope can be used to assist placement, with practice an operator can detect differences in resistance to tube passage that indicate successful placement. To confirm successful placement, condensation of breath on a cold surface or movement of a few rabbit hairs placed at the end of the tube, can be observed. Whichever method of intubation is used, it is recommended that the rabbit is allowed to breath 100% oxygen for 1–2 minutes before carrying out the procedure.

Cardiovascular function

Pulse oximetry will provide some indication of cardiovascular function, and cardiac function can also be monitored using a suitable electrocardiograph. As with pulse oximetry, an instrument capable of detecting low signal strengths and high frequencies is needed. Clinical assessment of circulatory function can be made using capillary refill time, but palpation of peripheral pulses is not practicable except in large rabbits.

Techniques for supporting the circulation or treating cardiac arrest are similar to those described in large animals (see Chapter 24). One practical problem is the difficulty of venous access and the small quantities of drug required. When the anaesthetist is more familiar with animals weighing more than 2 kg, calculation of the dose required for a rat weighing 200 g can easily lead to errors. It is helpful to keep a card stored with the emergency drugs, listing doses as dose/100 g, dose/kg and dose/20 kg, so that the correct quantity of drug can be calculated accurately and rapidly. Once venous access has been established, fluid therapy can be provided using the same general principles applied to larger species.

POSTOPERATIVE CARE

Providing continued monitoring and support in the postoperative period can be of critical importance in small mammals. A suitable recovery area should be established as part of the preoperative preparations, so that it can be stabilized at an appropriate temperature. Small mammals will continue to be susceptible to hypothermia until they regain normal activity, so initially a temperature of approximately 35°C should be maintained. This can be lowered to 26–28°C as the animal recovers consciousness. Animals should be provided with warm, comfortable bedding. Sawdust is not suitable. A layer of specialized bedding should be provided for the initial recovery period, and once the animal has regained activity it can be transferred to a cage or pen containing either shredded paper (for small rodents and ferrets) or good quality hay or straw (rabbits and guinea pigs). This type of bedding allows the animal to surround itself with insulating material, which provides both warmth and a sense of security.

Animals should be provided with water, but care must be taken that they do not spill water bowls because if the animal becomes wet it will lose heat rapidly. Small rodents are usually accustomed to using water bottles, so this is rarely a problem, but it can present difficulties with rabbits, guinea pigs and ferrets. With all species it is usually advisable to give warmed (37°C) subcutaneous or intraperitoneal dextrose/saline at the end of surgery to provide some fluid supplementation in the immediate postoperative period.

Animals should be encouraged to eat as soon as possible after recovery from anaesthesia. Rats and mice may prefer a softened diet and other species should be given their preferred foods.

It is particularly important that good postoperative analgesia is provided for small rodents, since pain can cause inappetence and prolong the adverse effects of surgery. The analgesics available for use in other companion animal species can be given safely to small mammals, and suggested dose rates are given in Figure

isoflurane
    birds 291
    cerebral vasodilation 233
    haemodynamic effects 164
    liver effects 204
    minimum alveolar concentration (MAC) 102
    physicochemical properties 100
isoprenaline, preoperative, in heart failure 159
isopropamide, preoperative, in heart failure 159

Jackson-Rees modification of Ayre's T-piece 33
    advantages/disadvantages 33
    gas flow rate 33

ketamine 67, 84, 91–3
    birds
        bodyweight, dosage rates 289
        combinations 289–90
    cat/dog sedation 92–3
    caution 208
    in chest trauma 188
    contraindications 212
    and diazepam 240, 241
    haemodynamic effects 164
    induction of anaesthesia 201
    and medetomidine (cats only) 82
    and midazolam, in caesarian section 218, 221
    and NSAIDS administration 68
    paediatric patients 249
    and propofol, paediatric patients 250
    rabbits, rodents, ferrets 298, 299–300
    reptiles 276, 278
ketoprofen 65, 215
    birds 288
    cat 65
    dog 66
    rabbits, rodents, ferrets 300
    reptiles 277

Lack non-rebreathing system 31–2, 32
    advantages/disadvantages 31–2
    gas flow 31
    parallel 32
lactated Ringer's 121, 237
laparoscopy and laparoscopic surgery 203–4
laryngoscopes 39–40
legal aspects (UK) 4–5
    consent 5
    duty of care 5
    negligence 5
lignocaine
    bolus injections 259
    in caesarian section 218
    CPR 262
    dogs 242
    preoperative, in heart failure 159
    rapid haemodynamic control 160
liver
    hepatic circulation 204–6
    hepatic effects, inhalant anaesthetics 104
    hepatic encephalopathy 204, 206
    paediatric patients 248
    volatile anaesthesia effects 204
liver biopsy, anaesthesia for ultrasound imaging 206
liver disease 12
liver dysfunction 161
liver surgery
    diaphragmatic hernia 188–9
    induction of anaesthesia 205–6
    intravenous fluids 205–6
    premedication 205
lizards, injection sites 274
local anaesthesia 4
local analgesic administration 62, 67
lumbosacral extradural, analgesia 206

Magill non-rebreathing system 30–1, 31
    advantages/disadvantages 31
    gas flow 31
Magill pattern endotracheal tubes 38
magnesium sulphate, emergency dose 127
mandibular nerve block 150–1
mannitol, cerebellar herniation 234
Mapleson D, E and F non-rebreathing systems 33, 34
masks, breathing systems 40
maxillofacial trauma and surgery 150–3
    elective tracheotomy 151–2
    endotracheal tube placement 152
    feeding tubes 152
    indwelling nasogastric intubation 152
    mandibular nerve block 151
    maxillary nerve block 150–1
    nasal oxygen catheter placement 150–1
    oesophagostomy tube 153
    pharyngostomy tube 152–3
    pharyngotomy for ETT diversion 151
    recovery and analgesia 150
medetomidine
    and butorphanol 82
    in caesarian section 220
    cerebroprotection 234

epileptic activity 234–5
    and ketamine (cats only) 82
    and midazolam 82
    paediatric patients 249
    premedication 164, 80–1
    rabbits, rodents, ferrets 297–8
    reptiles 278
megaoesophagus
    induction of anaesthesia 189
    preoperative 236
meloxicam 65
    cat 65
    dog 66
    reptiles 277
meninges, schema 232
meperidine hydrochloride see pethidine
metaclopramide, in caesarian section 220
methadone 64
    and diazepam 241
    dog/cat 63
    haemodynamically unstable cats/dogs 242
methohexitol, in caesarian section 221
methohexitone sodium (methohexital) 89–90
methotrimeprazine
    contraindications in cats 218, 219
    premedication 73–4
methoxyflurane 67
    contraindications 211, 290
    liver effects 204
    minimum alveolar concentration (MAC) 102
    physicochemical properties 100
metomidate, fish 269
midazolam
    and buprenorphine 82
    and butorphanol 82
    and fentanyl (dogs only) 82
    haemodynamic effects 164
    and ketamine, in caesarian section 218, 221
    and medetomidine 82
    and oxymorphone 82, 241
    paediatric patients 248–9
    premedication 164, 197, 74
    rabbits, rodents, ferrets 297–8
    reptiles 276
    and xylazine 82
minimum alveolar concentration (MAC)
    factors affecting 103
    inhalant anaesthetics 102–4
    and N$_2$O 104
minor procedures, sedation 82–4
mitral valve incompetence 169
mitral valve stenosis 169–70
mivacurium 112
monitoring 43–55
    anaesthesia 116
        birds 291–2
        reptiles 291–2
    neuromuscular blockade 112–13
monitors 43–8
    buying and choosing 55
    physiological variables dog/cat 43
morphine
    and acepromazine (dogs only) 82
    dog/cat 63
    haemodynamic effects 164
    paediatric patients 249
    premedication 76–7
    rapid haemodynamic control 160
mucolytics, preoperative, pulmonary disease 179
Murphy pattern endotracheal tubes 38
muscle relaxant drugs 110–12
    action 114–15
        acid–base balance 115
        anaesthetic agents 114
        antibiotics 114
        electrolyte disturbance 115
        hepatic and renal disease 115
        muscle disease 114
        temperature 114
    age of patient 114
    clinical use 116–17
        intermittent positive-pressure ventilation 116
        monitoring anaesthesia 116
    depolarizing and non-depolarizing, interaction 111, 112
    indications/contraindications 115
    see also neuromuscular blockade
myasthenia gravis 236
    thymomas 189
myelography, epileptic activity 234
myocardial contractility, inhalant anaesthetics 104
myocardial contusions 242
myocardial oxygen balance, factors affecting 161
myocarditis, traumatic 170–1

nalbufine, rabbits, rodents, ferrets 300
nalorphine 79
naloxone
    dog/cat 63, 79
    paediatric patients 249
nasogastric intubation 152
nebulizers and humidifiers 40–1